Demystifying and Preparing for Advanced Practice

A Guide for Healthcare Professionals

Demystifying and Preparing for Advanced Practice

A Guide for Healthcare Professionals

JONATHAN THOMAS, RN (ADULT), DIPN, BSC, PGCTHE, PGDIP, MSC

Associate Professor,
Department of Nursing, School of Health and Social Care,
Swansea University, Swansea, United Kingdom

MELANIE ROGERS, RGN, BSC, MSC, PHD

Professor, Department of Nursing and Midwifery,
School of Human and Health Sciences,
University of Huddersfield, Huddersfield, United Kingdom

ANGELA BANKS, RN, RNT, DIPPNS, BMEDSCI (HONS), MA (ED)

Associate Head of School: Health & Social Care (Advancing Practice),
School of Health & Social Care,
Sheffield Hallam University, Sheffield, United Kingdom

ANNA JONES, RN (ADULT), BN (HONS), MSC, PHD, SFHEA

Reader, School of Healthcare Sciences,
Cardiff University, Cardiff, United Kingdom

COLETTE HENDERSON, MSC, PGCERT HELT, PGCERT NURSE PRACTITIONER, BSC (HONS) NP, RN, RNT, NISP

Associate Dean, School of Health Sciences,
University of Dundee, Dundee, United Kingdom

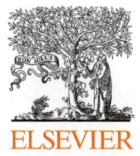

ELSEVIER

Notice

Practitioners and researchers must always rely on their own experience and knowledge in evaluating and using any information, methods, compounds or experiments described herein. Because of rapid advances in the medical sciences, in particular, independent verification of diagnoses and drug dosages should be made. To the fullest extent of the law, no responsibility is assumed by Elsevier, authors, editors or contributors for any injury and/or damage to persons or property as a matter of products liability, negligence or otherwise, or from any use or operation of any methods, products, instructions, or ideas contained in the material herein.

ISBN: 978-0-443-11758-9

Content Strategist: Robert Edwards
Content Project Manager: Abdus Salam Mazumder
Design: Greg Harris
Marketing Manager: Deborah Watkins

Printed in India

Last digit is the print number: 9 8 7 6 5 4 3 2 1

Working together
to grow libraries in
developing countries

www.elsevier.com • www.bookaid.org

Advanced practice is now a firmly embedded feature of healthcare delivery across many different services and types of settings ranging from acute care, community care, primary care and mental health care. The proliferative success of the advanced practice story in many countries is because it did not originate from a transient initiative imposed top-down on healthcare services by policymakers—instead it is an energised practitioner-led movement emerging from the ground upwards, which has grown over six decades of global developments via healthcare professionals innovating in practice by making best use of their experience, knowledge and expertise to improve care outcomes for the people they interact with on an everyday basis within the services they are employed. These grassroots origins of advanced practice have given its subsequent developments a pervasive influence accreted over time in healthcare settings, which has emboldened policy makers, professional bodies and universities to support its success with investments, guidance and education programmes. Consequently, a remarkable confluence of practitioner-based, policy-based and academic-based support for advanced practice has been generated, which has gradually cemented advanced practitioners in the architecture of contemporary healthcare provision.

Whilst this embeddedness of advanced practice has occurred over time with an ever-increasing awareness of multiprofessional advanced practitioner roles amongst healthcare professionals and policy makers, the corresponding awareness of the development of advanced practice amongst patients and the wider public has not occurred at the same expansive pace. It is clear that there is still work to be done to ensure a wider awareness of advanced practitioner roles amongst the public. Accordingly, it is important that those healthcare professionals entering advanced practice education and training are aware of the long history of advanced practice developments, and also of the need to clearly and unequivocally explain their discrete and distinct advanced practitioner roles to patients, carers and families so they can easily understand who it is that is providing care for them and making key decisions for their assessment and management.

With the expansion of advanced practice implementation within services has come a corresponding growth in advanced practice education and training offered by universities working in partnership with practice partners. Associated with this growth are increasing numbers of experienced healthcare professionals from multiprofessional registrant backgrounds across nursing, allied health, pharmacy and midwifery, training to become advanced practitioners. It is with the educational needs of those multitude of multiprofessional trainees that the genesis of this book, *Demystifying and Preparing for Advanced Practice: A Guide for Healthcare Professionals, arises.*

As such, this book presents the worldview of advanced practice developments to advanced practitioner trainees, as is mostly seen by those educators who have had a long-term involvement with advanced practice developments and innovations for the majority of their registrant careers. Accordingly, the book is designed for those starting or considering an MSc advanced practice programme, and this aim of orientation to the discourse of advanced practice is evident throughout the chapters. Reflecting the multiprofessional dimension of advanced practice in the United Kingdom (UK), contributors hail from various professional backgrounds, offering a UK-wide perspective, with an exception in the last chapter, which has an international focus. The book reviews the development of advanced practice, highlighting differences across the UK's four nations. The evolution of advanced practice from its early stages to the present day is outlined. Subsequent chapters explore each pillar of advanced practice, targeting those newcomers and students, with a mostly UK-centric viewpoint. Guidance is offered for aspiring advanced practitioners, acknowledging the varying approaches in advanced practice education, training and workforce development across the UK and different professions. From a more clinical perspective, one of the later chapters discusses common pathological processes and concepts, which is applicable to some MSc advanced practice programmes. In relation to study skills, the key components of academic reading and writing at level 7 are introduced. Advanced practice involves key decisions from the perspective of ethics, so the ethical and legal dimensions of advanced practice, relevant to all professions, are also examined in the book. Educators are not the only contributors to the book—Chapter 11 importantly shares experiences from trainee advanced practitioners across the UK, showcasing diverse professional contributions in this chapter written by advanced practitioner trainees from nursing (primary care, emergency medicine, paediatrics, mental health), physiotherapy, dietetic and orthoptic registrant backgrounds. Suitable supervision is key to a successful outcome as an advanced practice trainee, and supervisory perspectives are the focus of one of the later chapters covering assessment and supervision in practice, with core concepts applicable to all professions involved in advanced practice developments. For the development of trainee education and subsequent continuing professional development, portfolios are increasingly essential, and the book provides guidance on developing a professional portfolio, drawing on various professional body requirements. The penultimate chapter focuses on emotional well-being, emphasising its importance for all to ensure personal professional resilience. The concluding chapter presents an international perspective, with links to the longstanding work of the International Council of Nursing on advanced practice, so has a mostly nursing emphasis, contrasting with the UK's more multiprofessional approach to advanced practice.

Throughout the book runs the conceptual theme of autonomy when thinking of advanced practice as a level of practice. In essence, it is acknowledged that all professions possess some degree of autonomy upon registration, and this autonomy grows as practitioners gain seniority and experience in their roles. However, this autonomy is particularly evident and privileged for advanced practitioners because of their responsibilities for assessing and leading and managing patient care, hence why the quality of their postregistration advanced practice education and training is so important, as is emphasised by the learning to be gained from engaging with this book.

Writing this Foreword has enabled an opportunity to reflect on how far the work on advancing practice has progressed over an extended period of time, transforming services, by expediting access to care and improving experiences and outcomes for patients, families and carers. This book offers the opportunity for those new to advanced practice to begin to engage with the perspectives of the advancing practice community, to share its experiences, insights and innovations in this sphere, and to develop the necessary knowledge, skills and expertise required of advanced practitioners, so they too can begin to similarly optimise experiences and outcomes for their own patients.

——

Professor Julian Barratt
Head of Centre for Advancing Practice
Workforce, Training & Education
NHS England

Honorary Professor
Aston Medical School
Aston University

Honorary Research Fellow
Faculty of Education, Health and Wellbeing
University of Wolverhampton

Birmingham, England, UK
January 2025

PREFACE

In the rapidly evolving landscape of healthcare, the role of advanced practice professionals has become increasingly pivotal. This book, *Demystifying and Preparing for Advanced Practice: A Guide for Healthcare Professionals*, aims to provide a comprehensive and insightful resource for those aspiring to or advancing their journey in advanced practice.

The chapters in this book are meticulously crafted by leading experts in the field, each bringing a wealth of knowledge and experience. Our contributors, hailing from various regions of the UK and beyond, offer diverse perspectives and in-depth analyses on the multifaceted aspects of advanced practice.

Chapter 1 introduces the evolution of advanced practice within the UK, providing a broad overview of policy and regulatory frameworks across the four nations. This foundational chapter sets the stage for understanding the complexities and variations in advanced practice roles and titles.

Chapter 2 delves into transformative practice in the UK, exploring current developments, new roles and future directions. It critically examines the relevance of advanced practice pathways and discusses credentialing, prescribing and other key components.

The four pillars of advanced practice are thoroughly explored in Chapters 3 to 6, covering Education, Clinical Practice, Leadership and Research. Each chapter highlights the origins, development and current practices within these pillars, emphasising their importance in shaping competent and autonomous practitioners.

Chapter 7 provides practical guidance for aspiring advanced practitioners, focusing on the essential steps and considerations for starting this journey. This chapter is particularly valuable for those new to the field, offering insights into participatory research and development of a workbook hosted by the Association of Advanced Practice Educators UK (AAPE UK).

In Chapter 8, the importance of anatomy and physiology (A&P) is discussed, providing an introduction and overview that underscores its significance for clinical practice, and understanding disease process and managing care in advanced practice.

Chapter 9 offers a guide to critical writing at MSc level, with tips and exemplars to help practitioners develop their academic writing skills.

Chapter 10 addresses the moral and ethical issues faced by advanced practitioners, presenting real-world examples and vignettes to illustrate these challenges.

Chapter 11 shares survival tips from current trainees/students, offering a candid look at the experiences and strategies that can help new practitioners navigate their training programmes.

Chapter 12 focuses on supervision and assessment, providing insights from both student and supervisor perspectives. It covers various forms of supervision and the importance of effective assessment methods.

Chapter 13 discusses portfolio development, highlighting the opportunities and challenges associated with demonstrating competency and capability through portfolios.

Chapter 14 explores emotional and spiritual well-being and resilience, drawing on recent research to offer strategies for improving these crucial aspects of professional life.

Finally, Chapter 15 places advanced practice in an international context, comparing practices and developments across different countries and regions.

This book is a collaborative effort, and we are deeply grateful to all the contributors for their dedication and expertise. We hope that this guide will serve as a valuable resource for healthcare professionals at all stages of their careers, providing the knowledge and inspiration needed to excel in advanced practice.

Andrew Martin, RN, BSc, MA
Deputy Head of School, School of Health and
Social Care
College of Health, Wellbeing and Lifesciences
Sheffield Hallam University
Sheffield, United Kingdom

Angela Windle, RGN, MSc
Subject Area Lead – Advancing Practice
Department of Nursing
School of Human and Health Sciences
University of Huddersfield
Huddersfield, United Kingdom

Angie Banks, RN, RNT, DipPNS, BMedSci(Hons), MA (Ed)
Associate Head of School: Health & Social
Care (Advancing Practice)
School of Health & Social Care
Sheffield Hallam University
Sheffield, United Kingdom

Anna Jones, RN(Adult), BN(Hons), MSc, PhD, SFHEA
Reader, MSc Advanced Healthcare Practice
Programme Lead, School of Healthcare
Sciences, College of Biomedical Life Sciences,
Cardiff University
Cardiff, United Kingdom

Annabella Gloster, RGN, Dip PSN, BSc (Hons), PGCE, MSc
Regional Lead Advanced Practice
NHS England – North West
Manchester, United Kingdom

Caz Crossland, BN(Hons), RSCN, MSc ACP
Advanced Paediatric Nurse Practitioner,
Paediatric Emergency Unit
Cardiff and Vale University Health Board
Cardiff, United Kingdom

Charlotte Barker, RN, BSc, MSc, PGCert
Senior Lecturer
Department of Nursing, School of Human
and Health Sciences
University of Huddersfield
Huddersfield, United Kingdom

Claire Manderson
Advanced Clinical Practitioner
ACP Calderdale and Huddersfield NHS Trust
Huddersfield, United Kingdom

Clare Butler, RN, BSc, MSc, SFHEA
Programme Lead; Advanced, Enhanced and
Specialist Practice
Faculty of Health, Science and Technology
Oxford Brookes University
Oxford, United Kingdom

Colette Henderson, MSc, PGCert HELT, PgCert Nurse Practitioner, BSc(Hons) NP, RN, RNT, NISP
Associate Dean, School of Health Sciences
University of Dundee
Dundee, United Kingdom

Deborah Harding, PhD, MSc, BMedSci (Speech), PGCert LTHE, HCPC, RCSLT, FHEA
Professor
NHS England/ St. George's University,
London
London, United Kingdom

Donna McConnell, PhD, MSc, PG Cert, BSc, Dip NP, RN, FHEA
Retired – former Lecturer in Nursing
Course Director, MSc Advanced Nursing
Practice
Ulster University
Belfast, United Kingdom

Elisabeth Gulliksen, MBChB(hons)
Senior Lecturer, Department of Nursing and
Midwifery, School of Human and Health
Sciences
University of Huddersfield
Huddersfield, United Kingdom

Geinor Bean, RN, Dip Nursing, PgCE, BSc, MSc
Adult Nursing Lecturer, MSc Advanced
Clinical Practice Programme Lead
School of Healthcare Sciences, College of
Biomedical and Life Science
Cardiff University
Cardiff, United Kingdom

Gillian Morris, RN, BA, MSc, PGDip
Lecturer, Programme Lead Advanced Practice
University of Dundee
Dundee, United Kingdom

Helen Francis-Wenger, MSc, PGCAP, BSc, DipHE (RN)
Lecturer in Advanced Clinical Practice
Faculty of Health, School of Nursing and
Midwifery
University of Plymouth
Plymouth, United Kingdom

Helen Rushforth PhD, BA, RGN, RSCN, Recorded Nurse Teacher qualification.
Senior Lecturer in Advanced Practice
University of Southampton
Southampton, United Kingdom

James Taylor, BSc, PGCert, FHEA
Lecturer in Anatomy and Physiology
Faculty of Medicine, Health and Life Science
Swansea University
Swansea, United Kingdom

John Knight, BSc, PhD
Associate Professor, Department of
Healthcare Science, School of Health and
Social Care
Swansea University
Swansea, United Kingdom

Jonathan Drury, BSc, MMedSci, MSc
Advanced Clinical Practitioner in
Ophthalmology
University of Huddersfield/ Calderdale and
Huddersfield NHS Foundation Trust
Halifax/Huddersfield, United Kingdom

Jonathan Thomas, RN(Adult), DipN, BSc, PgCtHE, PgDip, MSc
Associate Professor
Department of Nursing, School of Health and
Social Care
Swansea University
Swansea, United Kingdom

Julie-Ann Hayes, RN, PhD, MRes, MA, PGCert, BSc(Hons)
Senior Lecturer (Law and Ethics) PGR
Co-ordinator, Programme Lead, Professional
Doctorate in Health
Liverpool John Moores University
Liverpool, United Kingdom

Kim Manley CBE, RGN, DipN (Lon), RCNT, PGCEA, BA, MN, PhD
Emeritus Professor, Practice Development
Faculty of Medicine and Health Sciences
University of East Anglia Organisation
Norwich;
Emeritus Professor, Practice Development,
Research & Innovation
Faculty of Medicine, Health & Social Care
Canterbury Christ Church University
Canterbury, United Kingdom

Marianne Jenkins, RGN, RSCN, MSc, IP, PGCert, Doctorate in Advanced Healthcare Practice
Consultant Nurse Practitioner – Emergency
and Acute Medicine
University Hospital of Wales
Cardiff and Vale University Healthboard
Cardiff, United Kingdom

Melanie Clarkson, BSc(Hons), PGCE, MSc, SFHEA
Senior Lecturer in Advancing Practice
Radiotherapy and Oncology
Sheffield Hallam University
Sheffield, United Kingdom

Melanie Rogers, RGN, BSc, MSc, PhD
Professor
Department of Nursing and Midwifery
School of Human and Health Sciences
University of Huddersfield
Huddersfield, United Kingdom

Nicola Assassa, MSc
Advanced Clinical Practitioner
Mid Yorks Hospital Trust
United Kingdom

Rebecca Britton, BSc, MSc
Advanced Clinical Practitioner in Mental
Health
University of Huddersfield / South West
Yorkshire Partnership NHS Foundation Trust
Huddersfield, United Kingdom

Sarah Fisher, RN, Adv Dip, BMedSci, MSc
Professional Lead for Advancing Practice
South Yorkshire Integrated Care Board
Sheffield, United Kingdom

Sandie Haigh, RGN, ACP, BSc, MSc
Consultant Practitioner, Remote Patient Care
Yorkshire Ambulance Service
Wakefield, United Kingdom

**Zubeyde Bayram-Weston, BSc, MSc, PhD,
SFHEA, FAS**
Senior Lecturer, School of Health and Social
Care
Swansea University
Swansea, United Kingdom

ACKNOWLEDGEMENTS

We would like to thank the following for their support and help when writing this book:

Dr Clair Graham for the MAP section in Chapter 1 and to Kathy Haigh, for her support in developing Chapter 3 alongside Annabella Gloster and Professor Kim Manley.

Any omissions or errors are ours as editors.

We'd like to thank our families, friends, colleagues and students for their patience and support whilst we have written and edited this book. Thank you all.

Dedication

To all of our students, past, present and future.

CONTENTS

CHAPTER 1

Introduction to Advanced Practice

Colette Henderson ■ Anna Jones ■ Jonathan Thomas ■ Melanie Rogers
■ Angie Banks ■ Donna McConnell

CHAPTER OUTLINE

This chapter provides the background details surrounding the development of advanced practice (AP) across the United Kingdom (UK). We begin by revisiting the history of AP within the UK, and specifically, we consider the unique UK multiprofessional approach to AP development. The policy framework for each of the UK countries is discussed and an update of the work surrounding AP regulation is provided. The chapter concludes with a debate about the challenges to UK AP development. Many of the book chapters will touch upon the themes discussed here; however, this chapter will provide a foundation that supports the rest of the book.

Background to the Evolution of Advanced Practice Within the UK

DEVELOPMENTS IN THE UNITED STATES

Nurse practitioner (NP) roles first emerged in the United States in the 1960s driven by a shortage of physicians, reductions in junior doctor working hours, changing healthcare needs and economic challenges (Silver et al., 1968). In 1965, Dr. Loretta Ford and Dr. Henry Silver developed the first NP programme, which led to the development of more NP programmes. In 1971, the University of Washington launched their family NP programme and in 1973 the National Association of Paediatric Nurse Practitioners was established. At the start of 1980, more than 200 NP programmes were available and 1985 saw the establishment of the American Academy of Nurse Practitioners (AANP). By 1989, many programmes were offered at master's level. Over the decades, the United States has witnessed the strategic development of and an increase in the number of NPs, with there being more than 385,000 NPs reported in 2023 (Black, 2023).

PIT STOP!

AANP provides a timeline from the birth of the NP to current date. Please have a look at this resource:

https://www.aanp.org/about/about-the-american-association-of-nurse-practitioners-aanp/historical-timeline

DEVELOPMENTS IN THE UK

The 1980s saw the importation of these roles to the UK, initially in primary care settings. Barbara Stillwell is credited with introducing NPs to the UK and supporting the development of the original accredited postregistration undergraduate NP degree programmes taught by the Royal College of Nursing (Barton et al., 2012); Chapter 3 discusses the birth of NP education in more detail.

The 1986 Cumberledge Report (Department of Health and Social Security, 1986) promoted expansion of these roles in primary care, and with ensuing support from government, it was in the 1990s that NPs became more evident in the UK. Following the publication of The Scope of Professional Practice by the United Kingdom Central Council for Nursing, Midwifery and Health Visiting, nurses were liberated to take on roles that were previously in the domain of medicine and were encouraged to make decisions much more independently (United Kingdom Central Council, 1992). The parallel development of the NP role and advancing practice may have contributed to the confusion and distinction between nurses who took on extended roles and advanced practice (AP) roles.

Subsequently, role development has been influenced by drivers such as the European Working Time Directive (EWTD) (2003), which preceded and inspired government policy such as Modernising Medical Careers (UK Health Departments, 2004) and Modernising Nursing Careers (Scottish Executive, 2006), the latter being the main driver for the development of NPs across the UK. Consequently, NP roles were developed to bridge the gap that materialised from the reduction in medical staff availability and saw nurses taking on many of the traditional medical roles. The role was seen to combine characteristics of nursing and medicine, holistic assessment and clinical decision-making skills.

At this time, and like the international focus, the NP role was limited to the nursing profession. There were no regulatory requirements beyond the regulation required for prescribing for Nursing and Midwifery Council (NMC) registrants. Initial regulation was seen to provide sufficient governance (NMC, 2009). The nursing profession pursued NMC regulation, and in 2004, a consultation was initiated which was supported by an influential UK body of educators known as the Association of Advanced Nursing Practitioner Educators UK (AANPE UK). The results of this consultation led to the adoption of the term 'advanced nurse practice'. In 2009, a report to the Department of Health from the Committee for Healthcare Regulatory Evidence (CHRE) advised that additional regulation for NMC registrants was unnecessary as this advanced nurse role did not suggest an additional clinical risk (NMC, 2009). This lack of regulation has led to the organic development of the advanced practitioner role across the four UK countries, and national variation is known to exist. Rogers and Gloster (2020) advise this variation limits the ability to portray the magnitude of AP development in the UK.

As advanced nursing practice moved into the 21st century, the breadth of roles and titles continued to develop with a current picture of many roles, titles and job descriptions related to clinical nurse specialist (CNS), NP and other advanced practitioner titles. Within the UK a multiprofessional focus began to emerge for

AP, with the development of multiprofessional AP frameworks. Examples which will be discussed further in the chapter include the Framework for Advanced Nursing, Midwifery and Allied Health Professional Practice in Wales (National Leadership and Innovation Agency for Health Care (NLIAH), 2010), updated in 2023 (Health Education and Improvement Wales (HEIW), 2023), and the Multiprofessional Framework for Advanced Practice (Health Education England (HEE), 2017), which has further been updated in 2025 (NHS England, 2025). Whilst many allied health professionals might have been working at an advanced level of practice, such frameworks provided greater recognition for these professions.

AP Development Across the UK

Work is gathering pace across the four UK nations in relation to AP and there is now clear recognition of the need for an AP workforce that is clinically governed (Hardy et al., 2021; NMC, 2024a). The differences highlighted in the next sections demonstrate the lack of cohesive structure and format of education programmes and variation in strategic direction, partially arguably due to different funding mechanisms that impact the scope of development of services.

> **PIT STOP!**
>
> Across the UK, the four nations have different names for the organisations that manage hospital and primary/community services. For clarification, in England, these are referred to as National Health Service (NHS) Trusts; in Scotland, these are referred to as NHS Boards; in Northern Ireland, these are referred to as Health and Social Care Trusts; and in Wales, these are NHS Health Boards and NHS Trusts.

SCOTLAND

In 2008, the Scottish Government (SG) indicated their unease with the diversity in titles, citing confusion from the public regarding the anticipated level of care. They stipulated that the title would be advanced nurse practitioner (ANP) and individuals in these roles would require master's-level education (NHS Education for Scotland (NES), 2018). The Advanced Practice Toolkit was developed as a resource to support the development of these roles (NES, 2018). The toolkit provided detail about educational preparation (master's-level education) and the four pillars of AP: clinical practice, research, leadership and education. Although terminology relating to these pillars varies across the UK, the content was seen as pertinent and the chief nursing officers of the four nations approved the application of the toolkit across the UK (NES, 2018). The SG produced guidance for NHS boards in 2010 where master's level thinking was articulated as a requirement for these roles (SG, 2010). Interestingly, this guidance stopped short of stipulating a master's level qualification, whilst internationally a master's degree was detailed as a requirement for ANPs in 2001 (AAPE UK 2024).

The Transforming Roles programme was introduced in 2017 with the aim of ensuring a national and consistent approach to role transformation. One of the first roles to be considered was ANPs. It was recognised at the time that the focus would be on ANP development but subsequently there would be a multiprofessional focus to AP. To ensure this consistency, ANPs were defined as:

> *'experienced and highly educated registered nurses who manage the complete clinical care of their patients'.*

(SG, 2017)

Funding was allocated by the Chief Nursing Office Directorate of the SG to progress this role development. The funding supported an additional 500 ANPs to complete the required postgraduate diploma in AP, although exact figures indicate that more ANPs were funded due to some staff having already completed some core modules. Scottish universities (higher education institutes (HEIs)) responded to this and developed programmes to align to the SG and NES requirements. Educational programmes included topics such as clinical assessment and decision-making, prescribing and workplace learning (NES, 2018). Specific competencies were agreed for ANPs working in acute care, primary and community care, mental health, paediatrics and neonatology (NES, 2018; SG, 2021a). The NHS boards approach was to develop trainee posts which included time for learning and supervision. Work was undertaken to align terminology and titles with use of ANP as the confirmed title.

In 2021, two key papers were published in the Transforming Roles programme. Paper 7 (SG, 2021a) provides further detail about the progression of AP reflecting the move to a multiprofessional focus on AP development. The paper also determines the requirement for impact assessment and provides specific detail about metrics that can be used. Requirements for focus on nonclinical pillars are detailed and indicate that this should be 10% pro rata. Scotland was the first country to stipulate this in a policy document (SG, 2021a), but Wales has now identified the requirement for a minimum of 20% of the advanced practitioner's time to be dedicated to supporting research, education and leadership (HEIW, 2023). Paper 8 of the Transforming Roles programme focuses on the review of CNS roles and provides definitions, competencies and recommendations for both governance and education for the CNS and advanced CNS roles (SG, 2021b).

Three AP academies have been established in Scotland to support governance. These virtual organisations are multidisciplinary collaborations between regional NHS boards and HEIs, and they cover the North, West and East of Scotland. The aim of the academies is to strengthen and facilitate governance and continuous professional development (CPD) of AP. An agreement across the academies regarding communication of developments has led to the publication of a twice annual national AP newsletter.

In 2021, the Scottish Advanced Practice Educators Network (SAPEN) was established. This network is multiprofessional and is comprised of AP programme leads, the Open University, AP nurse consultants in Scotland, NHS 24, the Scottish Ambulance Service (SAS), allied health professions and pharmacy representation.

The network aims to provide a coordinated approach to the development of AP education in Scotland.

Subsequently, two other networks have been established. First to be established was an advanced practice mental health support network, which is also multidisciplinary and comprises nurse and pharmacist colleagues from mental health practice areas who work together to raise the profile and achieve coordination in approach to mental health AP. A doctoral support network that comprises nurse and allied health professional colleagues from across Scotland who are undertaking doctoral studies with a focus on AP meet on a monthly basis for both organised and supportive sessions. The invitation to join this network has recently been extended to include colleagues from England who are undertaking doctoral studies.

The current direction for role development has moved away from a centrally funded approach to a service-led approach requiring individual service areas to determine the need and business case for advanced practitioners. Some of the ongoing challenges currently faced in Scotland will be similar across the UK, the continued evolution of the roles and inclusion of relevant content into programmes, the impact of COVID-19 and the availability of practice supervisors.

Medical Associate Professions in Scotland

The NHS Recovery Plan was published on 25 August 2021 (SG, 2021c), committing over £1 billion of targeted investment for the recovery and renewal of the health service. A key requirement to delivering the Recovery Plan is having the right workforce in place at the right time. Medical associate professions (MAP) roles were identified as potential alternative workforce options to build in flexibility and resilience to teams and to contribute to the increase in clinical capacity that is essential to meet current and future demand.

Based on the requirement within the Recovery Plan, the SG has appointed NES to undertake commissioning to map current and future demand and opportunities arising for MAP roles across Scotland. The MAP roles under consideration are physician associate (PA), anaesthesia associate (AA), surgical care practitioner (SCP) and advanced critical care practitioner (ACCP).

The objectives of the commission service and educational needs analysis will inform the outcomes of the commission. The objectives are to deliver national workforce scoping for the four MAP roles under consideration, including understanding of the potential for additionality of workforce and national educational scoping for these four MAP roles, and itemisation of any potential benefits anticipated, and the benefits appraisal will include identification of opportunities to adapt and collaborate with existing educational providers.

The findings will be documented and reported to the SG Health Directorate, Capacity Building and Recruitment Strategy Unit. This will inform and provide significant contribution to ongoing workforce and service consideration. In addition, findings and recommendations will inform options to mobilise greater MAP integration to the Workforce Plan, enabling flexibility and resilience in service delivery.

MAP roles support NHS Scotland Boards to deliver flexible and resilient workforce plans. They will contribute to the increased clinical capacity required by the NHS Recovery Plan (SG, 2021c) by enabling the right workforce in place at the right time.

WALES

Wales followed in the footsteps of Scotland with the adoption of the key principles outlined within the Scottish Toolkit, as highlighted earlier. This work was led by the former NLIAH, an organisation with a focus to develop NHS service redesign, innovations and improvement. This led to the creation of the Framework for Advanced Nursing, Midwifery and Allied Health Professional Practice in Wales (NLIAH, 2010), with the aim to create a more consistent approach to AP across Wales. Within this framework, it recognised that AP was a 'level of practice' as opposed to a specific role. Like Scotland, it recognised that master's-level education should underpin AP and adopted the four pillars. The framework was developed by a multidisciplinary team and placed emphasis on employers to ensure appropriate evaluation of AP roles were in place.

On the cessation of NLIAH, the responsibility for supporting and hosting AP in Wales was then carried by the Welsh Education and Development Service (WEDS). In 2018, HEIW was established, and this brought together WEDS, the Wales Deanery and the Wales Centre for Pharmacy Professional Education. In 2023, HEIW undertook a 'refresh' of the existing AP framework which resulted in the launch of the Professional Framework for Enhanced, Advanced and Consultant (EAC) Clinical Practice in Wales (HEIW, 2023). This new framework adopted and incorporated many key principles from the former framework and retained the four pillars of AP. It also drew upon the Guidance for Appointing Nurses, Midwives and Allied Health Care Professionals to Consultant Posts document (Welsh Government, 2014), which supported the consultant level practice of the framework.

The EAC framework now recognises enhanced level practice, this being a level of practice that develops over time through consolidation and development of competencies. This level of practice has been linked to both level 6 (degree level) and level 7 (master's level) education (HEIW, 2023).

PIT STOP!

The higher education system in the UK is based on levels, known as the Framework for Higher Education Qualifications (FHEQ), which highlights that bachelor's degree with honours is level 6 and master's degree is level 7. However, in Scotland, they have the Scottish Credit and Qualifications Framework (SCQF), which places bachelor's degree with honours at level 10 and master's degree at level 11.

There is the recognition that those working at an enhanced level may wish to progress to advanced level practice or continue to work at their current level. The creation of a roadmap within the EAC framework provides a clear visual journey for any practitioner from registrant to consultant level practice. Like any road map, there can be many twists and turns in the road that can resemble a career journey.

In relation to advanced level practice, HEIW (2023) has retained the former NLIAH (2010) definition (note that the 'clinical' remains in the AP title) and states:

'A role, requiring a registered practitioner to have acquired an expert knowledge base, complex decision-making skills, and clinical competencies for expanded scope of practice, the characteristics of which are shaped by the context in which the individual practices. Demonstrable, relevant master's level education is recommended for entry level'.

(NLIAH, 2010)

Despite the retention of the 'advanced clinical practice' definition, the EAC framework (HEIW, 2023) recognises that many practitioners might be advancing their practice but not within a clinical role. With the new framework, there is a shift in focus from the former NLIAH (2010) suggestion that AP is a level of practice to now suggesting it can be both a role and a level of practice.

In relation to education, the EAC framework recognises master's-level education and the achievement of an MSc AP, and the maintenance of a portfolio aligned to the four pillars; see Chapter 13 for work around portfolios. Currently, six Welsh universities deliver AP education, with five offering generic MSc AP programmes which are open to all registered healthcare professionals, whilst one delivers bespoke AP education aimed at allied health professionals such as podiatry and dietetics. A function of HEIW is that of commissioner of health education at both undergraduate and postgraduate. At the time of writing, HEIW is undertaking a 5-year commissioning exercise for postgraduate education including AP programmes. This will change the current funding process, which currently, for MSc AP programmes, is via the Welsh Health Boards and Welsh NHS Trusts who submit annual funding requests to HEIW.

Similarly to Scotland, in 2020, the Welsh Advanced Practice Educators Network (WAPEN) was formed which consists of the six universities that deliver AP education. Alongside this, the Welsh Advanced Clinical Practice Group Multi-Professional Advanced Practice Group Wales was created, which includes advanced practitioners from a breadth of specialties and areas and members of WAPEN.

ENGLAND

England has adopted a multidisciplinary approach to AP development, and in recognition of this, titles have evolved from ANP to advanced clinical practitioner (ACP) with similar moves from HEIs who now offer MSc Advanced Clinical Practice programmes (HEE, 2017; Rogers & Gloster, 2020).

These programmes follow the typical NP curricula seen in many countries with established NP roles. Completion of these programmes leads to the title 'advanced clinical practitioner' (ACP), although many nurses who undertake these courses still use the title of ANP as advocated by the Royal College of Nursing (Rogers &

Gloster, 2023). Joint education and training of nurses and allied health profession-als as ACPs are now the norm in England.

The government body HEE provided national leadership and coordination for educating and training the health workforce in England until 2023, when it was integrated into NHS England (NHSE) (NHSE, 2023a). As mentioned, NHSE has identified that AP is not the remit of nurses alone (NHSE, 2024). Through extensive consultation across the nursing and allied health professions, they developed the Multi-Professional Framework for Advanced Clinical Practice to set out a vision for developing the AP workforce to ensure safety, quality and effectiveness (HEE, 2017). This framework was developed across the whole of the healthcare system, including primary care, community care, acute hospital, mental health, learning disabilities, hospices and prisons, and covers public, independent, private and charity sectors. The framework has been adopted throughout England and aims to ensure a common understanding of advanced clinical practice to support individuals, employers, educa-tors and commissioners to improve patient experience and outcomes (HEE, 2017). In 2025, NHSE published a revised Multi-Professional Framework.

The publication of the Multi-Professional Framework supports the approach of attempting to clarify and standardise AP development (HEE, 2017, NHSE, 2025).

AP in England is defined as:

'Advanced clinical practice is delivered by experienced, registered health and care practitioners. It is a level of practice characterised by a high degree of autonomy and complex decision-making. This is underpinned by a master's level award or equiva-lent that encompasses the four pillars of clinical practice, leadership and management, education and research, with demonstration of core capabilities and area specific clin-ical competence. Advanced clinical practice embodies the ability to manage clinical care in partnership with individuals, families and carers. It includes the analysis and synthesis of complex problems across a range of settings, enabling innovative solutions to enhance people's experience and improve outcomes.'

(HEE, 2017)

HEE has established the Centre for Advancing Practice, which provides gover-nance and quality assurance to AP developments through setting and monitoring standards of education, accrediting AP programmes and supporting the transition and development of AP (HEE, 2017; NHSE, 2024).

Investment for AP development in England historically came from a variety of sources, including self-funding, employer funding and from HEE for areas that have considerable challenges with delivery of healthcare (Rogers & Gloster, 2020). How-ever, recent developments in England have seen an apprenticeship model being made available to all health and social care employers to support the training of advanced practitioners. AP apprenticeships are unique to England and allow a com-bination of study (off-the-job training) and workplace learning (on-the-job training) funded by tax to be reclaimed against training for employers (Rogers & Gloster, 2020). Many AP master's degrees are defined by an apprenticeship standard that defines an occupational role and sets out the knowledge, skills and behaviours required to fulfil it across four domains. The standard was developed in collaboration with multiple stakeholders, including employers, HEE and the Association of Advanced Practice Educators UK (AAPE UK) (Institute for Apprenticeships and Technical Education, 2018). AAPE UK is discussed further along in this chapter.

A large body of work is currently in progress across numerous arms of AP in England, including end point assessment (EPA) for apprenticeships, programme accreditation with either the Royal College of Nursing or the Centre for Advancing Practice and individual supported portfolio review for access to a national directory/digital badging for AP (NHSE, 2024). Aspects of work streams undertaken by the Centre for Advancing Practice are referred to in various chapters within the book.

NORTHERN IRELAND

Within Northern Ireland, education provision for AP is undertaken on a uniprofessional basis. However, in 2024, a change to the uniprofessional stance has been observed, with multiprofessional advanced practice programmes being developed in Northern Ireland. Education for advanced nursing practice, advanced clinical practice for Allied Health Professionals (AHP) and the PA role is undertaken separately with no multiprofessional provision.

The first graduate NP education programme was provided by the Royal College of Nursing Institute and commenced in 1995. This programme moved to Ulster University and was subsumed as a pathway under the Specialist Practice Qualification (SPQ), due largely to low numbers of students. Graduates from this programme were mainly from a general practice background initially; however, secondary care services soon saw the value of these nursing roles in providing nurses with expanded clinical skills. A lack of formal recognition, definition and standards for the role meant new nursing roles were introduced in the absence of meaningful guidance. There was little standardisation in terms of titles and scope of practice, and they appeared to be shaped by the context in which the NP was employed and were contingent on service demand (McConnell et al., 2013).

To provide clarity about the ANP role, the Department of Health developed Northern Ireland's first Advanced Nursing Practice Framework in 2014. It was further revised in 2016 and details the strategic approach to the development of, and education for, the ANP role in Northern Ireland (Department of Health, Social Services and Public Safety (DHSSPS), 2016). The framework provides a definition of advanced nursing practice and identifies the core competencies and learning outcomes essential for the role around the four pillars of direct clinical practice, leadership and collaborative practice, education and learning and research and evidence-based practice, setting the standard for education for the role.

According to the ANP Framework,

'The ANP will undertake comprehensive health assessments and will manage a range of illnesses and conditions that frequently present in the care settings within which the individual works. S/he will:
- *practise autonomously within an expanded scope of practice*

- *demonstrate a person-centred approach to care delivery*
- *develop and sustain partnerships and networks to influence and improve healthcare outcomes and healthcare delivery*
- *educate, supervise or mentor nursing colleagues and others in the healthcare team*
- *contribute to and undertake activities, including research, that monitor and improve the quality of healthcare and the effectiveness of practice.'*

(DHSSPS, 2016, p. 6)

In an attempt to protect the ANP title, they further state that

'only those who meet the requirements of the role and who are employed as Advanced Nurse Practitioners, will be able to use the title.'

(DHSSPS, 2016, p. 6)

As with the former Welsh Framework (NLIAH, 2010), the Northern Ireland Framework identifies the distinguishing characteristics between advanced and specialist nursing practice and identifies AP as a level beyond specialist practice. The current EAC framework (HEIW, 2023) now recognises the specialist practice can be at an advanced level.

Both Ulster University and Queens University currently provide programmes of education of ANPs, based on the competencies from the ANP framework. The programmes provide pathways for primary care, emergency care, adult medical and older people, mental health across the lifespan, children's nursing and critical care. These first cohort of ANPs graduated in 2018 in Northern Ireland.

The Advanced Allied Health Professions framework was published by the Department of Health in June 2019 and this framework supports the transformation of the 13 AHP disciplines in Northern Ireland (Department of Health, 2019) and provides consistency and understanding of roles and detailed competencies required for these role developments. It encompasses the four pillars of advanced clinical practice, leadership and management, education of self and others and research. The AP AHP role is defined as:

'A role, requiring a registered experienced practitioner to have acquired an expert knowledge base, complex decision-making skills and clinical competencies for expanded/extended scope of practice, the characteristics of which are shaped by the context in which the individual practices. Demonstrable, relevant education is recommended for entry level to the advanced practice role which is to be at master's level or equivalent and which meets the education, training and Continuous Professional Development (CPD) requirements for ACP as identified within the framework.'

(Department of Health, 2019, p. 20)

The first PAs were appointed in Northern Ireland in 2019 in an attempt to move forward the transformation of health and social care (Department of Health, 2019).

The MSc in PA Studies is undertaken at Ulster University and provides education and training in line with requirements of the national curriculum. These students are trained in the medical model to work with the medical team to deliver medical care to patients, and work under the supervision of a doctor in a range of specialities in both primary and secondary care. PAs are trained to take medical histories, carry out physical examinations, formulate diagnosis, request and interpret tests and investigations, undertake procedures and develop treatment and management plans (Ulster University, 2023).

MAPs—Differentiating Between MAPs and Advanced Practitioners

Within the UK, there has been the development and implementation of MAPs working across the NHS, which includes PAs, SCPs and AAs, with the number set to increase (British Medical Association (BMA), 2024). SCP training requires applicants to be a registered healthcare professional such a nurse or operating department practitioner. Hence, their professional accountability can lie with either the NMC or Health and Care Professions Council (HCPC). In contrast to this, the AA training requires applicants to be either a registered healthcare professional or a graduate with a biomedical degree. Clearly, those applicants coming from a biomedical degree pathway will not have professional regulation. Similarly, PAs are recruited to training from the same paths as those for the AAs. The lack of regulation has led to concerns with the Department of Health and Social Security (DHSS (2019) highlighting a need for regulation of the MAPs, specifically PAs and AAs. Legislation was passed through the House of Lords in February 2024 for the regulation of both PAs and AAs, and the General Medical Council (GMC) is undertaking work around the framework regulation for both PAs and AAs. Until regulation is implemented, both PAs and AAs have a voluntary register.

Currently, regulation appears to be a significant difference between advanced practitioners and PAs/AAs. Although advanced practitioners are regulated through their profession, AP is currently not regulated, although the NMC (2024a) has announced their intention to regulate AP within the nursing profession, which is discussed later.

In relation to PAs, they can undertake a range of tasks under the direction and supervision of a medical practitioner, unlike advanced practitioners, who are accountable and autonomous practitioners through their professional body regulation. PAs can undertake patient consultations which encompasses history taking, examination, formulation of a provisional diagnosis and management plans (Royal College of Physicians, 2020). However, Feinmann (2024) argues that PAs and AAs should not be diagnosing patients, basing their conclusion on documented cases where both PAs and AAs have incorrectly diagnosed patients, resulting in harm. The advanced practitioner can undertake all these components of a patient consultation (history taking, examination and independent decision-making), and they are also able to formulate a diagnosis and management plan.

Currently, the existing prescribing legislation and regulations do not allow any PA or AA to prescribe. It could be argued that those PAs or AAs with a professional registration background (nurse, paramedic, etc.) who have maintained their professional registration could prescribe through this route. However, if someone is employed as a PA or an AA, then prescribing would not be in their job description. The GMC recognises this scenario but refrains from commenting upon this within their website, as highlighted in the Pitstop.

PIT STOP!

Current GMC guidance on AAs and PAs prescribing.
https://www.gmc-uk.org/professional-standards/the-professional-standards/good-practice-in-prescribing-and-managing-medicines-and-devices
https://www.nmc.org.uk/standards/standards-for-post-registration/standards-for-prescribers/useful-information-for-prescribers/

Another feature that PAs and AAs cannot currently undertake is the requesting of investigations that contain ionising radiation; again, this is due to the lack of current regulation (Williams & Adhiyaman, 2022). Unlike PAs and AAs, certain clinical areas and NHS organisations allow the advanced practitioner to request investigations that contain ionising radiation. This often remains a key component of a clinician's work such as those working in emergency care or musculoskeletal services.

Whilst plans are in place to regulate PAs and AAs, they remain a recognised role within the current NHS, whether this be in community, primary or secondary care services. Many advanced practitioners will work alongside their PA and AA colleagues to support and deliver improved patient outcomes. The MAP workforce is set to remain, and some might view this as a threat to AP; however, with the existing workforce challenges within the health and social care sectors, this can only be viewed as a good measure to address these challenges.

AP Regulation

In 2021, the NMC committed to a review of postregistration standards for specialist community health nurses (SCPHNs) and SPQs. This review and publication of proficiencies (which is what registrants need to know and be able to do) and education and training standards, which include programme standards (for universities and practice partners), were completed in 2022. The published standards were subsequently updated in 2023 (NMC, 2023). This regulatory work identified the autonomy and clinical complexity involved in community nursing work. A result of this engagement work undertaken to develop these proficiencies and standards was the need to consider AP. The setting of SCPHN and SPQ postregistration standards was consequently described as a bridge to AP. Simultaneously, the chief nursing officers of the four UK countries proposed and promoted a need to review AP regulation. Subsequently, the NMC commissioned the Nuffield Trust to undertake a review of AP. This led to production of the Nuffield Trust report which highlighted a latent risk associated with diagnosis (Palmer et al., 2023).

Update on NMC Developments

Advanced practitioners work within and across a breadth of health and social care settings, and across the four pillars of practice. The context of the advanced practitioner's practice is important; that is, the environment in which they deliver care provides the context in which the intervention is delivered. Settings such as primary and community care, mental health, first contact and maternity services offer such contexts, and employers span a range of care providers such as the NHS, general practitioners, social care and independent sectors. Advanced practitioners can work as part of multidisciplinary teams or as an individual, lone practitioner within such settings.

It is important to recognise agency in the individuals who access care; they will have differing degrees of vulnerability and autonomy from those requiring, for example, urgent mental healthcare or care required at the end of life. Care can be delivered by advanced practitioners as the sole providers of care. They can care for individuals in their own homes, which increases the risk of vulnerability for and of the individual receiving care. There is, in addition, recognition that the public appreciation and understanding of AP roles is limited. This can impact on informed consent given by individuals needing care, and also influence decision-making by advanced practitioners (NMC, 2024a). This creates an element of risk, the proportion of which is dependent on the size of the individual groups who access services and the size of the group of practitioners who care for the individuals.

There are limited data available on the number of advanced practitioners who work within the UK, as this is not currently recorded by Professional, Statutory and Regulatory Bodies (PSRBs). The NMC does not currently maintain a record of the number of nurses and midwives who practice as ANP or advanced midwifery practitioners (AMPs) within the UK. A lack of agreed and joint definition of AP across professions and bodies hinders the collection of data and accuracy of recognition and management of risk. Current estimates of AP numbers are 8000 ANPs in England and 800 ANPs in Scotland, and there is a lack of data in Wales and Northern Ireland. The numbers of registrants practising as AMP is small, with an estimated 27 titles in England (NMC, 2024a). The Long-Term Working Plan (NHSE, 2023b) has identified the development of education and training for a further 6300 advanced practitioners by 2031/32 in England. The scale of any potential risk will therefore increase; it is currently managed by employer governance and local practice. There does, however, remain a lack of standardisation of role, scope, experience required, educational level and titles of advanced practitioners across the UK.

Phase 1 of the NMC Advanced Practice Regulatory Review has now concluded. The NMC Council on the 27th of March 2024 approved the development of standards of proficiency for advanced level practice (and associated programme standards), adopting a collaborative approach to develop a UK-wide AP principles framework incorporating a shared position or definition of advanced level practice. It will also ensure that advanced level practice requirements are included in both the review of revalidation and the NMC Code, which are scheduled to be undertaken in 2025/26. The AP regulatory work will now move to phase 2 of the project;

timeframes for outcomes from a regulatory perspective are currently unavailable (NMC 2024c).

PIT STOP!

A link to the current NMC AP review can be found here:
https://www.nmc.org.uk/about-us/our-role/advanced-practice-review/

What Is Standard Setting, Collaborative Practice and Revalidation?

DEVELOPING STANDARDS OF PROFICIENCY FOR ADVANCED LEVEL PRACTICE (AND ASSOCIATED PROGRAMME STANDARDS)

The NMC has previously set standards for nurses and midwives for postregistration practice (NMC, 2023). With the pace of change in healthcare and clinical practice, standards should reflect the changes to ensure that patient safety is maximised and clinical practice risks are minimised. The changes to the previously published postregistration standards have reflected the progress of practice and enabled care to be delivered safely to people receiving care in such contexts and communities as care homes, nursing homes and prison and social care settings (NMC, 2024b).

ADOPTING A COLLABORATIVE APPROACH TO DEVELOP A UK-WIDE AP PRINCIPLES FRAMEWORK INCORPORATING A SHARED POSITION OR DEFINITION OF ADVANCED LEVEL PRACTICE

PSRBs are and will continue to work collaboratively with the NMC; however, the HCPC is currently not considering aligning to the NMC move to regulate, as indicated in their 2021 report (Hardy et al., 2021). There is ongoing work to develop a joint statement or description of AP, which again will be published and shared via the NMC website. There are, however, precedents set, with the Independent Prescribing programme being aligned to the General Pharmaceutical Council (GPhC), NMC and HCPC via the Royal Pharmaceutical Society (RPS) framework (RPS, 2021). This may offer PSRBs a framework and baseline from which to work.

REVALIDATION

To maintain registration with the NMC, registrants such as nurses, midwives and nursing associates (England, and with work commencing from March 2024 in Wales) are required to revalidate. Registrants are currently asked to revalidate every 3 years to enable continual reflection of individual practice against the Code of practice of registrants, to support practice development and maintain standards (NMC, 2024b).

The implications of regulation are widespread, which may require individual countries to review current practice around accreditation and digital badging

(NHSE, 2024). Commissioning processes, although separate to any regulatory frameworks and standards, will need to be met, whilst specialist and professional bodies' input could be instrumental in the shaping of standards and revalidation.

Impact on the Health and Care Sector

There is the potential to influence and restrict individual practitioners' access to AP roles. This could have a beneficial impact on risk, whilst potentially restricting the practice of practitioners who have been practising for a number of years who do not have the requisite qualifications and accreditation. In contrast, attraction to the roles and clarity of accountability and responsibilities of advanced practitioners, through the creation of clearly defined career pathways, may positively reinforce and improve the understanding of AP roles and responsibilities by the public, whilst improving retention. This may complement the government-driven increase in AP roles to support health and social care.

In terms of quality, the regulation of AP could improve care quality through the setting of education standards and revalidation requirements. The increase in accountability would reinforce public safety. However, this could be tempered by a potential increase in cost to the registrant practitioners, the NMC and employers, resulting in potential disincentivising of uptake of AP roles. Impacts on wider PSRBs and professional groups may ensue, with individual practitioners who practice within their primary professional scope of practice developing elements of their roles which overlap with AP. The four country approaches, with the different frameworks and definitions, also have implications for regulation and standard setting.

The Association of Advanced Practice Educators UK

The AAPE UK has been a key ally for the developmental and regulatory work ongoing within the UK. This association brings together educators from across the four UK countries. The NMC has previously recognised this network of educators for their influence (Jones et al., 2023). The change of name from the Association of Advanced Nursing Practice Educators UK to AAPE UK in 2015 reflected the commitment to multiprofessional AP (Jones et al., 2023). AAPE UK's terms of reference include *inter alia* to serve as a forum in the development of curricula across the four nations of the UK, in a collaborative manner, sharing resources for AP research, education, contemporaneous clinical practice and leadership, lobbying government bodies where appropriate and responding to consultations from PSRBs, for example. AAPE UK promotes debate on advanced clinical practice education and issues, and priorities in health and social care. AAPE UK is a not-for-profit organisation, and the time invested in the roles and responsibilities of the committee members is entirely voluntary (AAPE UK, 2024).

AAPE UK continues to be involved in AP developments having more recently supported AP curriculum development frameworks for the RPS (2022), who took a UK-wide approach to supporting the development of AP pharmacists. AAPE

UK is committed to continuing to support the development of AP and as such provide an annual conference and annual general meeting, which you are encouraged to attend. Please visit the AAPE UK website for more information.

PIT STOP!

The AAPE UK website can be accessed via this link: https://aape.org.uk/

Conclusion

In conclusion, the development of the NP role within the United States migrated over to the UK in the early 1990s and this laid the foundations for AP, initially focusing on the nursing profession, with the adoption of the titles of NP and ANP, although some healthcare professionals might have been working at an advanced level at that time but did not gain this recognition. With workforce challenges and political drivers, the development and recognition of advanced level practice soon started to be embedded into the practices of other healthcare professions across the UK. With the development of AP frameworks, initially within Scotland, the other nations of the UK soon followed. The four pillars of AP underpin all such frameworks across the UK, with advanced practitioners working across these pillars. AP has witnessed a significant growth since the early 1990s and continues to develop. With the NMC plans to regulate advanced level practice for the nursing and midwifery profession, this is now leading AP into new unchartered waters.

References

AAPE UK. (2024). *Advanced Nursing Practice.* Available at: https://www.aape.org.uk/about/advanced-nursing-practice/. (Accessed January 20, 2025)

Barton, T., Bevan, L., & Mooney, G. (2012). The development of advanced nursing roles. *Nursing Times, 108*(24), 18–20.

Black, B. (2023). *Nurse practitioner profession grows to 385,000 strong.* https://www.aanp.org/news-feed/nurse-practitioner-profession-grows-to-385-000-strong#:,:text=The%20ranks%20of%20NPs%20grew, strengthen%20the%20health%20care%20system (Accessed April 8, 2024)

British Medical Association. (2024). *Safe scope of practice for medical associate professionals (MAPs).* https://www.bma.org.uk/media/tkcosjt1/maps-scope-of-practice2024-web.pdf (Accessed April 5, 2024)

Department of Health. (2019). *Advanced AHP practice framework.* Belfast: Department of Health.

Department of Health and Social Security (DHSS). (1986). *Neighbourhood nursing: A focus for care.* London: DHSS.

Department of Health and Social Security (DHSS). (2019). *Consultation outcome: The regulation of medical associate professions in the UK.* London: DHSS. https://www.gov.uk/government/consultations/regulating-medical-associate-professions-in-the-uk (Accessed January 10, 2024)

Department of Health, Social Services and Public Safety (DHSSPS). (2016). *Advanced nursing practice framework.* Belfast: Northern Ireland Practice and Education Council for Nursing and Midwifery.

European Working Time Directive. (2003). *European working time directive.* https://employment-social-affairs.ec.europa.eu/policies-and-activities/rights-work/labour-law/working-conditions/working-time-directive_en (Accessed April 1, 2023)

Feinmann, J. (2024). Physician associates should not diagnose patients, says BMA guidance. *The BMJ.* 384, q589. https://doi.org/10.1136/bmj.q589

Hardy, M., Snaith, B., Edwards, L., Baxter, J., Millington, P., & Harris, M. (2021). *Advanced practice: Research report.* https://www.hcpc-uk.org/globalassets/resources/policy/independent-research-report-advanced-practice-27th-january-2021.pdf (Accessed April 7, 2024)

Health Education and Improvement Wales (HEIW). (2023). *Professional framework for enhanced, advanced and consultant clinical practice in Wales.* https://heiw.nhs.wales/files/enhanced-advanced-and-consultant-framework/ (Accessed April 7, 2024)

Health Education England. (2017). *Multi-professional framework for advanced clinical practice in England.* https://www.hee.nhs.uk/sites/default/files/documents/multi-professionalframeworkforadvancedclinical-practiceinengland.pdf (Accessed April 6, 2023)

Institute for Apprenticeships and Technical Education. (2018). *Advanced clinical practitioner (integrated degree) standard.* Institute for Apprenticeships and Technical Education. https://www.instituteforapprenticeships.org/apprenticeship-standards/st0564-v1-0 (Accessed April 15, 2024)

Jones, A., Maclaine, K., Henderson, C., & Thomas, J. (2023). UK advanced practice educators networks. *International Journal for Advancing Practice, 1*, 3.

McConnell, D., Slevin, O. D., & McIlfatrick, S. J. (2013). Emergency nurse practitioners' perceptions of their role and scope of practice: Is it advanced practice? *International Emergency Nursing, 1*(2), 76–83.

National Leadership and Innovation Agency for Health Care (NLIAH). (2010). *Framework for advanced nursing, midwifery and allied health professional practice in Wales.* https://aape.org.uk/wp-content/uploads/2015/02/NLIAH-Advanced-Practice-Framework.pdf (Accessed October 6, 2024).

NHS Education for Scotland. (2018). *Advanced practice toolkit.* https://www.advancedpractice.scot.nhs.uk (Accessed March 31, 2023)

NHSE. (2023a). *Health Education England and NHS England complete merger.* https://www.england.nhs.uk/2023/04/health-education-england-and-nhs-england-complete-merger/ (Accessed April 7, 2023)

NHSE. (2023b). *NHS long term workforce plan.* https://www.england.nhs.uk/publication/nhs-long-term-workforce-plan/ (Accessed April 7, 2023)

NHSE. (2024). *Centre for advancing practice portal.* https://advanced-practice.hee.nhs.uk/resources/portal/ (Accessed April 4, 2024)

NHS England. (2025). *Multi-professional framework for advanced Practice in England.* Birmingham: Centre for Advancing Practice.

Nursing and Midwifery Council. (2009). *NMC statement re CHRE report.* http://aape.org.uk/nmc-statement-re-chre-report-2009/ (Accessed September 26, 2023)

Nursing and Midwifery Council. (2023). *Standards for post-registration programmes.* https://www.nmc.org.uk/globalassets/sitedocuments/standards/2023-pre-reg-standards/new-vi/standards-for-post-registration-programmes.pdf (Accessed April 22, 2024)

Nursing and Midwifery Council. (2024a). *Advanced practice review.* https://www.nmc.org.uk/about-us/our-role/advanced-practice-review/ (Accessed April 7, 2024)

Nursing and Midwifery Council. (2024b). *Why we reviewed our post-registration standards.* https://aape.org.uk/wp-content/uploads/2015/02/NLIAH-Advanced-Practice-Framework.pdf (Accessed October 6, 2024)

Nursing and Midwifery Council. (2024c). *Revalidation overview.* https://www.nmc.org.uk/revalidation/overview/what-is-revalidation/ (Accessed April 4, 2024)

Palmer, W., Julian, S., & Vaughan, L. (2023). *Independent report on the regulation of advanced practice in nursing and midwifery.* https://www.nuffieldtrust.org.uk/research/independent-report-on-the-regulation-of-advanced-practice-in-nursing-and-midwifery (Accessed April 4, 2024)

Rogers, M., & Gloster, A. (2020). Advanced practice nurse development in the United Kingdom. In S. Hassmiller & J. Pulcini (Eds.), *Advanced practice nursing leadership: A global perspective* (pp. 167–180). Switzerland: Springer; 2020.

Rogers, M., & Gloster, A. (2023). The evolution of the nurse practitioner role and practice in the United Kingdom. In S. Thomas & J. Rowles (Eds.), *Nurse practitioners and nurse anesthetists: The evolution of the global roles* (pp. 167–180). Springer.

Royal College of Physicians. (2020). *Focus on physician associates: Census 2020.* RCP. www.fparcp.co.uk/about-fpa/fpa-census (Accessed April 5, 2024)

Royal Pharmaceutical Society. (2021). *A competency framework for all prescribers.* https://www.rpharms.com/resources/frameworks/prescribing-competency-framework/competency-framework (Accessed April 7, 2024)

Royal Pharmaceutical Society. (2022). *Core advanced curriculum.* https://www.rpharms.com/about-us/news/details/new-rps-core-advanced-curriculum-published (Accessed April 7, 2024)

Scottish Executive. (2006). *Modernising nursing careers: Setting the direction.* https://www.gov.scot/publications/modernising-nursing-careers-setting-direction/ (Accessed April 1, 2023)

Scottish Government. (2010). *Advanced nursing practice roles guidance for NHS boards*. https://www.advanced-practice.scot.nhs.uk/media/614/sg-advanced-practice-guidance-mar10.pdf (Accessed September 26, 2023)

Scottish Government (SG). (2017). *Transforming nursing, midwifery and health professions roles: Introduction*. https://www.gov.scot/publications/transforming-nursing-midwifery-health-professions-roles-introduction/ (Accessed April 1, 2023)

Scottish Government. (2021a). *Advanced nursing practice—Transforming nursing roles: Phase two*. https://www.gov.scot/publications/transforming-nursing-roles-advanced-nursing-practice-phase-ii/ (Accessed October 6, 2024).

Scottish Government. (2021b). *Transforming nursing, midwifery and health profession (NMaHP) roles: Review of clinical nurse specialist and nurse practitioner roles within Scotland*. https://www.gov.scot/publications/transforming-nursing-midwifery-health-profession-nmahp-roles-review-clinical-nurse-specialist-nurse-practitioner-roles-within-scotland/ (Accessed April 4, 2023)

Scottish Government. (2021c). *NHS recovery plan*. https://www.gov.scot/binaries/content/documents/gov-scot/publications/strategy-plan/2021/08/nhs-recovery-plan/documents/nhs-recovery-plan-2021-2026/nhs-recovery-plan-2021-2026/govscot%3Adocument/nhs-recovery-plan-2021-2026.pdf (Accessed April 4, 2023)

Silver, H. K., Ford, L. C., & Day, L. R. (1968). The pediatric nurse-practitioner program expanding the role of the nurse to provide increased health care for children. *JAMA, 204*(4), 298–302.

UK Health Departments. (2004). *Modernising medical careers the next steps*. https://webarchive.nationalar-chives.gov.uk/20110929193948/; http://www.dh.gov.uk/prod_consum_dh/groups/dh_digitalassets/@dh/@en/documents/digitalasset/dh_4079532.pdf (Accessed April 1, 2023)

Ulster University. (2023). *Physician associate studies – MSc*. https://www.ulster.ac.uk/courses/202324/physi-cian-associate-studies-30695 (Accessed May 3, 2023)

United Kingdom Central Council (UKCC). (1992). *Scope of professional practice*. UKCC.

Williams, L., & Adhiyaman, V. (2022). What do physician associates think about independent prescribing? *Future Healthcare Journal, 9*(30), 282–285.

CHAPTER 2

Transformative Practice in the UK for Demystifying and Preparing for Advanced Practice

Helen Rushforth

CHAPTER OUTLINE

This chapter builds on the scene setting in Chapter 1 and starts by further exploring the historical evolution of advanced practice (AP) in the UK, focusing in particular on issues key to its potential future regulation and development. It then explores in some depth the current UK position in respect of its various mechanisms of voluntary regulation and considers the position of AP in terms of the extent to which it is a level of practice and/or a role. These issues are then contextualised by consideration of the 'debate so far' in respect of the potential formal regulation of AP in the UK and concludes by linking this debate into some of the wider issues influencing the future of UK AP.

Introduction

The purpose of this chapter is to build upon Chapter 1, which presents the developments of advanced practice (AP), to debate and demystify some of the key contemporary issues currently affecting AP in the UK. In doing so, it will identify important considerations and ways forward for the future development of AP, so that its potential transformative impact on healthcare across the UK can be fully realised.

This book comes at an important time in the history of the development of AP, with the current Nursing and Midwifery Council (NMC) review having determined that AP should be formally regulated (NMC, 2023a). It also comes at a time when the value of advanced practitioners as a vital part of the healthcare workforce is being increasingly recognised, with, for example, the recent National Health Service (England) (NHSE) Long-Term Workforce Plan (NHSE, 2023) advocating a doubling of the number of trainees from the current 3000 per year to 6300 per year by 2031/32. This recognition of the considerable value that advanced practitioners bring to the workforce was also thrown into sharp focus by the COVID-19 pandemic (Morley et al., 2022; NHSE, 2022) and anecdotally by the 2023 junior and consultant doctor strikes.

PIT STOP!

National Health Service (NHS) England has been cited as recognising the need for advanced practitioners in their workforce, but what are the other countries' workforce strategies for advanced practitioners?

As noted by Lewis (2022), to influence the future direction of travel for AP it is first important to understand its evolution. Therefore, it is pertinent to start by considering the international and then UK perspectives on the evolution of AP, building on Chapter 1, but, in the context of this chapter, with a particular focus on regulation. This will inform the reasons behind the current position of AP within the UK, the key issues influencing the regulatory debate and the potential future direction of travel for AP in terms of both threats and opportunities.

International Perspectives on AP

The international perspective on AP differs from the UK in a number of important ways. One key differentiator, as noted in Chapter 1 (albeit variable even across the four countries of the UK), is that of viewing AP in a multiprofessional context (Health Education and Improvement Wales (HEIW), 2023; National Health Service England (NHSE) 2024). National Health Service (England) (NHSE) 2025. Internationally, an explicit focus on AP beyond nursing and midwifery is very hard to identify. Countries with well-established models of AP tend to focus largely on nursing (typically referred to as advanced practice nursing, and often using the role title nurse practitioner or clinical nurse specialist)—early adopters include the United States, Canada, Australia, New Zealand, Republic of Ireland, Botswana and Oman (International Council of Nurses (ICN), 2020; Palmer et al., 2023); to date, around 80 countries have some form of model of AP. It is sobering and important to note that a key influencer of the extent of the development of advanced nursing practice roles in each country is the sufficiency or otherwise of its medical workforce (Cooper & Lidster, 2021; Palmer et al., 2023; Williams, 2017). Midwifery features in different ways in a small number of these countries; this includes formal recognition of advanced midwifery practice in Ireland, and the status of midwifery itself as an advanced nursing role for 'nurse midwives' in the United States, where they form one of the four roles for 'advanced practice nurses' alongside nurse practitioners, clinical nurse specialists and nurse anaesthetists.

Within many countries where AP nursing is well developed, there is also some form of regulation of AP. The models to a greater or lesser extent often include some form of title/role protection, often restricting title use to those who have completed appropriate training and competency assessment (ICN, 2020). However, as noted by Wheeler et al. (2022), the exact nature and extent of regulation is internationally very variable, including in respect of the titles used and their protection, and other aspects of regulatory development and barriers to certain aspects of practice.

PIT STOP!

For further discussions on AP internationally, please see Chapter 15.

Historical Development of AP in the UK

In contrast to the international described in in Chapter 1, despite a 30-year history there has until recently been no statutory regulation of the AP role or title in the UK. However, as discussed in Chapter 1, the NMC's governing council accepted recommendations for the regulation of AP. This work will take time to implement; thus, until this regulation comes into effect, an employer can endorse a practitioner holding a title such as nurse practitioner, advanced clinical practitioner, clinical nurse specialist or any such variation of these titles without the practitioner ever having undertaken any formal education or assessment to demonstrate the knowledge and skills that the title might reasonably suggest. Indeed, the practitioner could have undertaken such training but not successfully completed it and still hold the title (Leary et al., 2017; Nadaf, 2018). Leary et al. (2017) also identified a concerning number of examples of 'nonregistered' practitioners holding AP titles. And more recently, Mann et al. (2023) reported title confusion and misuse as one of the key findings in their survey of 63 AP stakeholders. The potential risk to public protection that arises from these observations is arguably considerable.

Drawing upon Lewis (2022) regarding the value of looking back to help us move forward, it is helpful to consider how AP in the UK got to this point. Of initial relevance perhaps is the 1992 Scope of Professional Practice document (United Kingdom Central Council for Nursing, Midwifery and Health Visiting (UKCC), 1992), which replaced the need for certification for what were known as 'extended roles', instead enabling individual practitioners to make judgements regarding their own competency to undertake enhancements to the scope of their professional practice (Rushforth & McDonald, 2004). This opened opportunities in respect of advanced nursing and midwifery practice, and in 1994 the UKCC did define advanced nursing practice, but did so in a very broad, inclusive way, referring to the notion of 'adjusting boundaries for the development of future practice' (UKCC, 1994, p. 8). However, following a subsequent 1996 'listening exercise' (Rolfe, 2014), the NMC decided not to set formal standards for AP. Key to the decision, as Rolfe (2014) notes, there was a dichotomy of viewpoints, wherein one group saw advanced nursing practice as medical 'role substitution', whilst others saw it as more 'holistic and nursing centric'. In contrast, the UKCC did choose to set the Standards for Specialist Practice, although the nomenclature was (and remains) confusing, as this was primarily in respect of Health Visiting, School Nursing and Community Nursing.

In 1999, the Department of Health (DH) laid out its vision for the development of healthcare in 'Making a Difference' (DH, 1999). The document introduces the consultant nurse, midwife and health visitor roles as the pinnacle of clinical careers for these professions and situates consultant practice as the level above registered senior practitioners. But, the report was silent on the notion of AP and makes only one passing reference to nurse practitioners. However, a year later the original National Health Service (NHS) Plan (DH, 2000) laid out their vision of how nurses, midwives and therapists might work across traditional boundaries and in expanded roles to better meet patient needs. With regards to nursing in particular, it laid out its '10 Key Roles for Nurses', stating:

> *'NHS employers will be required to empower appropriately qualified nurses, midwives and therapists to undertake a wider range of clinical tasks including the right to make and receive referrals, admit and discharge patients, order investigations and diagnostic tests, run clinics and prescribe drugs.'*
>
> (DH, 2000, p. 83)

This work was a catalyst for further development of the emerging nurse practitioner roles (albeit titles rarely included the word 'advanced' at this point), and in particular for the development of nonmedical prescribing. Of note at this point is the focus on tasks that were traditionally the remit of medical practice, in marked contrast to the more inclusive UKCC definition of advanced nursing practice noted earlier.

Meanwhile, the application of 'advanced practitioner' titles to allied health professionals (AHPs) didn't emerge until many years later, although physiotherapy widely used the notion of 'extended scope practitioner' to describe a similar level of practice, attributed perhaps in its first articulation to Byles and Ling (1989). However, other allied health professions didn't at this time tend to use formal titles for AP, although via role expansion, a number of roles did evolve which began to further 'blur the boundaries' between the different healthcare professions, as visioned by DH (2000).

Fast forward a few years and within nursing in particular, there was a growing lobby to the NMC that the nurse practitioner role should be regulated, leading to the 2004/05 NMC Formal Consultation on the issue. Importantly, midwifery opted out of this Consultation, suggesting that many of the hallmarks of AP as they were then articulated were already conferred on midwives at the point of registration, and seeing no clear place for AP within midwifery at that time.

Three key aspects of the Consultation on Nurse Practitioner regulation were as follows:

1. Whether the 'nurse practitioner' role should be regulated;
2. If so, whether the title 'specialist nurse practitioner' or 'advanced nurse practitioner' (or something else) should be the regulated title; and
3. What the definition of the chosen title/role should be.

The Consultation offered strong support for regulation, and within that preferred the 'advanced nurse practitioner' title. However, the consultation largely rejected the original proposed definition of the nurse practitioner which had been derived from the ICN 2001 (see ICN, 2008, and ICN, 2020, p. 6) definition, which was as follows:

> *A registrant who "has command of an expert knowledge base and clinical competence, is able to make complex clinical decisions using expert clinical judgement, is an essential*

member of an interdependent health care team and whose role is determined by the context in which s/he practices.'

In contrast, the final definition put forward by the NMC (2006) for its proposed regulation of Advanced Nursing Practice in 2006 (cited by Association of Advanced Practice Educators (AAPE), 2006) was:

'Advanced nurse practitioners are highly experienced and educated members of the care team who are able to diagnose and treat your healthcare needs or refer you to an appropriate specialist if needed.'

Various key skills were then listed as part of the definition, echoing the 10 key roles for nurses, including:

- *Take a comprehensive patient history.*
- *Carry out physical examinations.*
- *Use their expert knowledge and judgement to identify the potential diagnosis.*
- *Refer patients for investigations where appropriate.*
- *Make a final diagnosis.*
- *Decide on and carry out treatments, including the prescribing of medicines, or refer the patient to an appropriate specialist.*

This important 'shift' of emphasis in the way in which advanced nursing practice was viewed in the NMCs 2004/05 consultation and subsequent report echoed the dichotomy in the UKCC 'listening exercise' a decade earlier and crucially offered important insight for the current regulatory debate. Arguably, the original definition, and indeed the well-established ICN 2001/08 definition which underpinned it, could be seen as more akin to nursing 'expertise', or put another way, a higher 'level' of practice. The final agreed NMC definition, in contrast, offered something that could tangibly differentiate the advanced nurse practitioner from those in other senior, experienced nursing roles. However, at its heart sits a list of medical tasks, and in particular the notion of making and responding to a diagnosis. Various terms have been used over many years to recognise this 'medical model' perspective on AP, including 'role substitution', 'task shifting' and 'gap filling' (Lawler et al., 2022; Leary & Maclaine, 2019; Maier et al., 2018; Nadaf, 2018). This is something that proponents of a more inclusive perspective on AP have found difficult to accept (Rolfe, 2014). But, and herein lies an important point which it seems likely influenced the agreed final NMC definition; arguably, a clear, role-focused definition with quantifiable defining attributes is much more amenable to regulation.

However, despite the support for regulation in the NMC 2004/05 consultation, and subsequent support in the key DH (England) (2007) document 'Trust, Assurance and Safety' (clause 2.3), it never happened. The reasons for this stem from the need for government endorsement of changes to regulation, reflective of its considerable cost. Thus, the case was referred to the Privy Council, who asked the then Council for Healthcare Regulatory Excellence (CHRE—now the Professional Standards Authority) to offer their perspective on the issue.

Timing wise, this review happened separate to, but alongside, the UK-wide work of Agenda for Change/Skills for Health in respect of the 'banding' of most healthcare practitioners, the bands 1 to 9 with which many healthcare practitioners will be familiar. This work is significant in the evolution of AP for two key reasons. Firstly, it moved the notion of AP from a nursing-centric to a multiprofessional context. Secondly, in its original iteration, it aligned band 7 with AP (Skills for Health, 2007).

Essentially what this work did was to revert the focus back to a more inclusive notion of AP as reflected in the initially proposed NMC (2005) definition, seeing it as something that all experienced practitioners might aspire to as they moved up the clinical career ladder, i.e., situating it not only multiprofessionally but also as a 'level of practice' rather than a clearly defined 'role' with specific responsibilities. And the conclusions that the CHRE drew in its key paper on AP—also taking a multiprofessional focus on the issue—very much reflected this perspective. They concluded (CHRE, 2009, pp. 2–3):

> '...advanced practice is a level of practice along a continuum in which practitioners develop their professional knowledge, skills and behaviours to a high level, at which they are capable of safe and effective practice in more complex situations and with greater autonomy, responsibility and clinical accountability...it can only be understood in the context of a particular profession at a particular time....relative to the ordinary scopes of practice of members of a profession.'

This paper effectively stated that the CHRE could see no clear case for regulation of AP, also making clear that there was insufficient evidence of the 'risk' of not regulating AP.

Paradoxically though, during the same decade as these debates were ongoing, 'Non-Medical Prescribing' *was* regulated via the NMC, the General Pharmaceutical Council (GPhC) and the Health and Care Professions Council (HCPC), underpinned by associated changes to legislation. From a regulator perspective, recognition of prescribing authority takes the form of a recordable qualification rather than being on a separate part of the register (so not requiring government endorsement in the same way as changes to registration). This started with supplementary prescribing for nurses in 2003, with pharmacists added a year later, and was shortly followed by the endorsement of independent nurse and pharmacist prescribing in 2006. Subsequently, some, but not all, allied health professions were given prescribing authority (see NMC, 2023b; GPhC, 2022; and HCPC, 2023). But interestingly, these regulatory developments within what is arguably a key aspect of AP, and the contrasting view taken regarding the need to regulate AP more generally, were not closely 'joined up' as the professional debates unfolded, despite considerable similarity in some of the attendant risks. Indeed, there remains ongoing uncertainty regarding the extent to which prescribing authority should be viewed as an indicator of AP (Evans et al., 2021).

The NMC did then have one further attempt to achieve its mandate to regulate AP in 2010, achieving support from the then Labour government in its final days for a requirement that advanced nursing practice 'must be regulated' and regulation of advanced midwifery practice 'considered' (Front Line Care, DH (England), 2010). However, the Conservative/Liberal Coalition was in power within days of the report being published, and in a climate of economic austerity and a lack of evidence of the 'risk' of not regulating AP, the coalition concluded in its 2011 white paper that the CHRE perspective was correct, and that there was insufficient evidence of risk associated with not regulating AP. Clause 2.8 (DH, 2011, p. 11) stated:

'...the health professions regulators will need to demonstrate that measures such as advanced practice registers, which have some professional support but where a compelling case for further regulatory action has yet to be made, are an appropriate and proportionate use of registrants' fees.'

Voluntary Regulation of UK AP

What thus emerged from these definitive decisions regarding the regulation of AP was a mandate for 'self' or 'voluntary regulation', which remains at the time of writing until the NMC implements their regulatory plans. These regulatory plans are for nursing and midwifery only, and at time of writing, there are no plans for other professional bodies to regulate AP.

2008 onwards saw the development of the country-specific AP frameworks as summarised in Chapter 1, common to which were the four pillars of AP (albeit slightly differently articulated) and the requirement for master's level education (Department of Health, Social Services and Public Protection (Northern Ireland) (DHSSPS), 2016; HEE, 2017; HEIW, 2023; Scottish Government, 2021). However, the variability between the four countries, particularly in terms of the extent of the multiprofessional status of AP and its different levels of inclusivity, is an ongoing concern in relation to the potential for geographical movement between the four UK countries by staff (Palmer et al., 2023), and potentially by service users.

Furthermore, despite the important development of AP guidelines since 2008, a key area of concern remains their voluntary nature, with, as previously noted, practitioners and employers free to appoint advanced practitioners without any assurance that they have demonstrated their country-specific AP competencies/ capabilities or successfully completed the recommended master's level education (Gloster & Leigh, 2021; Nadaf, 2018). This has resulted in a marked variability in the underpinning qualifications, competency assessment and experience of those holding AP roles, and the education programmes by which they are prepared (Lawler et al., 2022; Palmer et al., 2023). It has also resulted in a wide proliferation of AP titles (Evans et al., 2021; Leary et al., 2017). The risks of this situation for both public understanding of the role and public protection are clear, as have been recently recognised by the NMC-commissioned 'Nuffield Report' in relation to nursing and midwifery in particular (Palmer et al., 2023).

One of the most formalised responses to this concern has come within England, in its establishment of the HEE Centre for Advancing Practice (CfAP). (N.B. from

1 April 2023, this sits under the auspices of the NHS England Workforce, Training and Development Directorate.)

Established as a means of implementing the HEE (2025) 'Multiprofessional Framework', CfAP roles include:

The Centre oversees the workforce transformation of advanced level practice, by: establishing and monitoring standards for education and training including in specific areas of high priority need; accrediting advanced practice programmes offered by universities via 'programme accreditation'; supporting and recognising educational and training equivalence via the ePortfolio (supported) Route; and growing and embedding the advanced and consultant practice workforce.

It is too early to know what traction the Digital Badge will gain as an employer prerequisite for future AP roles. The Digital Badge is also currently a 'one-off' endorsement at a given point in time, with no current formal infrastructure for renewal, revalidation or indeed discontinuation, thus currently sitting some way from the rigour that formal regulation will hopefully confer.

Also key to note, CfAP also offers supportive documents for the levels above and below AP, namely, consultant practice and enhanced practice. For consultant practice, it offers its 2022 Multiprofessional Consultant Practice Framework (HEE, 2022). With regards to the level below AP, it advocates the notion of enhanced practice (Leary, 2022), and within this work also sits some important articulation of career progression from newly qualified to consultant-level practitioner. Importantly, the recently published Welsh 'Professional Framework for Enhanced, Advanced and Consultant Clinical Practice' (HEIW, 2023) uses the same terminology, with similar definitions and career progression, helpfully articulated in a single framework document. Meanwhile, the formal policy focus in Scotland and Northern Ireland remains somewhat more nursing and AP centric, but with some parallel development in relation to the Advanced Allied Health Practice guidance in Northern Ireland (DH Northern Ireland, 2019), and an active 'AHP Education and Workforce Policy Advanced Practice' group in Scotland.

Whilst much focus is currently on the NMC as the regulator who has actively engaged in the consultation for AP regulation, it is pertinent to note the work of two other UK professional statutory regulatory bodies of healthcare practitioners: the General Pharmaceutical Council (GPhC) and the Health and Care Professions Council (HCPC). The GPhC of itself doesn't regulate or formally endorse AP but has been part of the current NMC AP review. However, there is a well-established Royal Pharmaceutical Society (RPS) 'Advanced Pharmacy Framework' (RPS, 2013) and underpinning the more recently published 'core curriculum' (RPS, 2022). The HCPC position is somewhat more complex as the regulator of 15 health and care professions, a position considered in a 'deep dive' review published in January 2021 (Hardy, 2021). Despite the support of 78% of respondents to their consultation in favour of regulation, the review failed to find evidence of sufficient risk of not regulating, concluding that:

'no evidence, with respect to HCPC regulated professions, was found to support the premise that additional regulation is needed to protect the public as is the purpose of regulation',

(Hardy, 2021, p. 57)

Thus the current focus for HCPC's work in this space is on an agreed definition (the lack of which was another key finding from the work) and higher-level guiding principles (HCPC, 2021. Importantly, whilst the NMC decision to regulate Advanced Nursing and Midwifery Practice hasn't at time of writing changed the HCPC perspective, they are collaborating with the NMC as part of the current review (HCPC 2024).

It is also interesting to contrast the perspectives of the HCPC work with the initial research commissioned to support the current NMC review, undertaken by the Nuffield Trust (Palmer et al., 2023). This review again found explicit evidence of the risk arising from AP to be small (albeit citing more evidence than Hardy, 2021), but in contrast, this work took a different view of the potential or latent risk, leading it to support the potential value of regulation, noting:

'the risk of harm to patients receiving advanced practice care has increased and that additional regulation might be useful in improving patient safety.'

(Palmer et al., 2023, p. 58)

The findings of this report are key in terms of informing the NMC's review of AP. Interestingly though, what the HCPC review also throws into sharp focus in contrast to the NMC work are the particular challenges of the multiprofessional agenda. The HCPC is where most of the professions that sit within the UK AP regulatory debate are regulated, and it is the sheer diversity of these different professions that is perhaps central to the challenges of achieving an agreed definition of AP, even within HCPC.

In terms of other key professional bodies with oversight of AP, of note is the Royal College of Nursing (RCN) 'Advanced Level Nurse Practitioner', which it refers to as a 'credential' (RCN, 2023). Built on a long history of RCN programme accreditation, the RCN credential offers another route to underpin voluntary regulation. However, from its inception in 2018 (RCN, 2018), for a number of years the credential offered 'grandparenting rights' to those who could evidence the RCN Advanced Level Nursing Competencies, which included those with little or no formal master's level education. This was a process more akin to the NHSE 'e-portfolio (supported) route', but with less extensive requirements to demonstrate evidence of master's level study and academic writing. In contrast, from a clinical competency perspective, the credential has included from its inception clear requirements with respect to advanced health assessment, diagnosis and pharmacology/prescribing, situated in the context of holistic care delivery. Thus, the credential has afforded some employers a valuable mechanism for verifying the level of practice of their advanced nurse practitioner employees with important assurances of clinical competency, but less certainty regarding the extent of underpinning master's level attainment in many instances. There is also much that can be learned from the RCN's experience of developing and delivering this credentialing process, as indeed there can from the work of CfAP, in terms of informing the implementation of any future mandatory regulation.

Then to complete the picture, it is important to briefly note other profession- or role-specific frameworks within the AP space. Early 'adopters' were some profession-specific AP frameworks, including the RPS (2013), as previously noted, and also the College of Radiography (CoR) accreditation scheme launched in 2010 (College of Radiographers, 2023). Also, relevant here is the College of Paramedics (CoP) (2023) career framework, which articulates AP as a level of practice between consultant-level and specialist-level practice, arguably a confusing use of the term 'specialist' as a level below enhanced practice, albeit congruent with the nomenclature used in the earlier iterations of the Knowledge and Skills Framework (Skills for Health, 2007). Helpfully though, the CoP 5th edition (2023) does refer to 'specialist/*enhanced*' practice to describe the level below AP, hopefully suggesting a shift towards the use of the term 'enhanced practice' as an arguably less confusing descriptor of the level below AP. Notably, a similar albeit slightly more fluid career framework is offered by the College of Podiatry (2021).

Indeed, of note here is that each of the HCPC-regulated professions has its own professional body, most of which offer their own stance on AP, within which some have more recently chosen to direct practitioners to the country-specific frameworks rather than developing their own (notably the Chartered Society of Physiotherapists, 2023; Royal College of Occupational Therapists, 2023).

In contrast, also key to note are two early Medical Royal College-affiliated frameworks: the Faculty of Intensive Care Medicine (FICM, 2015) 'Advanced Critical Care Practitioner' framework and the Royal College of Emergency Medicine (RCEM) 'Advanced Emergency Care Practitioner' framework launched in 2017 and revised in 2022 (RCEM, 2022). Both frameworks were developed under 'medical college/faculty' leadership, in large part mirroring the medical curricula for registrars within the speciality. These curricula perhaps have the strongest emphasis towards 'medical role substitution' of any of the AP initiatives—with their key focus on preparing their practitioners for specific 'advanced practitioner roles' to practice on a junior and increasingly middle grade medical rota. Importantly, whilst these frameworks are both multiprofessional, they do restrict access to particular professions.

Other speciality-specific credentials have also been developed or are in development, several with the formal endorsement of NHSE (e.g., acute medicine, older people and mental health). Note that from the end of 2024, to avoid confusion with other types of credentials, these credentials were renamed Multi-Professional Area Specific Capabilities and Guidelines.

PIT STOP!

Review the current area of specific capabilities in England.
https://advanced-practice.hee.nhs.uk/our-work/credentials/

However, joint working with relevant medical royal colleges means some of this work has potential four country application. These additional credentials are designed to contextualise the core capabilities laid out in NHSE (2024/5) with the requisite speciality-specific capabilities. Again, several of these credentials, especially in acute physical healthcare or primary care settings, include requirements for advanced health assessment, diagnosis and therapeutic intervention in their articulation of the requisite-specific clinical pillar capabilities. Importantly though, they balance this with strong endorsement of the added value brought by the other three pillars and the broader professional perspectives within the clinical pillar. It is important to note that it will be all but impossible to ensure speciality-specific credentials that cover all specialities, given the huge diversity of AP roles and specialities which exist (Nielsen, 2018).

Finally, the picture would not be complete without mention of the first contact practitioner (FCP) role (HEE, 2023). This England-specific, AHP-specific and primary care-specific role applies to five professions—musculoskeletal (usually physiotherapy), dieticians, paramedics, podiatrists and occupational therapists. They are seen as 'diagnostic clinicians' working as a first point of contact to 'assess and manage' people with 'undifferentiated and undiagnosed conditions' in primary care (HEE, 2021, p. 12). Articulated via a series of 'FCP Roadmaps' (HEE, 2023), the FCP is in one sense articulated as a level below AP and in some way aligns with Enhanced Practice. However, with recognition that the clinical competencies achieved by FCPs are congruent with the Clinical Pillar of the HEE (2017) Multiprofessional AP framework (HEE, 2021, p. 15), it could be argued that these practitioners 'straddle the transition zone' between the two levels of practice. Given their scope of practice particularly in respect of diagnosis, it is vital that this practitioner group is not overlooked in any future requirements for AHP regulation.

Thus, to bring this summary of voluntary regulation together, what emerges is an extremely complex landscape of guidance and opportunities for recognition of advanced practitioner 'status' that individual practitioners have open to them, and also the inequality of opportunity across the UK dependent on country, professional registration and speciality. This leaves some UK practitioners with more than one route to formal recognition as an advanced practitioner (several in some cases—both generic and speciality specific) and yet others have none. When this is considered alongside the complexity and variability within the different frameworks, it is not surprising that Evans et al., (2021, p. 8) describes AP as having a *'lack of clarity for organisations and stakeholders regarding preparation, role definition and scope of practice'*, a perspective endorsed by several other contemporary UK authors (Gloster & Leigh, 2021; Hardy, 2021; Lawler et al., 2022; Mann et al., 2023; Palmer et al., 2023; Wallis et al., 2022). This level of inequity and complexity requires a coordinated approach to finding a solution that perhaps only the professional regulators can offer.

The Level vs Role Debate

One of the other important observations that emerge from consideration of the previously mentioned frameworks is that most key UK frameworks from the past 15 years refer to AP as a 'level of practice' (including DH (England) 2010; NHSE 2024/5; HEIW, 2023; RCN, 2018). The notion of AP as a level of practice as opposed to a specific role arguably emerges in part from the widespread variability between all the different roles overseen collectively by the NMC, HCPC and GPhC, and the corresponding need for inclusivity. However, the RCN is a uniprofessional organisation and still advocates the notion of advanced level practice, so it is also perhaps reflective of the diversity of AP currently evident within some professions such as nursing. Almost certainly, the 2009 CHRE assertion that AP was a level of practice has also been influential in this respect. Yet others articulate AP as a 'role' (Brook & Rushforth, 2011; Evans et al., 2021; Imison et al., 2016). It could also be argued that this isn't an 'either/or' debate, and that within 'advanced level practice', there are numerous AP roles. However, several authors recognise the importance of this issue in relation to the discussion surrounding the complexity and confusion of the UK position on AP (Evans et al., 2021; Lawler et al., 2022). And the question of regulation arguably throws the issue into sharp focus. Indeed, going back to CHRE (2009), it was precisely because CHRE argued that AP was a level of practice, and a part of natural career evolution, that they also argued that it didn't require regulation. And more recently within the current NMC review of the requirement for regulation, it was noted anecdotally in early discussions that the NMC had never previously regulated a level of practice, only specific roles.

Also pertinent to this discussion is the notion of autonomy or 'independence' to act (Keenan, 1999), identified in Mantzoukas and Watkinson's (2007) seminal work as the overarching defining attribute of 'advanced nursing practice'. Indeed, nearly all definitions of AP cite autonomy as a key aspect of AP. However, whilst some refer to autonomy in the absolute, e.g., RCN (2018, p. 3), '...*they have the freedom and authority to act, making autonomous decisions...*', several other recent definitions refer to autonomy in the relative, most commonly as a higher degree of autonomy, e.g., NHSE (2025) p14, '...*characterised by a high degree of autonomy*'. This latter conceptualisation of autonomy in relative terms is arguably more helpful, in that having 'full control of all aspects of a role' as absolute autonomy arguably requires (Kaplan & Brown, 2006, p. 37) is rare in any role in healthcare. The reality is that all professions arguably have a certain level of autonomy at point of registration, and that level of autonomy increases as the practitioner becomes more senior and experienced in their role. And thus, whilst those practicing at an advanced level invariably practice with a notably higher level of autonomy than that conferred on them by their initial professional registration, all AP roles, as any others, have their appropriate scope and boundaries of professional practice. Such a way of viewing autonomy also addresses the concern of professions such as midwifery who have historically not aligned themselves with AP due to their autonomy at point of registration.

Therefore, in bringing these two debates together, whether AP is a level or a role, and whether it is characterised by absolute or higher levels of autonomy, there may be a different way of viewing things that might be helpful to the debate surrounding regulation. It could be suggested that when we refer to AP as a level of practice, we are saying that AP is practiced with a significantly higher level of autonomy than that conferred at professional registration. And within this higher level of autonomous practice, there are numerous different AP roles, all of which are characterised by higher levels of autonomy in relation to the skills and capabilities conferred at point of registration, but which vary markedly in many other respects.

The Current NMC Debate

It is in the context of all the challenges described in the preceding sections that the NMC (2023a) reentered the regulatory debate. The catalyst for the current NMC review, as explained in Chapter One, is the recently completed review of the NMC Standards for Specialist Practice, the recordable qualifications for those undertaking education and role endorsement as 'Specialist Practice Public Health Nurses', i.e., health visitors, school nurses and occupational health nurses, and 'Specialist Practice Community Nursing', including district nursing and other community nursing roles (N.B. these roles are largely distinct from the role of the clinical nurse specialist more usually aligned with AP, and another potential source of titular confusion in the debate). These new standards, the first revision for 20 years, were published in July 2022 (NMC, 2022a, 2022b). But key throughout the consultation process were recurrent comments that consideration of specialist practice couldn't and shouldn't be viewed as separate from the debate surrounding AP, with various stakeholders suggesting that the risks arising from the lack of regulation of AP were as great or greater than the risks from specialist practice that *is* regulated (Mitchell, 2019; Queens Nursing Institute, 2021).

Relevant also to discussion is the statement within both new sets of 'Standards' (NMC, 2022a, 2022b, p. 3) that the NMC reserves regulation,

'For those areas where ensuring consistency of standards of proficiency, and standards for education and training, is needed to achieve a higher level of quality and safety in order to mitigate risk and to reassure the public.'

Thus, in the current NMC work on regulation, consideration has centered on those aspects of practice that form the greatest areas of risk, and thus the clearest mandate for regulation (Palmer et al., 2023).

Looking back at the CHRE's conclusions in 2009, and the subsequent decision in 2011 not to regulate AP, this was based on the premise that advanced level practice is a natural evolution of a career as someone develops greater expertise. However, there is another important but much less frequently cited clause within CHRE (2009, p. 10), where it states in clause 7.3 that a case for regulation would exist where regulators:

'...identify clear risks to patient safety and associated standards of proficiency that go far beyond those of the ordinary scope of a profession's practice.... It is only where a practice is so significantly out with the ordinary scope of profession's practice, such that the level of public protection from its associated standards become inadequate... that further standards – clearly different from the ordinary ones – would be a coherent basis for controlling professional practice.'

This then seemingly fits with the NMC's (2022a, 2022b) assertion regarding the case for additional regulation. Therefore, the situation that starts to emerge from the collective picture of the evolution of AP in the UK to date is arguably a need for some, but not all, of those roles currently articulated as sitting under the auspices of advanced level practice to be regulated. This is because it seems rightly reasonable to suggest that someone working at a senior, expert level, often with a higher degree of autonomy and complex decision-making, but in a role which builds on the natural evolution of their own original professional standards and competencies, doesn't need regulation (Brook & Rushforth, 2011). Conversely, it is exceptionally difficult to put forward the same argument for someone who has taken on significant elements of traditional medical practice and incorporated these advanced health assessment, diagnostic and therapeutic 'medical skills' into their own practice, sometimes to the point of being able to work on a medical rota or otherwise substitute for a medical practitioner. Thus, such practitioners become, as Brook and Rushforth (2011) argue, effectively 'hybrid practitioners'. Such practitioners are still founding their practice in their own professional registration but are taking on significant elements of traditional medical practice that have had little or no part in their previous training and sit beyond what might reasonably be regarded as 'natural career evolution'.

And indeed crucially, Palmer et al. (2023) identified medical diagnosis and intervention as the greatest area of risk to public protection in the recent

NMC-commissioned Nuffield Report. Thus, the risk associated with not having regulation that requires such advanced practitioners to have successfully completed appropriate education and competency assessment could be viewed as considerable; indeed, the equivalent diagnostic role within the field of medical practice requires several years of mandatory education and assessment. In other words, whilst AP is rightly much more than 'role substitution' (or 'task shifting' or 'gap filling') (Nadaf, 2018), the extent to which roles and/or tasks that are predominantly situated within the domain of medicine form part of a practitioner's AP role, particularly in relation to medical diagnosis and the actions arising from it, is arguably the nub of the issue when it comes to risk, and thus to regulation.

Also of key relevance here are the Bolam Principles on which suboptimal practice will typically be judged. Legally, as most advanced practitioners will be aware, this states:

'The standard of care expected is the standard of the ordinary skilled man exercising and professing to have that special skill.'
(Bolam vs Friern Hospital Management Committee, 1957, cited in Liddell et al., 2022, p. 37)

This means that where activities normally undertaken by one healthcare professional are delegated/transferred to another healthcare professional, the new practitioner is expected to meet the same standard as that required of the professional who previously performed the task (Dimond, 2011). In other words, the standard of care that the patient is entitled to and can expect to receive is the same, irrespective of who delivers it. And arguably, wherever we equip nurses, midwives, AHPs and pharmacists to undertake roles or skills that are predominantly the domain of medical practitioners (or indeed predominantly the domain of any other profession other than their own), arguably we must have assurance that these practitioners have been educated and assessed to the same standard as the professional group whom they supplement or replace.

With the plans for the NMC to regulate AP, it remains challenging to identify those practitioners whose practice falls significantly out with the ordinary scope of the person's own professional registration (CHRE, 2009). However, within nursing at least, the identification of 'tasks such as diagnosis and interventions' as being associated with the highest level of latent risk (Palmer et al., 2023) could be a very helpful starting point.

To develop this debate a little further, it is interesting to consider the most recent AP frameworks from each of the four UK countries. These four documents are NHSE (2025) and HEIW (2023) from England and Wales, respectively, both multiprofessional in focus, and the Scottish Government (2021) and DHSSPS (2016), which are respectively the uniprofessional Scottish and Northern Irish frameworks for advanced nurse practitioners. Scrutinising the nursing-specific documents first, there is a clear and explicit focus on the role of the nurse practitioner in undertaking (with a high degree of autonomy) advanced health/clinical assessment, diagnosis/differential diagnosis and prescribing/therapeutic intervention. The more recent and more detailed Scottish Government (2021) document, offering greater detail than its

Northern Irish counterpart, also includes specifics regarding investigations, nonpharmacological treatment and specific conditions/situations which the advanced nurse practitioner can independently manage. In contrast, the NHSE 2025 document for England includes in capabilities 1.4, 6 and 7 the notions of advanced history taking, diagnosis, undertaking/interpreting diagnostic tests and prescribing, but does so by way of examples, suggesting these *may* characterise AP alongside other arguably lower-risk alternatives such as conducting health needs assessments and giving lifestyle advice and care, different aspects of practice presumably offered to ensure multiprofessional inclusivity. Interestingly, the most inclusive document from HEIW (2023) has no mention of advanced clinical assessment, diagnosis or prescribing/therapeutic intervention anywhere in its section on AP.

Further consideration of the professions regulated by HCPC brings this aspect of the debate into sharper focus. What does advanced health assessment and diagnosis mean for an art therapist? How can a speech and language therapist embrace notions of 'diagnostics' and 'therapeutic intervention' as a hallmark of AP when these skills are fundamental requirements at point of registration? And how do we unravel the scope and boundaries 'diagnosis and intervention' in the context of 'regular' vs 'advanced roles' for a diagnostic vs a therapeutic radiographer? Arguably, there are several HCPC-regulated professions whose AP is largely congruent with developing professional expertise within their own profession and chosen speciality, and thus representing much lower risk. In contrast though, a growing number of physiotherapists and paramedics, in particular, and a smaller group of practitioners from some other HCPC-regulated professions (in particular some occupational therapists, radiographers, dieticians and podiatrists), alongside a growing number of GPhC regulated pharmacists, are undertaking 'hybrid practitioner' roles which cross over the boundaries into medical practice; these roles thus pose similar levels of risk to those of their nursing counterparts. It seems clear that the challenges for the future in terms of defining, let alone potentially regulating, AP are particularly tricky for HCPC. In contrast, within nursing, this is somewhat less problematic, with notions of medical diagnosis and therapeutic intervention easier to differentiate, thus making nursing in this regard a helpful starting point for the regulatory debate. That being said, defining the scope and boundaries of advanced practice for midwifery regulation may be somewhat more challenging.

Where this arguably leaves us is with a need to recognise two important points. Firstly, any attempt to find a 'one-size-fits-all' definition of AP or regulatory framework inclusive of all the professions regulated by the NMC, HCPC and GPhC would be so broad as to be potentially meaningless. Secondly, to meaningfully take forward any moves towards regulation that can offer the intended additional public protection, we may well have to consider these in a profession-specific way. The key here is recognition that professional registration confers an individual with a unique set of knowledge, skills and competences in the context of a particular profession, and thus what sits within that profession as its 'natural career evolution' versus what constitutes practice significantly out with the ordinary scope of a profession's practice (CHRE, 2009) will also inevitably vary from one profession to the next. Indeed,

CHRE's (2009, p. 3) assertion that AP '...*can only be understood in the context of a particular profession at a particular time...relative to the ordinary scopes of practice of members of a profession*' is also very relevant in this context. What all this means for the future of the currently inclusive 'advanced clinical practitioner' title and its variants is also of course key to the debate.

However, that is not to suggest that a complete U turn on the multiprofessional AP agenda is required. There remains much in common across the three nonclinical pillars in particular that are key and pivotal to any AP role definitions. Notions of higher-level autonomy, complex clinical judgement and decision-making, and the need for master's level education as key recurrent hallmarks of contemporary AP definitions (DHSSPS, 2016; NHSE 2025; HEIW, 2023; RCN, 2018; Scottish Government, 2021), remain an important starting point and context for such work. But to move forward, arguably, we need to balance our consideration of the common hallmarks of AP across the various professions and roles with a closer consideration of the differences and, in particular, the aspects of each AP role which constitute the greatest risk to public protection, and how that risk can best be mitigated.

Conclusion

The consideration of the various issues outlined in this chapter leaves us with a recognition of the enormity and complexity of the current situation regarding AP. It is a situation underpinned by considerable good endeavour by numerous individuals and organisations to maximise the benefits that AP can confer. But it is also currently an exceptionally difficult area of practice for many practitioners, employers, educators and service users to navigate, with potential shortfalls that constitute an increasingly recognised latent risk to public protection.

What is also clear is that, at the time of writing, AP currently sits at a crossroads. The decisions made over the next few years as regulators progress the complex debate surrounding the regulation of AP and will be key to its future. In this context the current work of the NMC surrounding the regulation of advanced nursing and midwifery practice is warmly welcomed, as is its inclusion of other regulators in this work going forward. But in a climate of austerity, this may be the last opportunity for a generation to enable AP regulation to happen.

Arguably though, much of the influence on the outcome of the current regulatory debate sits in our own hands, in our roles as key stakeholders—as trainees, practitioners, managers, educators and researchers who are involved in the field of AP. It is beholden on us to learn the lessons from the past, to recognise the complexity of the debate and to move beyond our individual agendas and career aspirations to focus firmly on patient best interest and ensuring public protection. If we get this wrong, the very sustainability of AP as we currently know and understand it could be in question. But if we approach this debate wisely, we can help to facilitate an outcome that will have immensely important benefits for the people that we care for, and for the potential transformative impact of AP on the future of healthcare delivery.

References

Bolam vs Friern Hospital Management Committee (1957), cited in Liddell, K., Skopek, J., Gallez, I., & Fritz, Z. (2022). Differentiating negligent standards of care in diagnosis. *Medical Law Review, 30*(1), 33–59.

Brook, S., & Rushforth, H. (2011). Why is the regulation of advanced practice essential? *British Journal of Nursing, 20*(16), 996–1000.

Byles, S. E., & Ling R. S. M. (1989). Orthopaedic out-patients – a fresh approach. *Physiotherapy, 75*(7), 435–437.

Chartered Society of Physiotherapists. (2023). *Advanced practice physiotherapists.* https://www.csp.org.uk/careers-jobs/advanced-consultant-practice-physiotherapy/advanced-practice-physiotherapists

College of Paramedics. (2023). *Paramedic career framework* (5th ed.). https://swastcpd.co.uk/wp-content/uploads/Sept-23_Paramedic_Career_Framework_5th_edition_REVISED-2023-FINAL.pdf

College of Podiatry. (2021). *Podiatry career framework.* https://rcpod.org.uk/workforceprogramme/modernisation-and-reform/the-career-framework

College of Radiographers. (2023). *Advanced practitioner accreditation.* https://www.collegeofradiographers.ac.uk/education/accreditation/advanced-practitioner-accreditation

Cooper, J., & Lidster, J. (2021). Perceptions of competency in advanced clinical practice. *British Journal of Nursing, 30*(14), 852–856.

Council for Healthcare Regulatory Excellence. (2009). *Advanced practice: Report to the four UK health departments.* London: CHRE. http://www.professionalstandards.org.uk/docs/default-source/publications/advice-to-ministers/advanced-practice-2009.pdf?sfvrsn=6

Department of Health. (1999). *Making a difference: Strengthening the nursing, midwifery and health visiting contribution to health and healthcare,* London: DH. http://www.nursingleadership.org.uk/publications/nurstrat.pdf

Department of Health. (2000). *The NHS Plan: A plan for investment, a plan for reform.* London: DH. https://navigator.health.org.uk/theme/nhs-plan-2000

Department of Health. (2011). *White paper: Enabling excellence: Autonomy and accountability for health and social care staff.* Leeds, Professional Standards Division, DH. http://www.dh.gov.uk/en/Publicationsandstatistics/Publications/PublicationsPolicyAndGuidance/DH_124359

Department of Health (England). (2007). *Trust, assurance and safety – The Regulation of health professionals in the 21st century.* London: The Stationary Office. https://assets.publishing.service.gov.uk/government/uploads/system/uploads/attachment_data/file/228847/7013.pdf

Department of Health (England). (2010). *Advanced level nursing: A position statement.* https://assets.publishing.service.gov.uk/government/uploads/system/uploads/attachment_data/file/215935/dh_121738.pdf

Department of Health Northern Ireland. (2019). *Advanced AHP Practice Framework: Guidance for supporting advanced allied health professions practice in Northern Ireland.* https://www.health-ni.gov.uk/sites/default/files/publications/health/AHP-Framework.pdf

Department of Health, Social Services and Public Protection (Northern Ireland). (2016). *Advanced Nursing Practice Framework.* Belfast: Northern Ireland Practice and Education Council. https://www.health-ni.gov.uk/sites/default/files/publications/health/advanced-nursing-practice-framework.pdf

Dimond, B. (2011). *Legal aspects of nursing and healthcare* (6th ed.). London: Pearson.

Evans, C., Poku, B., Pearce, R., Eldridge, J., Hendrick, P., Knaggs, R., et al. (2021). Characterising the outcomes, impacts and implementation challenges of advanced clinical practice in the UK: A scoping review. *British Medical Journal* Open, *11*, e048171. https://bmjopen.bmj.com/content/11/8/e048171

Faculty of Intensive Care Medicine. (2015). *Curriculum for training for advanced critical care practitioners.* https://www.ficm.ac.uk/careersworkforceaccps/accp-curriculum

General Pharmaceutical Council. (2022). *Pharmacist independent prescriber.* https://www.pharmacyregulation.org/education/pharmacist-independent-prescriber

Gloster, A., & Leigh, J. (2021). The knowledge and skills required for advanced level practitioners for accreditation and safe practice. *British Journal of Nursing, 30*(3), 168–171.

Hardy, M. (2021). *Advanced practice: Research report.* University of Bradford/Health and Care Professions Council. https://www.hcpc-uk.org/globalassets/resources/policy/independent-research-report-advanced-practice-27th-january-2021.pdf?v=637483937140000000

Health and Care Professions Council. (2021). *Advanced Practice Project: An update on important developments.* https://www.hcpc-uk.org/news-and-events/blog/2021/advanced-practice-project-an-update-on-important-developments/

Health and Care Professions Council. (2023). *Our professions' medicines and prescribing rights.* https://www.hcpc-uk.org/standards/meeting-our-standards/scope-of-practice/medicines-and-prescribing-rights/our-professions-medicines-and-prescribing-rights/

Health Education and Improvement Wales. (2023). *Professional framework for enhanced, advanced and consultant advanced clinical practice in Wales.* Cardiff: HEIW. https://heiw.nhs.wales/files/enhanced-advanced-and-consultant-framework/

Health Education England. (2017). *Multi-professional framework for advanced clinical practice in England.* London: HEE. https://www.hee.nhs.uk/sites/default/files/documents/multi-professionalframeworkforadvancedclinicalpracticeinengland.pdf

Health Education England. (2021). *First contact practitioners and advanced practitioners in primary care (musculoskeletal): A roadmap to practice.* https://www.hee.nhs.uk/sites/default/files/documents/MSK%20July21-FILLABLE%20Final%20Aug%202021_2.pdf

Health Education England. (2022). *Multi-professional consultant-level practice capability and impact framework.* England: HEE. https://www.hee.nhs.uk/sites/default/files/documents/Sept%202020%20HEE%20Consultant%20Practice%20Capability%20and%20Impact%20Framework.pdf

Health Education England. (2023). *First contact practitioners: Roadmaps to practice.* https://www.hee.nhs.uk/our-work/allied-health-professions/enable-workforce/roadmaps-practice/first-contact-practitioners-roadmaps-practice

Imison, C., Castle-Clark, C., & Watson, R. (2016). *Reshaping the workforce to deliver the care that patients need.* London: Nuffield Trust/NHS Employers. https://www.nuffieldtrust.org.uk/sites/default/files/2017-01/reshaping-the-workforce-web-final.pdf

International Council of Nurses (ICN). (2020). *Guidelines on advanced practice nursing.* https://www.icn.ch/system/files/documents/2020-04/ICN_APN%20Report_EN_WEB.pdf

International Council of Nurses. (2008). *The scope of practice, standards and competencies of the advanced practice nurse.* Geneva: ICN.

Kaplan, L., & Brown, M. (2006). What is 'true' professional autonomy? *The Nurse Practitioner, 31*(3), 37.

Keenan, J. (1999). A concept analysis of autonomy. *Journal of Advanced Nursing, 29*(3), 556–562. https://onlinelibrary.wiley.com/doi/pdf/10.1046/j.1365-2648.1999.00948.x

Lawler, J., Maxwell, E., Radford, M., & Leary, A. (2022). Advanced clinical practitioners' experience of establishing a workplace jurisdiction. *International Journal of Healthcare Management, 15*(3), 246–254. https://www.tandfonline.com/doi/full/10.1080/20479700.2020.1870368

Leary, A. (2022), *The principles of enhanced level practice.* London: Health Education England. https://www.hee.nhs.uk/sites/default/files/documents/The%20Principles%20of%20Enhanced%20Level%20Practice.pdf

Leary, A., & Maclaine, K. (2019). The evolution of advanced nursing practice: Past, present and future. *Nursing Times, 115*(10), 18–19.

Leary, A., Maclaine, K., Trevatt, P., Radford, M., & Punshon, G. (2017). Variations in job titles within the nursing workforce. *Journal of Clinical Nursing.* https://onlinelibrary.wiley.com/doi/epdf/10.1111/jocn.13985

Lewis, R. (2022). The evolution of advanced nursing practice: Gender, identity, power and patriarchy. *Nursing Inquiry. 29*, 12489. https://www.ncbi.nlm.nih.gov/pmc/articles/PMC9787357/pdf/NIN-29-e12489.pdf

Maier, C., Koppen, J., Busse, R., & MUNROS Team. (2018). Task shifting from physicians to nurses in primary care in 39 countries: a cross-country comparative study. *Human Resources for Health, 16*, 24. https://academic.oup.com/eurpub/article/26/6/927/2616280?login=true

Mann, C., Timmons, S., Evans, C., Pearce, R., Overton, C., Hinsliff-Smith, K., & Conway, J. (2023). Exploring the role of advanced clinical practitioners and their contribution to health services in England: A qualitative exploratory study. *Nurse Education in Practice, 67*, 103546 https://www.ncbi.nlm.nih.gov/pmc/articles/PMC9872859/

Mantzoukas, S., & Watkinson, S. (2007). Review of advanced nursing practice: The international literature and developing the generic features. *Journal of Clinical Nursing, 16*, 28–37.

Mitchell, G. (2019). NMC considers advanced nurse regulation as part of review. *Nursing Times.* https://www.nursingtimes.net/professional-regulation/nmc-considers-advanced-nurse-regulation-as-part-of-review-12-06-2019/

Morley, D., Kilgore, C., Edwards, M., Collins, P., Scammell, J., Fletcher, K. and Board, M. (2022). The changing role of advanced clinical practitioners working with older people during the COVID-19 pandemic: A qualitative research study. *International Journal of Nursing Studies*, 130: 104235. https://www.ncbi.nlm.nih. gov/pmc/articles/PMC8956343/

Nadaf, C. (2018). Perspectives: Reflections on a debate: When does advanced clinical practice stop being nursing? *Journal of Research in Nursing*, 23(1), 91–97.

National Health Service (England). (2022). *How did advanced clinical practitioners respond to COVID-19?* https://www.hee.nhs.uk/coronavirus-covid-19/how-did-advanced-clinical-practitioners-re-spond-covid-19

National Health Service (England). (2023). *Long term workforce plan.* London: NHSE. https://www.england. nhs.uk/wp-content/uploads/2023/06/nhs-long-term-workforce-plan-v1.2.pdf

NHS England. (2025) *Multi-professional framework for advanced Practice in England.* Birmingham: Centre for Advancing Practice.

Nielsen, F. (2018). *Advanced clinical practice education in England.* London: Council of Deans for Health.

Nursing and Midwifery Council. (2005). *The proposed framework for the standard of post registration nursing.* London: NMC.

Nursing and Midwifery Council. (2006). *Outcomes of consultation on the proposed framework.* London: NMC, cited in Association of Advanced Practice Educators. (2006). *Regulation of Advanced Nursing Practice.* https://aape.org.uk/regulator-updates/.

Nursing and Midwifery Council. (2022a). *Standards of proficiency for specialist practice public health nurses.* London: NMC. https://www.nmc.org.uk/standards/standards-for-post-registration/standards-of-profi-ciency-for-specialist-community-public-health-nurses2/

Nursing and Midwifery Council. (2022b). *Standards of proficiency for community nursing specialist practice qual-ifications.* London: NMC. https://www.nmc.org.uk/standards/standards-for-post-registration/stand-ards-of-proficiency-for--community-nursing-specialist-practice-qualifications/

Nursing and Midwifery Council. (2023a). *Advanced practice review.* London, NMC. https://www.nmc.org.uk/ about-us/our-role/advanced-practice-review/#:~:text=Over%20the%20years%20there%20have,our%20 2020%2D25%20corporate%20strategy

Nursing and Midwifery Council. (2023b). *Standards for prescribers.* London: NMC. https://www.nmc.org.uk/ standards/standards-for-post-registration/standards-for-prescribers/

Nursing and Midwifery Council. (2024). *Advanced practice review.* https://www.nmc.org.uk/about-us/our-role/advanced-practice-review/. Accessed April 4, 2024.

Palmer, W., Julien, S., & Vaughan, L. (2023). *Independent report on the regulation of advanced practice in nursing and midwifery.* London: Nuffield Trust. https://www.nuffieldtrust.org.uk/sites/default/files/2023-05/Ad-vanced%20practice%20report%20FINAL%5B69%5D.pdf

Queens Nursing Institute. (2021). *QNI response to NMC consultation on post registration standards* (open letter). https://www.qni.org.uk/wp-content/uploads/2021/07/QNI-Response-to-NMC-Consultation-on-Post-Registration-Standards-July-2021.pdf

Rolfe, G. (2014). Understanding advanced nursing practice. *Nursing Times*, 110(27), 20–23. https://www. nursingtimes.net/clinical-archive/public-health/understanding-advanced-nursing-practice/5072428.article

Royal College of Emergency Medicine. (2022). *Advanced clinical practitioner curriculum.* https://rcem.ac.uk/ acp-curriculum/

Royal College of Nursing. (2023). *Advanced Practice Standards.* London: RCN. https://www.rcn.org.uk/Pro-fessional-Development/Advanced-Practice-Standards

Royal College of Nursing. (2018). *Royal College of Nursing standards for advanced level nursing practice.* Lon-don: RCN. https://www.rcn.org.uk/Professional-Development/publications/pub-007038

Royal College of Occupational Therapists (2023). *Advanced practice.* https://www.rcot.co.uk/advanced-practice

Royal Pharmaceutical Society. (2013). *Advanced Pharmacy Framework.* London: RPS. https://www.rpharms. com/Portals/0/RPS%20document%20library/Open%20access/Frameworks/RPS%20Advanced%20Phar-macy%20Framework.pdf

Royal Pharmaceutical Society. (2022). *Core advanced pharmacist curriculum.* https://www.rpharms.com/devel-opment/credentialing/core-advanced-pharmacist-curriculum

Rushforth, H., & McDonald, H. (2004). Decisions by nurses in acute care to undertake expanded practice roles. *British Journal of Nursing*, 13(8), 482–490.

Scottish Government. (2021). *Transforming nursing roles – Advanced nursing practice. Phase Two.* https://www.gov.scot/binaries/content/documents/govscot/publications/advice-and-guidance/2021/04/transforming-nursing-roles-advanced-nursing-practice-phase-ii/documents/transforming-nursing-roles-advanced-nursing-practice-phase-ii/transforming-nursing-roles-advanced-nursing-practice-phase-ii/govscot%3Adocument/transforming-nursing-roles-advanced-nursing-practice-phase-ii.pdf

Skills for Health. (2007). *Key elements of career framework.* London: Skills for Health.

United Kingdom Central Council (UKCC). (1992). *The scope of professional practice.* London: UKCC.

United Kingdom Central Council (UKCC). (1994). *The future of professional practice: The Council's standards for education and practice following registration.* London: United Kingdom Central Council for Nursing, Midwifery and Health Visiting (UKCC), cited in Rolfe, G. (2014). Understanding Advanced Nursing Practice. *Nursing Times, 110*(27), 20–23. https://www.nursingtimes.net/clinical-archive/public-health/understanding-advanced-nursing-practice/5072428.article

Wallis, L., Locke, R., Sutherland, C., & Harden, B. (2022). Assessment of advanced clinical practitioners. *Journal of Interprofessional Care, 36*(6), 946–950.

Wheeler, W., Miller, M., Pulcini, J., Gray, D., Ladd, E., & Rayens, M. K. (2022). Advanced practice nursing roles, regulation, education and practice: A global study. *Annals of Global Health, 88*(1), 42. https://annalsofglobalhealth.org/articles/10.5334/aogh.3698

Williams, K. (2017). Advanced practitioners in emergency care: A literature review. *Emergency Nurse, 25*(4), 36–41.

CHAPTER 3

Four Pillars of Advanced Practice — Education: Foundations and Future

Kim Manley ■ Annabella Gloster

Recognition to Kathy Haigh for her contribution to this chapter

CHAPTER OUTLINE

This chapter explores the historical foundation of advanced practice (AP) education in the United Kingdom (UK) and how the education pillar became a core requirement through the capabilities required of the role. The current education capabilities and how they are developed in advancing practice provide the backdrop for considering future direction with an emphasis on (1) learning in, from and for practice and (2) the developmental pathway from advanced towards multiprofessional consultant level practice.

Introduction

Education is an integral pillar of advanced practice (AP) for optimising both patient learning and growing the workforce. Education in AP encompasses learning and development activities that enable self and others to learn, embedding learning cultures in the workplace and more formal approaches to support patient pathways, health and education provider organisations with their education and workforce priorities.

This chapter first explores the historical foundation of AP education in the United Kingdom (UK) and how the education pillar became a core requirement. Current education capabilities and how these capabilities are developed then pave the way for future considerations with an emphasis on learning in, from and for practice and the developmental pathway from advanced towards multiprofessional consultant level practice.

The Historical Context of the Education Pillar

AP evolved in the UK from a nursing origin with nurse practitioner roles that developed in the late 1980s in response to the changing needs of the population and a desire to advance the nursing profession. The first training programme was established in the UK by the Royal College of Nursing (RCN) in conjunction with the

University of London and was delivered at diploma level. Subsequently franchised, the programme became available to education institutions on a commercial basis as an accredited programme benchmarked to nationally agreed standards (RCN, 2012).

The RCN standards defined the level of AP as embracing health education, leadership and consultancy functions and teaching skills, which is consistent with the UK frameworks:

> *'developing with the patient an ongoing nursing care plan for health, with an emphasis on health education and preventative measures'*
> *'providing a leadership and consultancy function as required'*
>
> (RCN, 2012, p. 4)

Non-RCN-accredited education programmes began to emerge in UK universities in the 1990s with programme content initially replicating a North American conceptual model (Hamric et al., 2009). University programmes reflected the complexity of the role and included key topic areas such as the consultation, ethical decision-making, research, expert guidance, coaching and leadership.

Developments across the four nations included the publication of 'The Advanced Practice Toolkit' (NHS Education for Scotland, 2008) and a position paper in England by the Department of Health (2010) with the expectations that advanced level practice is more than direct clinical practice, but also requires the development of self and others through 'education' competencies and capabilities. Table 3.1 provides an overview of the UK frameworks; however, please see Chapter 1 for a breakdown of the approach to AP in each of the UK countries.

The multiprofessional framework for advanced clinical practice in England (Health Education England (HEE), 2017 and revised version by NHS England (NHSE, 2025)) both acknowledged and built on previous frameworks to link the education pillar with specific capabilities required for health and care professionals practicing at the level of AP.

The HEE multiprofessional framework definition of advanced level practice sets the tone for AP programmes and the level of education required integrating the education pillar with core and area-specific clinical capabilities. The language used to describe the capabilities (Table 3.2) maps to the master's level taxonomy, making it clear that practitioners working at this level should have developed and can evidence the capabilities required (Box 3.1). The requirement of a master's graduate who has in-depth knowledge and understanding of their subject area informed by current practice, scholarship and research is required across all four pillars. The education pillar detailed in the NHSE (2025) framework lists the expectations of practitioners to critically assess and address their own learning needs and that of others, acknowledging health literacy, understanding individuals' motivation and developmental stage and enabling empowerment and participation in decisions to maximise health and well-being. Facilitating learning or education is important for supporting patients, staff and advanced practitioners' self-awareness to assess and meet their own learning needs (Gloster & Leigh, 2021).

TABLE 3.1 ■ UK Frameworks Illustrating the Education Focus of AP

Publication/Frameworks	Education Requirement as Part of Advanced Level Practice
Transforming Nursing, Midwifery and Health Professions Roles – Advance Nursing Practice (Scottish Government, 2017)	Four pillars: 1. Clinical practice 2. Leadership 3. **Facilitation of learning** 4. Evidence, research and development
Department of Health Position Paper (Department of Health, 2010)	Four themes working at an advanced level required to have competencies in: 1. Clinical/direct care or practice 2. Leadership and collaborative practice 3. Improving the quality and developing practice 4. **The development of self and others**
Professional Framework for Enhanced, Advanced and Consultant Clinical Practice in Wales (Health Education and Improvement Wales, 2023)	Four pillars of practice: 1. Clinical practice 2. **Education** 3. Management and leadership 4. Research
Multiprofessional Framework for Advanced Clinical Practice in England (Health Education England, 2017)	Four pillars of practice: 1. Clinical practice 2. Leadership and management 3. **Education** 4. Research
Advanced Nursing Practice Framework: Supporting Advanced Nursing Practice in Health and Social Care Trusts (Northern Ireland Practice and Education Council for Nursing and Midwifery, 2018)	Four Pillars of Practice 1. Direct clinical practice 2. Leadership and collaborative practice 3. **Education and learning** 4. Research and evidence-based practice
Advanced AHP Practice Framework: Guidance for Supporting Advanced Allied Health Professions Practice in Health and Social Care (Department of Health—Northern Ireland, 2019)	Four pillars of practice: 1. Clinical practice 2. Leadership and management 3. **Education** 4. Research

AP, Advanced practice, *AHP,* Allied health professionals.

TABLE 3.2 ■ Three Domains of Learning as Identified by Bloom (1956)

Psychomotor	Skills concerned with dexterity, for example, the insertion of a central line. This requires underpinning knowledge but predominantly needs practice in the physical or manual skill.
Cognitive	The 'how' and 'why', knowledge and the thinking skills.
Affective	Concerned with attitudes. Deals with growth in feelings or emotional areas. For example, what attitude we would like the learner to display as a result of the learning.

BOX 3.1 ■ Capability Defined

'The attributes (skills, knowledge and behaviours) which individuals bring to the workplace. This includes the ability to be competent and beyond this, to manage change, be flexible, deal with situations which may be complex or unpredictable and continue to improve performance.'
(Health Education England, NHS England and Skills for Health, 2020, p. 9)

The ability to support the wider team to build capacity through work-based learning and acting as a role model, educator, supervisor, mentor and coach to others is also required at this level of practice.

HEE acknowledged the variation in regional and local practice and states that the framework is to be used as a standard for professionals whilst employers need to ensure good governance of AP. The development of the Centre for Advancing Practice (CfAP) in England in 2021 (see Chapter 2) saw programme accreditation introduced whereby education providers submit evidence about how their programmes meet the standards set out in the framework in addition to the Standards for Education and Training set by HEE (now NHSE). This process aims to standardise education and training across multiprofessional groups working at an advanced level of practice. How individual practitioners currently gain and evidence the required capabilities across this pillar is discussed next.

As illustrated in Table 3.1, all countries of the UK define levels of AP and the education that underpins them and provides support and guidance for employers, universities and clinical practitioners or those aspiring to practice at these levels. Master's programmes are provided in higher education institutes (HEIs) across each country, and these are increasingly embracing a multiprofessional approach to developing the workforce and its capabilities.

> **PIT STOP!**
>
> You need to be familiar with your country's AP framework, prior to applying for an MSc AP programme. Take time to read and understand the relevant framework.

Present Focus—The Education Capabilities and How They Are Developed

Having explored the development of education preparation for advanced practitioners and the pillars of practice, the underpinning education capabilities that advanced practitioners need to demonstrate and how they can be developed relate to the following four areas.

THEORIES OF LEARNING AND TEACHING

Advanced practitioners educate patients and other health professionals informally at the bedside, in patient's or client's own homes, in clinics and to other professionals either formally or informally in a variety of settings. The need to learn is often to make sense of new things around us. Patient education can support the self-management of long-term conditions and avoid hospital admission in addition to delivering health prevention strategies that can maintain health.

Learning is about change: change brought about by developing a new skill, understanding something new and changing an attitude, and is a relatively permanent change usually brought about intentionally. Educational theory has psychology, sociology and the study of behaviour as its foundation, and as educators, advanced practitioners need to understand how people behave in certain conditions so that learning can be optimised.

The main learning theories need to be understood in conjunction with how people learn: learning models, to maximise the likelihood of relating the learning to their needs and improving learning potential.

> **PIT STOP!**
>
> There are many learning theories and learning styles, which have debate surrounding validity and relevance. Take time to review some popular learning theories and styles.

The three domains of learning (Bloom, 1956) (Table 3.2) have a taxonomy within each domain, from the simplest behaviour, such as recall, to the most complex, this being synthesis and evaluation.

HEALTH LITERACY

Health literacy can be defined as the ability to which an individual has the capacity to obtain, process and understand the information and services being communicated to them to make appropriate decisions (von Wagner et al., 2009). Speaking, reading, writing and numeracy are particularly important for people with limited English proficiency, with some authors arguing that negotiation and navigation skills are also an element in the context of eHealth (Squiers et al., 2012).

When developing and giving information, advanced practitioners need to understand that low health literacy has been associated with poor general health status and a higher risk of hospitalisation. This is because external influences may influence or strengthen health literacy skills for patients and clients through community-based interventions or other learning opportunities. Health-related decisions often involve jargon, technical terms and multiple options which may need to be considered in terms of individual motivation to enact change and the ability to weigh the options presented with the importance associated to an individual's choice. Motivation alone is not the sole predictor for health action but practical barriers such as financial costs of action, influencing the translation of intention to act when considering health prevention strategies.

EFFECTIVE LEARNING ENVIRONMENT

The need to understand what makes an effective learning environment is often covered within undergraduate health professionals' education programmes; however, a synthesis of learning theories, motivation and behaviour, together with methods of teaching and an understanding of how adults learn, is required at an advanced level of practice.

What makes an effective learning environment? If we look back on our own experiences of learning, we may recall aspects of the learning environment: the teacher, the subject, the location (place) and perhaps the technology used. However, when we consider what was good about our learning experiences, we need to understand that the combination of all of these factors and the role of motivation to learn all influence our learning.

Knowles et al. (2005) identified six assumptions about adult learning:

1. The need to know—adults need to know **why** they need to learn something.
2. Self-concept—adults have a self-concept of being responsible for their own lives.
3. Experience—adults have a repository of experience they can draw from.
4. Readiness to learn—adults are motivated to learn what they need to know.
5. Orientation to learning—adults are motivated to learn when it will help real-life situations.
6. Motivation.

Understanding how adults learn and recognising the experiences they can draw from will help the advanced practitioner to adapt their patient education or training content to connect with those experiences and the desire to improve themselves.

COACHING, MENTORING AND ROLE MODELLING

Learning preferences and styles have been explored in the literature extensively and need to be critically understood when advanced practitioners are addressing the learning needs of their team, colleagues or patients and caregivers. However, there are other methods the advanced practitioner may use in learning, such as coaching and mentoring, which help others to take charge of their own development, realising their potential and to achieve results they value (Connor & Pokora, 2017).

To be an effective coach, there is a need for the individual to know themselves, to assess the benefits of coaching, clarifying their role, and to build and manage a productive learning relationship reflecting on the learning that occurs. The learning relationship is at the heart of change, with the context being work and the outcome being change. The client sets the agenda, and the coach uses skills to develop insight and release potential for the client. Various models and approaches to coaching can be explored, such as the GROW model (Whitmore, 2017) and the Skilled Helper (Egan & Reese, 2021)

Coaching is becoming part of the culture in many organisations, with research highlighting the benefits for a leader being a coach: coaching others and experiencing compassion through the development of others helps to balance the psychophysiological effects of the leadership role (Boyatzis et al., 2017). As advanced practitioners develop their leadership and education pillars, becoming a trained coach may be an area that they may choose to explore to formalise training within those pillars.

PIT STOP!

The NHS across the UK has coaching and mentoring resources; take a look at the four countries' websites.

England—https://www.leadershipacademy.nhs.uk/programmes/coaching-and-mentoring/
Scotland—https://learn.nes.nhs.scot/21457
Wales—https://nhswalesleadershipportal.heiw.wales/people-profession/opportunities/coaching-mentoring#:~:text=We%20offer%20a%20range%20of,across%20NHS%20Wales%20in%20their
Northern Ireland—https://leadership.hscni.net/

Various methods of social learning have been discussed in the literature to increase skill levels within clinical settings such as mentoring, demonstration and role modelling. Studies have demonstrated that experiential teaching through role modelling is essential to competence-based training and was successful in both changing attitudes and increasing skill. Role modelling can be a powerful method by which learning occurs in the clinical context because of the affective inspirational overtones observed by others and emphasises the art of practice (Tomlinson et al., 2002).

Advanced practitioners are expected to 'act as role model, educator, supervisor, coach and mentor seeking to instil and develop the confidence of others' (NHSE, 2025) and therefore need to progress along this continuum from developing the foundations and knowledge of the education pillar beyond training. Box 3.2 provides a narrative example of the integration of the education pillar into AP.

Future Focus—Learning in and From Practice: From Advanced Towards Multiprofessional Consultant Practice

Having explored past and present aspects of the education pillar relevant to AP, the focus of this section is future orientated and highlights the need for advanced practitioners to further develop:

1. Expertise in using the workplace as a key resource for integrating learning with developing and improving of self and others; and
2. The capabilities required for transitioning towards multiprofessional consultant practice (MPCP) with a focus on establishing learning cultures across systems.

BOX 3.2 ■ Integration of the Education Pillar Into Practice

David—Advanced Physiotherapy Practitioner in Primary Care

David is a 47-year-old advanced practitioner who undertook his master's degree 17 years ago. His day-to-day work encompasses all four pillars of practice.

David integrates the education pillar in several ways, through his own professional development and by developing his colleagues and clinically with patients. Clinically, he empowers his patients to have the knowledge to be able to make informed choices. He works hard to ensure patients' health and well-being are maximised through appropriately developed health literature and education. David is an honorary lecturer on an AP programme at a local university where he ensures those working in primary care have sessions focused on developing the capabilities required to meet the specific health needs within primary care and delivered by experts in the field.

David is part of a community of practice in primary care where he can access training and development for his own developmental needs. This is run by a collaboration of primary care providers. He has asked been asked to present at these events and to offer mentorship and support for other advanced practitioners who may be working in small practices with little support.

David is also developing his coaching skills by training to become a certified 'Institute of Leadership and Management' (ILM) coach.

Both areas require facilitation of an integrated approach to learning, development, improving, knowledge translation, inquiry and innovation (Martin & Manley, 2017), enhanced by all the domains of the MPCP (Manley & Titchen, 2016; Manley et al., 2019).

The need to focus on these two education-related priorities is required if the workforce and the communities served are to experience workplace cultures where everyone (both providers and users) can contribute to learning for improvement and experience benefit from its impact.

International and national healthcare strategies emphasise the provision of people-centred, integrated care and services (World Health Organisation, 2015). To this end, there is greater recognition of both the facilitation skills and the leadership required to break down barriers across silos and boundaries to develop place-based learning approaches across systems with people to address what matters to them (Germaine et al., 2022; Manley et al., 2016). Three key purposes build on the AP education pillar towards the MPCP domain of 'Learning, developing and improving' (HEE, 2020; Manley et al., 2016, 2019):

- Place-based learning through coproduction to focus on what matters to people
- Workforce transformation to develop the essential skills sets for sustaining person- and people-centred transformation
- Demonstrating the impact of learning and continuous professional development (CPD) to meet society's needs

PLACE-BASED LEARNING THROUGH COPRODUCTION AND A FOCUS ON WHAT MATTERS TO PEOPLE

Using the workplace as a key resource for learning requires skilled facilitators to enable learning in and from practice (Manley et al., 2009; Martin & Manley, 2017). This has huge potential for integrating learning with the multiple purposes of developing, improving, knowledge translation, inquiry and innovation, especially if the workplace, organisational and system cultures enable this. The ability to facilitate an integrated approach to achieve these purposes in practice are skills that advanced practitioners will need to develop so that no opportunity is lost for developing self and others, enabling the impact of learning to benefit service users, the communities served and the workforce—their growth, progression and retention. This holistic facilitation expertise is a key domain in MPCP (HEE, 2020) and has previously been recognised as: catalytic in enabling others to become more effective (Manley & Titchen, 2016); an attribute of work-based learning (Manley et al., 2009); and an enabler for getting evidence used in practice (Rycroft-Malone et al., 2013), place-based learning (Germaine et al., 2022), collaboration, inclusion and participation for coproduction (Hardy et al., 2021), effective workplace cultures that also embed safety (Manley et al., 2019) and system and workforce transformation (Manley et al., 2016; Manley & Jackson, 2020). A Delphi study (Martin & Manley, 2017) drew on experts across each of the facilitation purposes to develop the first integrated multiprofessional facilitation standards (Box 3.3). These standards have become the foundation for New South Wales (Australia) education strategy using 'facilitated learning as strategic intent' (Solman et al., 2021, p. 188).

Facilitating a learning culture in any setting is underpinned by person-centred learning involving all stakeholders (Germaine et al., 2022). This pivotal value, combined with cultures of learning and networks that enable learning, informs the purpose of place-based learning (Box 3.4), which resulted from cocreating a shared direction for place-based learning with all stakeholders across primary care networks at the heart of integrated health and care communities in England.

BOX 3.3 ■ Facilitation Standards for an Integrated Approach to Workplace Learning, Development, Improvement and Inquiry (Manley et al., 2015)

STANDARD 1: Negotiate, agree and sustain clarity of purpose for facilitation activity at the individual, team or organisational level in the context of developing person-centred cultures and improved health outcomes.

STANDARD 2: Optimise the external enablers and values necessary for successful facilitation practice.

STANDARD 3: Draw on the qualities necessary to build effective relationships for facilitation practice.

STANDARD 4: Demonstrate the skills required for integrated facilitation practice in health & social care.

STANDARD 5: Commence the facilitation journey with confidence at different starting points depending on where individuals and teams are at.

STANDARD 6: Use common strategies appropriately for effective facilitation practice.

STANDARD 7: Monitor and maintain effective facilitation practice using a range of methods.

STANDARD 8: Evaluate and evidence process outcomes, intermediate outcomes and impact that individuals or teams may experience using a range of approaches.

BOX 3.4 ■ Values and Purpose of Place-Based Learning (Germaine et al., 2022, pp. 6 and 8)

People-centred learning values all people, the workforce and people in communities, recognising their interdependence and what matters to them.

Cultures of teamwork enable learning and value the role of teamwork in enabling learning cultures, regardless of context.

Networks for learning together value everyone across communities and workplaces learning together to meet health and social care needs.

Purpose of place-based learning

'Grow, develop and sustain an effective health and social care workforce that evolves with changing needs, and is equipped with the skills, knowledge and expertise to deliver effective, safe, compassionate, consistent, holistic care with the aim of improving patient pathways and outcomes, and the wellbeing of the local population' (p. 8).

The key role of facilitation in place-based learning is summarised by Germaine et al. (2022) as:

- Providing collective leadership
- Embedding cultures of learning in teams
- Integrating learning and improving with other functions such as embedded research
- Nurturing and creating psychological safety modelling and challenging inappropriate behaviours

Whilst mentorship, coaching and supervision embrace aspects of facilitation, critical companionship is a model that embeds all its purposes through recognising mutual, reciprocal and shared learning based on reflection and coinquiry (Titchen, 2004). Critical companionship works with the challenges of the 'swampy lowlands' so deftly described by Schon (1984), its focus being to enhance practice by integrating both learning and inquiry, akin to the embedded researcher concept (Whitehouse et al., 2022), that draws on the workplace as its starting point. In critical companionship, both partners bring expertise in different areas; for example, advanced professional practice expertise may be brought by one person and systems transformation or embedded research by the other. Critical companionship is dedicated to person-centred learning and creating contexts and cultures where everyone can flourish. This is achieved through living the values of being person centred and recognising that each person brings different expertise as opposed to a more hierarchical or technical view associated with expert–novice relationships and instrumental approaches.

Integral to critical companionship is the role of facilitating creativity in helping us to be 'freed from the things we take for granted in our everyday practice'. This involves helping people to think 'outside of the box', to be imaginative and to do things differently. The metaphor of being 'a radical gardener' is used to express what matters and to find solutions collaboratively (Titchen & McMahon, 2013). A second metaphor, 'the hamster wheel', is often used to describe the feeling that there is no time to step off the hamster wheel to reflect and learn. Yet, taking time out to reflect and think is increasingly recognised as essential for work-based learning and to become more effective in our work (West, 2021) to innovate a different future. Taking time out does not always mean spending hours in a workshop setting but can also be as short as a few minutes in everyday practice when facilitators support colleagues to address workplace issues. Expert facilitators can help practitioners and others in the workplace to become aware of the things 'taken for granted' as these assumptions may deter us from thinking differently and more creatively. Skilled facilitators help people to become consciously aware of their behaviour, actions and decisions and the consequences of these on self and others using simple reflection. The 'Three Es' of critical theory illustrate this point when helping people to change the way they work intentionally in either the moment of practice or more formal learning sessions (Box 3.5).

As a facilitator of learning and the other integrated role functions, evaluating how challenging and how supportive we are in our relationships with others is

---

BOX 3.5 ■ **The Three Es (Fay, 1987)**

E for enlightenment—becoming aware of the things we take for granted and the consequences of our actions and decisions on self and others

E for empowerment—becoming motivated to want to change the way we are or act, having become self-aware of the things we take for granted and the consequences of our actions and decisions

E for emancipation—liberated to acting differently and intentionally to free ourselves from the things we take for granted in our practice

---

important for becoming more effective in facilitation practice. Achieving a high-support, high-challenge relationship fine-tuned through feedback from the people we work with is vital for optimising our effectiveness both as a facilitator and an enabler of others (Titchen et al., 2013). Facilitation strategies such as these are core to the integrated facilitation standards (see Box 3.3), as is the ability to enable creativity and innovation in a psychologically safe environment. The development of workplace cultures where everyone can flourish emphasises the link between facilitation and leadership, as facilitating person-centred relations as well as leadership are the key approaches through which workplace cultures can be changed.

Workforce Transformation: The Essential Skillsets for Sustaining Person-Centred Transformation

Facilitation skills for achieving multiple purposes, learning combined with leadership for culture change and skills as an embedded researcher in evaluating impact constitute the expertise required for transitioning from advanced MPCP, where integrated capabilities are recognised as a foundation for consultancy (Fig. 3.1).

To achieve sustainable person-centred workforce transformation, the Venus model (Manley & Jackson, 2020) identifies the integrated skillsets required derived from practice-based research and inquiry, namely:

- Facilitation skills integrating all the purposes highlighted previously
- Practice development skills with its focus on person-centred values and cultures where everyone can flourish through collaboration, inclusion and participative approaches and systematic inquiry (Hardy et al., 2021)
- Culture changes as without attention to workplace culture, no strategy will succeed
- Leadership at all system levels as it is through person-centred leadership and relationships that culture changes to enable everyone to feel valued and flourish based on collective leadership (Cardiff et al., 2021)
- Improvement and innovation—informed by coproduction, a focus on what matters and a psychological safe environment that supports experimentation with new ideas and creativity for innovation (Cardiff et al., 2021)

MPCP capabilities are underpinned by these integrated skillsets and, when combined with credibility from expertise in one's own professional practice, enable

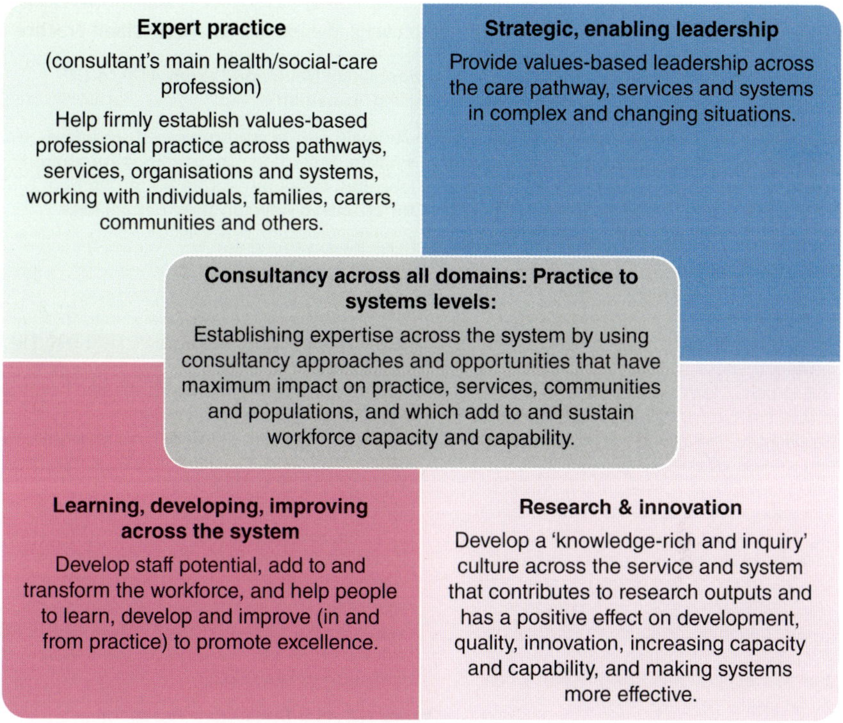

Expert practice

(consultant's main health/social-care profession)

Help firmly establish values-based professional practice across pathways, services, organisations and systems, working with individuals, families, carers, communities and others.

Strategic, enabling leadership

Provide values-based leadership across the care pathway, services and systems in complex and changing situations.

Consultancy across all domains: Practice to systems levels:

Establishing expertise across the system by using consultancy approaches and opportunities that have maximum impact on practice, services, communities and populations, and which add to and sustain workforce capacity and capability.

Learning, developing, improving across the system

Develop staff potential, add to and transform the workforce, and help people to learn, develop and improve (in and from practice) to promote excellence.

Research & innovation

Develop a 'knowledge-rich and inquiry' culture across the service and system that contributes to research outputs and has a positive effect on development, quality, innovation, increasing capacity and capability, and making systems more effective.

Fig. 3.1 The multiprofessional consultant practice capability and impact framework. *(From Health Education England (HEE) (2020).* Multi-professional consultant practice capability and impact framework. *https:// advanced-practice.hee.nhs.uk/consultant/consultant-level-practice-capability-and-impact-framework/)*

system transformation through breaking down silos and barriers (Manley et al., 2022). A Delphi study (Manley et al., 2021) has enabled each capability in the MPCP framework to be ranked according to the expectation that they are achieved at the following stages in the career development:

■ Transition from AP to consultant level practice
■ 1–3 years in consultant practice
■ 3–5 years in consultant practice

Table 3.3 illustrates the numbered MPCP capabilities from the learning, developing and improving domain that are specifically relevant to transition from AP towards consultant practice, and beyond.

The developmental pathway from AP to consultant practice is characterised by the very skills that have been introduced so far in this section—experiential, active learning and reflection; critical companionship; and shared learning focused on cocreation and what matters to people, combined with self-assessment and a focus on evaluation of impact as an embedded researcher (Manley & Crouch, 2022).

TABLE 3.3 ■ Domain: Learning, Developing, Improving: Multiprofessional Consultant Practice

Capabilities Expected at Transition Point	Capabilities Developed From ACP to CP During Transition
8. Stay effective through reflection and learning—and help others to do the same.	**9. Actively create a learning culture across the system, providing opportunities for shared learning, development and improvement and for others to develop their capabilities.**
8.1. Model • Asking for feedback about how your own behaviour and values affect others. • Reflecting on your actions, peer reviews and support for ongoing learning, increasing effectiveness and career planning. • Taking part in learning and development across the system to improve service users' experiences, safety and people's well-being and to pass on knowledge. • Using learning and development processes that support blended approaches to learning (for example, formal and informal, face-to-face, e-learning and so on) and promote learning together, and which are adapted to individual learning styles and motivation. 8.2. Take part in continuous professional development (CPD), valuing lifelong learning and peer support and being flexible when dealing with changing situations.	9.1 Use the workplace as a key resource for active learning, development and improvement, to support: • Quality learning cultures and placements; • Giving and receiving feedback and critical review; • Reviewing quality and safety data, including outcomes and experience; and • Practise transforming the workplace and how this can be sustained across the system. 9.2 Work as an effective facilitator, using different learning and development strategies across different situations to develop: • Person-centred, safe, effective workplace learning, from practice to system levels; and • Continued and effective ways of learning and working, including educational innovations and technology. (This should reflect good teamwork, a clear purpose, agreed priorities, a high level of support and challenge, learning from mistakes and building on what works.) ***Years 1–3 As a Consultant Practitioner*** 9.3 Motivate and coach or mentor individuals and teams to: • Perform better and more effectively; • Meet future workforce demands through cross-sector working; • Develop individual and group independence; • Improve career progression within and beyond traditional boundaries; and • Develop capacity and capability across the health economy and sectors at regional and national levels.

10. Take the lead in putting in place peer reviews and learning and development systems, and in developing the workforce so that it can maintain consistent professional standards, helping career progression, systems learning and transformation.

Years 1–3 As a Consultant Practitioner
10.1. Lead peer learning reviews and ongoing learning and development systems and evaluate their effect on service users and their families, carers and staff, and services.
10.3. Work with higher education to make sure professional curriculums reflect excellence, the needs of the service, current evidence and ways of working that inspire students and academic staff to contribute to future health and care, regionally and nationally.

Years 3–5 As a Consultant Practitioner
10.2. Develop the workforce so that staff can fulfil their potential, make progress in their careers and meet the future needs of the system.

Numbered capabilities relevant to advanced practice and transitioning to consultant practice (Manley et al., 2021).
ACP, Advanced clinical practice; *CP,* consultant practice.

Demonstrating the Impact of Learning and Continuous Professional Development to Meet Society's Needs

Defining impact in the context of MPCP draws on the impact continuum of Belcher and Halliwell (2021), where research and other outputs as a theory of change define impact as a change in behaviour, attitudes, practice, policy, sustainability and benefits realisation for society.

It is important that capabilities are linked to purpose, to keep at the forefront our shared direction, and for this reason, the MPCP capability framework is aligned to impact (HEE, 2020). Consultant practice impact embraces a strong focus on both workforce and system transformation and draws on all integrated domains, not just learning developing and improving (Manley et al., 2022).

Demonstrating the impact of learning and CPD provides plenty for advanced practitioners to consider when thinking about the importance of transferring learning to practice (Illing et al., 2018). However, essential investment in CPD activities is required if positive impact is to be achieved. A realist synthesis of CPD strategies that work across health and care disciplines specified the main purpose of CPD to be 'service users' experiences of health and social care and that this is person centred, safe and effective' (Jackson et al., 2015, p. 102). This is linked to CPD that focuses on the individual's as well as the team's journey of transformation in their work and workplace, specifically the transformation of:

- The individual's professional practice
- Skills to meet a continually changing context
- Knowledge so that it is used and blended with other knowledge in practice through knowledge translation
- The workplace culture/context to enable everyone (those experiencing care and those providing it) to flourish and thrive

Transformation theories were developed that describe how the contextual factors in practice combine with specific mechanisms that work to achieve impact and outcomes through transformation. Box 3.6 identifies the links between the contextual factors which when combined with the mechanisms account for and explain the outcome and impact of CPD. The importance of expertise in facilitation of learning and its evaluation are evident whilst the detail is presented in other publications (Manley et al., 2018).

Increasingly, it is recognised that CPD needs to be commissioned with citizens to focus on what matters and combined with the transfer of learning into practice to have greater impact (Jackson & Manley, 2022).

Conclusion

The education role is both pivotal and integral to AP and subsequent career progression having been a key feature from the early development of AP to the present day and the future. Understanding the factors that impact on learning for self and

---

BOX 3.6 ■ Four Transformation Theories Explaining the Interaction Between Key Contextual Factors and the Mechanisms That Work With Outcomes and Impact (Jackson et al., 2015)

Workforce Transformation Focus Through CPD	*Relationships Between Contextual Factors Combined With Mechanisms to Achieve Outcomes*
Transformation of *individuals' professional practice*	CPD that is work-based within a context that is enabling, inquiring and supportive and learner driven, and centred on the provision of facilitated support and reflection and includes self-assessment and a focus on self-awareness will increase self-confidence, self-awareness, self-efficacy and role clarity, as well as create a positive attitude to change with opportunities for role and career development.
Transformation of *the skills required to meet society's changing needs*	CPD that focuses on the transformation of skills to meet society's changing healthcare needs embracing team and system assessment to identify gaps and expand skills to meet a changing healthcare context will be reflected in better service user experiences of continuity and consistency of service provision, better employability and opportunities for career progression for individuals, more effective teams, better organisational/systems outcomes around integration, partnerships and more effective use of human resources.
Transformation *to enable knowledge translation*	CPD in workplace contexts that both support and encourage engagement with and use of different types of knowledge in everyday practice and active sharing through CPD strategies that focus on using and blending multiple knowledge to inform professional decision-making; skills in facilitating dialogue, active enquiry and evaluation; and developing practical and theoretical knowledge fostering leadership, evaluation and culture will achieve knowledge-rich cultures recognised by knowledge use and development, active inquiry, innovation and creativity.
Transformation *of workplace culture to implement workplace and organisational values and purpose relating to person centred, safe and effective care*	CPD that takes place within contexts where there are shared values and purposes and organisational readiness that draws on CPD strategies which focus on developing and implementing shared values, evaluating the experiences of service users and staff in relation to these values and developing skills in developing effective workplace cultures through leadership will achieve improved service user and provider experiences, outcomes and impact, sustained person-centred, safe and effective workplace cultures and team effectiveness, increased employee commitment, organisational leadership and effectiveness.

CPD, Continuous professional development.

---

others is essential for optimising person-centred learning, workforce transformation and quality health and care across systems. The ability to draw on the workplace as the main resource for integrating learning, development and improvement as a facilitator of learning, in addition to participating in collaborative learning networks and developmental opportunities, will enable advanced practitioners to demonstrate both the centrality of learning to their practice and the impact of learning on people, communities, care and services.

References

Belcher, B., & Halliwell J. (2021). Conceptualizing the elements of research impact: Towards semantic standards. *Humanities and Social Sciences Communications, 8*, 183. https://doi.org/10.1057/s41599-021-00854-2

Bloom, B. S. (1956). *Taxonomy of educational objectives, handbook: The cognitive domain.* New York: David McKay.

Boyatzis, R. E., Smith, M. L., & Blaize, N. (2017). Developing sustainable leaders through coaching and compassion. *Academy of Management Learning & Education, 5*(1). https://journals.aom.org/doi/abs/10.5465/amle.2006.20388381

Cardiff, S., Sanders, K., Webster, J., & Manley, K. (2020). Guiding lights for effective workplace cultures that are also good places to work. *International Practice Development Journal, 10*(2). https://doi.org/10.19043/ipdj.102.002v2

Connor, M., & Pokora, J. (2017). *Coaching and mentoring at work: Developing effective practice* (3rd ed). London: Open University Press.

Department of Health. (2010). *Advanced level nursing: A position statement.* London: Department of Health.

Department of Health, Social Services and Public Safety (DHSSPSNI). (2018). *Advanced Nursing Practice Framework Supporting Advanced Nursing Practice in Health and Social Care Trusts.* https://www.health-ni.gov.uk/sites/default/files/publications/health/advanced-nursing-practice-framework.pdf

Department of Health—Northern Ireland. (2019). *Advanced AHP Practice Framework: Guidance for supporting advanced allied health professions practice in health and social care.* https://www.health-ni.gov.uk/publications/advanced-ahp-practice-framework

Egan, G., & Reese, R. J. (2021). *The skilled helper: A client centred approach* (3rd ed.). Andover: Cengage Learning EMEA.

Fay, B. (1987). *Critical social science.* Cambridge: Polity Press.

Germaine, R., Manley, K., Stillman, K., Nicholls, P. J. (2022). Growing the interprofessional workforce for integrated people-centred care through developing place-based learning cultures across the system. *International Practice Development Journal, 12*(1), Article 4. https://doi.org/10.19043/ipdj.121.004

Gloster, A., & Leigh, J. (2021). The knowledge and skills required of advanced level practitioners for accreditation and safe practice. *British Journal of Nursing, 30*(3), 168–171.

Hamric, A. B., Spross, J. A., & Hanson, C. M. (2009). *Advanced practice nursing: An integrative approach.* 4th ed. Philadelphia, PA: Saunders.

Hardy, S., Clarke, S., Frei, I. A., Morley, C., Odell, J., White, C., & Wilson, V. (2021). A global manifesto for practice development: Revisiting core principles. In K. Manley & V. Wilson (Eds.), *International practice development in health and social care* (2nd ed., 99–117). Chichester: Wiley Blackwell. https://doi.org/10.1002/9781119698463.ch8

Health Education and Improvement Wales. (2023). *Professional framework for enhanced, advanced and consultant clinical practice in Wales.* https://heiw.nhs.wales/files/eac-framework-consultation/

NHS England (2025) *Multi-professional framework for advanced Practice in England.* Birmingham: Centre for Advancing Practice. https://advanced-practice.hee.nhs.uk/multi-professional-framework-for-advanced-practice/

Health Education England (HEE). (2020). *Multi-professional consultant-level practice capability and impact framework.* https://www.hee.nhs.uk/sites/default/files/documents/Sept%202020%20HEE%20Consultant%20Practice%20Capability%20and%20Impact%20Framework.pdf

Health Education England, & NHS England and Skills for Health. (2020). *NHS Core capabilities framework for advanced clinical practice (nurses) working in general practice/primary care in England.* Royal College of General Practitioners and Skills for Health. https://www.hee.nhs.uk/sites/default/files/documents/ACP%20Primary%20Care%20Nurse%20Fwk%202020.pdf

Illing, J., Corbett, S., Kehoe, A., Carter, M., Hesselgreaves, H., et al. (2018). *How does the education and training of health and social care staff transfer to practice and benefit patients? A realist approach.* Newcastle University: Durham University: University of York.

Jackson, C., & Manley, K. (2022). Contemporary challenges of nursing CPD: Time to change the model to meet citizens' needs. *Nurse Open, 9*(2), 880–891. doi:10.1002/nop2.941

Jackson, C., Manley, K., Wright, T., & Martin, A. (2015). *Continuing professional development for quality care: Context, mechanisms, outcomes and impact. Final Report.* ECPD. ISBN 978-1-909067-39-4.

Knowles, M. S., Swanson, R. A., & Holton, E. F. III. (2005). *The adult learner: The definitive classic in adult education and human resource development* (6th ed.). California: Elsevier Science and Technology Books.

Manley, K., & Crouch, R. (2022, April). *Co-creating a developmental pathway for multi-professional consultant practice: Building on the outputs from the three care group workshops. Final report.* University of East Anglia and Health Education England.

Manley, K.; Crouch, R. and Furber, L. (2021, September). *The development pathway from advanced practice to consultant practice using a modified Delphi approach. Final Report.* University of East Anglia and Health Education England.

Manley, K., Crouch, R., Ward, R., Clift, E., Jackson, C., Christien, J., Williams, H., & Harden B. (2022). The role of the multi-professional consultant practitioner in supporting workforce transformation in the UK. *Advanced Journal of Professional Practice*, *3*(2), 1–26. https://doi.org/10.22024/UniKent/03/ajpp.1057, https://journals.kent.ac.uk/index.php/ajpp/article/view/1057/2082

Manley, K., & Jackson, C. (2020, January 20). The Venus model for integrating practitioner-led workforce transformation and complex change across the health care system. *Journal of Evaluation in Clinical Practice-International Journal of Public Health Policy and Health Services Research.* https://doi.org/10.1111/jep.13377

Manley, K., Jackson, C., & McKenzie, C. (2019). Microsystems culture change – A refined theory for developing person centred, safe and effective workplaces based on strategies that embed a safety culture. *International Journal of Practice Development*, *9*(2), Article 4. https://doi.org/10.19043/ipdj.92.004

Manley, K., Martin, A., Jackson, C., & Wright, T. (2016). Using systems thinking to identify workforce enablers for a whole systems approach to urgent and emergency care delivery: A multiple case study. *BMC Health Services Research*, *16*, 368. https://doi.org/10.1186/s12913-016-1616-y

Manley, K., Martin, A., Jackson, C., & Wright, T. (2015). *Developing standards for integrated facilitation in and about the workplace. Phase 2 report: Transforming urgent & emergency care together.* Canterbury: England Centre for Practice Development.

Manley, K., Martin, A., Jackson, C., & Wright, T. (2018). A realist synthesis of effective continuing professional development (CPD): A case study of healthcare practitioners' CPD. *Nurse Education Today*, *69*, 134–141. https://doi.org/10.1016/j.nedt.2018.07.010

Manley, K., & Titchen, A. (2016). Facilitation skills: The catalyst for increased effectiveness in consultant practice and clinical systems leadership. *Educational Action Research*, 24(2), 1–24. https://www.tandfonline.com/doi/full/10.1080/09650792.2016.1158118

Manley, K., Titchen, A., & Hardy, S. (2009). Work based learning in the context of contemporary healthcare education and practice: A concept analysis. *Practice Development in Health Care*, *8*(2), 87–127.

Martin, A., & Manley, K. (2018). Developing standards for an integrated approach to workplace facilitation for interprofessional teams in health and social care contexts: A Delphi study. *Journal of Interprofessional Care*, 32(1):41-51. https://www.tandfonline.com/doi/abs/10.1080/13561820.2017.1373080?journalCode=ijic20

NHS Education for Scotland. (2008). *Advanced practice toolkit.* https://learn.nes.nhs.scot/63343

Royal College of Nursing. (2012). *Advanced nurse practitioner – An RCN guide.* London: Royal College of Nursing.

Rycroft-Malone, J., Seers, K., Chandler, J., Hawkes, C., Crichton, N., Allen, C., Bullock, I., & Strunin, L. (2013). The role of evidence, context, and facilitation in an implementation trial: Implications for the development of the PARIHS framework. *Implementation Science*, *8*, Article 28. https://doi.org/10.1186/1748-5908-8-28

Scottish Government. (2017). *Transforming nursing, midwifery and health professions roles – Advance nursing practice.* https://www.gov.scot/publications/transforming-nursing-midwifery-health-professions-roles-advance-nursing-practice/

Schön, D. (1984). *The reflective practitioner: How professionals think in action.* Aldershot, UK: Ashgate.

Solman, A., Manley, K., & Christie, C. (2021). Systems leadership enablement of collaborative healthcare practices. In K, Manley, V. Wilson, & C. Oye (Eds.), *International Practice Development in Health and Social Care* (2nd ed., pp. 187–204.). Chichester: Wiley.

Squiers, L., Peinado, S., Berkman, N., Boudewyns, V., & McCormack, L. (2012). The health literacy skills framework. *Journal of Health Communication*, *17*, 30–54. https://doi.org/10.1080/10810730.2012.713442

Titchen, A. (2004). Helping relationships for practice development: Critical companionship. In B. McCormack, K. Manley, & R. Garbett (Eds.), *Practice development in nursing* (148–174). Oxford: Blackwell Publishing Ltd.

Titchen, A., Dewing, J., & Manley, K. (2013). Getting going with facilitation skills in practice development. In B. McCormack, K. Manley, & A. Titchen (Eds.), *Practice development in nursing and healthcare* (2nd ed., 109–129). Chichester: Wiley-Blackwell.

Titchen, A., & McMahon, A. (2013). Practice development as radical gardening: Enabling creativity and innovation. In B. McCormack, K. Manley, & A. Titchen (Eds.), *Practice development in nursing and health-care* (2nd ed, 212–232). Chichester: Wiley-Blackwell.

Tomlinson, P. S., Thomlinson, E., Peden-McAlpine, C., & Kirschbaum, M. (2002). Clinical innovation for promoting family care in paediatric intensive care: Demonstration, role modelling and reflective practice. *Journal of Advanced Nursing, 38*(2), 161–170.

Von Wagner, C., Steptoe, A. M., Wolf, M. S., & Wardle, J. (2009). Health literacy and health actions: A review and a framework from health psychology. *Health Education & Behaviour, 36*(5), 860–877. https://doi.org/10.1177/1090198108322819

West, M. (2021). *Compassionate leadership: Sustaining wisdom, humanity and presence in health and social care.* The Swirling Leaf Press.

Whitehouse, C.L., Tinkler, L., Jackson, C., Hall, H., Webster, J., Hardy, S., Coppoing, J., Morris, P., and Manley, K. (2022) Embedding research (ER) led by nurses, midwives and allied health professionals (NMHAPs): the NMAHP-ER model. *BMJ Leader.* Published Online 22 April 2022. https://doi.org/10.1136/leader-2021-000578

Whitmore, J. (2017). *Coaching for performance: The principles and practices of coaching and leadership* (5th ed). Boston USA: Nicholas Brealey Publishing.

World Health Organization (WHO). (2015). *WHO global strategy on people-centred and integrated health services. Interim report.* Geneva, Switzerland: World Health Organization. http://apps.who.int/iris/bitstream/10665/155002/1/WHO_HIS_SDS_2015.6_eng.pdf. Accessed January 20, 2020.

Four Pillars of Advanced Practice—Clinical

Anna Jones ■ Jonathan Thomas ■ Melanie Rogers

CHAPTER OUTLINE

This chapter will offer oversight of the clinical pillar of advanced practice. It begins with an exploration of some of the core elements underpinning a patient consultation in relation to communication skills, history taking and the consultation models that can provide structure to the consultation. This then leads into decision-making exploring models and influences upon decisions advanced practitioners can make in clinical practice.

Introduction

Across the UK and globally, clinical practice is a central feature within all the different advanced practice (AP) frameworks (Health Education and Improvement Wales (HEIW), 2023; National Health Service England (NHSE) 2025; Nursing and Midwifery Board Australia (NMBA), 2021; Nursing Council of New Zealand, 2017). Common components to the clinical practice pillar include:

- History taking
- Consultation skills
- Decision-making
- Examination skills

Universities that deliver AP education will offer various clinical modules; however, there is no standardisation in terms of module syllabus. Therefore, content and assessment strategies will vary greatly between each programme globally (Rushforth, 2008). Despite these variations, a core component of any AP learning is the need for bridging the taught theory into clinical practice gap through the support of robust clinical supervision in practice.

As highlighted from the previous three chapters, the clinical practice pillar forms one of the four pillars of AP. Chapter 3 focused on the education pillar, while Chapters 5 and 6 examine leadership and research, respectively. For those advanced practitioners who might be embarking on a clinically focused AP role, the clinical pillar will be more prominent within both their job plan and job description; however, all pillars are important and are essential for the AP role.

It would be impractical to examine each component of the clinical pillar in one chapter; therefore, the aim of this chapter is to examine the core components of a patient encounter, these being the consultation and communication skills, a history-taking format and the decision-making skills that underpin AP. It is intended that this will provide a foundation for the aspiring advanced practitioner to build upon during their AP journey.

The Consultation

A consultation could be compared to cooking:

'The fact is that food varies, and that is what makes it so interesting. Today's piece of cod may be slightly thicker, has larger or finer flakes or thicker skin, than yesterday's. One brand of butter may be different from another. Olive oil changes with every bottle; that is part of its joy. So how can anyone be so pedantic as to give exact timings? Each egg, each steak, each potato is different and will behave in a different way in the pan. That is what cooking is about, and that is why it is essential to understand what you are doing rather than just mindlessly following a recipe.'

(From *Appetite* by Nigel Slater, 2000, p. 34)

Applying the cooking analogy to clinical practice, the consultation will differ based on the clinical environment, the clinical speciality, the patient and the practitioner. Each patient that you review and consult with will present differently, with different needs and perspectives; what is important to one may be less so to another. Denness (2013) recognises the consultation as being a privilege, as you enter into the patient's life. It is therefore key that you develop the skills to ascertain what the patient's expectations are. The consultation is the central component to clinical practice (Silverman, 2017). It can, however, be a juggling act as there are many elements to manage such as history taking, being able to process what has been said and thinking where next to proceed, thinking about and reflecting on your decisions and considering how you then apply and demonstrate good interpersonal skills. Juggling these and many more factors can potentially lead the consultation down a chaotic path; however, consultation models have been developed to help provide a framework (Silverman, 2017). There are numerous consultation models you can review and utilise in your practice; some appear to have similar elements and stages. Many that emerged from early 1970s and 1980s will be doctor-centred, in that the 'doctor knows best', with a reductionist, disease focus and the doctor dominating the consultation (Dunn, 2003). This is in comparison to patient-centred care, which places the patient at the heart of the consultation through listening to their concerns, their feelings and their agendas and working with the patient towards shared decision-making (Bodegard, 2019).

MSc AP programmes will normally have taught sessions on how to consult and we recommend reflecting on which consultation model/s fit best in your area of practice, as no one model is superior to the other, but the more modern consultation models tend to adopt a more patient-centred approach. Table 4.1 provides some examples of consultation models that you may want to review and reflect upon, whether you currently use one or a mixture of models, to support and provide a framework for your consultation and assessment of your patients.

As we note from Table 4.1, the varied consultation models stem from medical practice and have a focus upon the doctor and the patient. The dates of when these models were developed reflect the development of AP in the UK (see Chapter 1), which has resulted in advanced practitioners adopting and using a combination of models for their own consultations.

TABLE 4.1 ■ **Summary of Consultation Models**

Model	Description
Byrne and Long (1976)	This model derives from the work of a general practitioner (GP) and a psychologist based on over 2000 patient consultations and is divided into six phases, which are: 1. The doctor establishes a relationship with the patient. 2. The doctor discovers or attempts to discover the reason for the attendance. 3. The doctor conducts a verbal and/or physical examination. 4. The doctor, the doctor and the patient or the patient (in that order of probability) considers the condition. 5. The doctor and occasionally the patient detail further treatment or investigation. 6. The consultation is terminated, usually by the doctor. This model provides a clear structure from start to finish and we can observe from the six steps that there is consideration of the patient. However, Moulton (2007) recognises that this is more doctor-focused, but in the 1970s, when this work was undertaken, patient centredness was not a common phenomenon. Byrne and Long (1976) studied more than 2000 consultations and identified that a main reason for a dysfunctional consultation was a failing at stage 2 or 4 of their model, that being, not identifying the problem or considering all elements to the presenting problem.
Stott and Davis (1979)	Stemming from primary care, the model focusses on four areas, which are: 1. Identification and management of presenting complaint 2. Modification of help-seeking behaviours 3. Management of continuing problems 4. Opportunistic health promotion Similarly to Byrne and Long (1976), this model appears to be doctor-centred, which reflects the era when the model was developed.
Helman (1981)	The 'Folk Model' developed by Cecil Helman, a medical anthropologist, suggests that the patient presents to the doctor seeking the answers to six questions, which are: 1. What has happened? 2. Why has it happened? 3. Why to me? 4. Why now? 5. What would happen if nothing was done about it? 6. What should I do about it or whom should I consult for further help?

TABLE 4.1 ■ Summary of Consultation Models—cont'd

Model	Description
Pendleton et al. (1984)	Derived from David Pendelton, a psychologist around a group of GPs, this is often referred to as the 'Pendleton Model'. The model sets out seven 'doctor's tasks' that must be achieved during the consultation. The tasks include: 1. Define the reason for attending. 2. Consider other problems. 3. Doctor and patient choose an action for each problem. 4. Share understanding. 5. Involve the patient in the management of problems and sharing appropriate responsibility. 6. Use time and resources appropriately. 7. Establish and maintain positive patient relationships. This is an interesting model as it encourages the clinician to consider appropriate use of time and resources, which is very prudent. The model also starts to involve the patient, which supports a patient-centred approach. However, Denness (2013) argues that this model might be impractical for use in a 10-minute consultation due to the number of steps to work through.
Neighbour (1987, 2004)	Based on the work by Roger Neighbour, a GP, this is a simpler model that suggests that the GP is working as both an organiser and a responder to achieve five set tasks. The organiser role is around keeping structure to the consultation and deciding the course of action, while the responder role responds to the patient, maintaining a patient-centred approach. The tasks provide 'checkpoints' and include: 1. Connecting 2. Summarising 3. Handing over 4. Safety netting 5. Housekeeping Neighbour's (1987) model is unique as this considers the practitioner's needs within the housekeeping task. The model is patient-centred as the rapport stage occurs within the connecting task; the handover task is where the patient and clinician formulate a plan and much of the decision-making is passed on to the patient (Neighbour, 1987). A criticism highlighted by Denness (2013) is that this model does not help with closure of a consultation.
Kurtz and Silverman (1996)	Kurtz and Silverman (1996) produced a guide for the teaching of communication in medical education programmes, this being 'The Calgary–Cambridge Observation Guide', and often referred to as the Calgary–Cambridge model. This provides a simple five-point plan with each step having a defined task. The set tasks include: 1. Initiating the session 2. Gathering information 3. Building the relationship 4. Giving information—explaining and planning 5. Closing the session Alongside these five tasks, two threads run in parallel which focus on building relationships and providing structure. This appears to be a common framework predominantly used in education and in clinical practice to teach consultation skills (Diamond-Fox, 2021) as this incorporates the physical, psychological and social aspects of a consultation (Kurtz et al., 2003).

PIT STOP!

If you were to design your own consultation model, what elements would this include and why would you include them?

Communication Skills

Underpinning any consultation model is the need for good communication skills, to ensure patient safety (Frain, 2017). A failure to apply good communication skills will impact upon the ability to extract patient information, which will influence the diagnosis and management and can lead to diagnostic error and potential clinical negligence (Frain, 2017). In addition to patient safety, good communication skills underpin patient-centred care and the four principles set by The Health Foundation (2012), which include:

1. Affording people dignity, compassion and respect
2. Offering coordinated care, support or treatment
3. Offering personalised care, support or treatment
4. Supporting people to recognise and develop their own strengths and abilities to enable them to live an independent and fulfilling life

Based upon effective communication skills and application of the patient-centred approach, this can lead to improved shared decision-making and improved patient education, allowing for better health outcomes (Frain, 2017). Improved communication skills can also benefit teamworking and the wider organisation. The clinician can also reflect and consider how a consultation went if effective communication skills have been used (Denness, 2013).

A discussion and analysis of all communication skills are beyond the scope of this chapter, since this would be a book on its own. However, some practical communication skills have been cited by Mahendran (2014) which are relevant to clinical practice and can be included in the consultation; these are discussed in Table 4.2.

PIT STOP!

Questioning styles are another key communication skill. Review the difference between open, closed, focused and leading questions and decide which styles support a more effective consultation.

Individual Expectations and Concerns

What you and what the patient see as concerns may differ; it is therefore important to ask what the patient's expectations are of the consultation and assessment. They may have expectations around treatment, for example, the prescribing of antibiotics, when antibiotic stewardship and nonprescribing would steer your treatment plan on a different course. Clear communication between you and your patient can support them and lessen their anxiety and offer opportunities to engage in health education (Dart, 2010).

TABLE 4.2 ■ **Practical Communication Skills**

Tip	Discussion
Language	In terms of language, the use of jargon and abbreviations is common within healthcare and can be misunderstood and misinterpreted by both patients and clinicians (Kumar et al. 2023). For example, LFT can mean liver function test, but it could also be an abbreviation for lung function test. Another example would be telling the patient they had an 'MI', but would the patient know what an MI meant? Furthermore, the patient's first language will need to be considered. For example, in Wales, some people only speak Welsh and may be more comfortable conversing in their first language. An example of this was when a patient consent was required for an immediate investigation, but the patient only spoke Welsh, and no clinician on duty spoke Welsh. Translation services are available; however, these can often act as a barrier to developing patient rapport.
Nonverbal communication	Nonverbal communication can be a very powerful sign to the patient displaying an array of responses and emotions from the clinician. Being mindful of open body language and facial expressions is important, along with avoiding distractions. For example, the wandering eye to look at a computer screen can indicate a lack of interest in the patient. Likewise, the clinician should recognise and respond to the patient's nonverbal cues such as closed body language (Denness, 2013) and lack of eye contact, which might suggest a potential problem that needs exploring, for example, anxiety.
Agenda setting	It is key to establish the patient's agenda from the outset as if this is not established by the clinician, then the patient may feel that their needs have not been met. For example, a patient might have a hidden agenda, such as a gentleman presenting with a sore throat but in reality wants to discuss their erectile dysfunction, or a patient presenting to the clinician with a verbal cue, such as 'my wife is concerned and made me come in today' but not responding and exploring to the verbal cue of the wife and the concerns (Denness, 2013). To respond to this verbal cue, the clinician could say 'so I understand your wife is concerned, do you share these concerns?' This allows the patient the opportunity to share their agenda.
Rapport setting	Rapport setting is essential as this will facilitate a relationship between patient and clinician, which underpins a good consultation (Silverman et al., 2008). As with the previous example, if the gentleman felt a good rapport had been established, they might be able to discuss their main concern of erectile dysfunction. Developing a rapport starts from the onset of the consultation and needs to continue and develop throughout the consultation as reflected within the Calgary–Cambridge model.
Empathy and listening	Being empathetic enables you to view the problem from the patient's perspective, 'putting yourself in their shoes', which can aid better understanding to guide your support. Listening and allowing the patient to tell their story is a powerful tool as this generates a wealth of information that aids decision-making.
Information	During a consultation, patients will need information to help them make an informed decision, which underpins the patient-centred approach. Information would need to be tailored in a format that the patient can understand and addresses their questions. It should be jargon free.
Empowerment	It is important to be receptive to patient choice, and to be knowledgeable around cultural differences. Being patient-centred and not stereotyping will lead to patient empowerment (Edwards et al., 2009).
Reflection	There are two components to reflection. First is reflecting the narrative and history taking back to the patient, as this will both demonstrate listening and can help in clarifying certain points. Secondly, critical self-reflection can be used by the clinician in reflecting on what went well with the consultation and what areas require development for future practice.

When conducting a consultation, consider the following questions:

- What part did the environment play?
- Did you have competing demands?
- Were you time restricted?
- Would it have been helpful to have more time?
- What did it mean to the patient/client?
- How did the patient/family member/carer perceive you?
- Were family members/care giver present?
- Do family members/care giver affect the consultation and, if so, in what way?

Clinical History Taking

AP has expanded to include undifferentiated and undiagnosed conditions, with patients presenting with myriad of issues and concerns. The consultation will be different and reflective of the patient's need; however, clinical history taking is the most fundamental and important part of the consultation. An accurate history provides key information required for a diagnosis. History taking should take a structured and sequential approach, underpinned by effective therapeutic communication skills (Peart, 2022). Stoeckle and Billings (1987) note that this timeless art has been established for centuries between the doctor and patient but has greatly evolved. Despite these developments over time and a shift from doctor focus to patient-centred focus, the means of structuring and obtaining the clinical history remains the same (Stoeckle & Billings, 1987). There are variations especially within specialities such as psychiatry and paediatrics (Craske et al., 2017), as certain components are added which are applicable to the speciality. For example, mental health history taking would include elements such as past mental health history and forensic history, while a paediatric history would explore birth history. However, these are additions to the traditional medical history take, which is captured within Box 4.1.

BOX 4.1 ■ Approaches to History Taking

Introductions

Introduction of self which would include name, role and seeking permission to undertake a clinical history. This would then be followed by checking of patient demographics.

Presenting Complaint

This is the initial and brief information the patient offers on why they have accessed healthcare services. It should be concise. To start the consultation with your patient, you can ask an open question, such as 'What has brought you to see me today?'

History of Presenting Complaint

The history of the presenting complaint should include most of the information, and should involve you as a practitioner in establishing the symptom/s. Some patients are poor historians, and it requires skill as a clinician to ascertain the specific details. Some examples of specific questions around each symptom include when the symptom started, its location, what alleviates the symptom, whether this has occurred before and how are they currently managing the symptom/s.

BOX 4.1 ■ Approaches to History Taking—cont'd

You can encourage your patient to share more details with the use of encouragement and good communication skills. There are mnemonics available for the exploration of the presenting complaint, many originating from pain assessments but have been adopted for other symptoms. Each university's master's programme will have their own ideas and views on the use of these mnemonics, so speak to your programme/module leader.

Red flags, that is, symptoms that may offer information into serious underlying conditions such as cancer, need to be asked and explored. Remember the importance of documentation of both positive findings (the patient has haemoptysis) and negative findings (the patient denies any weight loss). It would be essential to ask about all red flags applicable to the presenting symptom/system as well as generalised red flags.

Also consider and explore the impact the presenting symptom has upon the patient's daily living.

Past Medical History

Open questioning around previous medical history can sometimes be challenging, with patients denying that they have any medical history. This then requires you to hone and develop your skills to probe in more detail and, when appropriate, use closed questioning. Be mindful that there are specific mnemonics for exploring past medical history; however, used in isolation, these can lead to the practitioner missing vital information. Speak to your programme/module leader about how they want you to structure the past medical history.

Questions around medication can offer guidance around previous medical history. The use of electronic records will aid you in drawing a picture of the medical history of your patients, but be mindful these records might not be fully updated or accurate.

Medication and Any Allergic Reactions (Specifically Noting What These Allergic Reactions Are)

Gaining the medication history, and noting any reactions and how these manifest, is key. Asking whether the patient has any allergies in general may also provide indication of allergens important to avoid. A list of medications can be obtained, for example, from the patient's notes, or from the patient themselves. Take care to note that there are proprietary and generic drug names and to note any over-the-counter medication bought and self-administered. It is also important to ask whether any illicit drugs are taken. A nonjudgemental approach, through the building of a rapport with your patient, is important to gain trust and potentially a more honest and complete account of their health history. Assessment of both compliance and concordance is also essential.

Family History

This can be highly relevant, depending on the presenting condition/s. For example, presentation and symptoms of breast cancer require the family history of the patient to be explored for other diagnoses of cancer (Peart, 2022).

Social History

Establishing any environmental or lifestyle factors that impact on health is key. This can include questions around family and support networks, occupation, alcohol, smoking and recent travel history.

Systems Review

Systems review is the final sieve to review each system and check nothing has been missed from the history take. This explores each system with some brief questioning; for example, the central nervous system (CNS) can be checked by asking questions around 'any fits, faints or funny turns'.

Application to Practice

Within their work, Kurtz and Silverman (1996) recognised the need for developing communication skills within medical education, resulting in the birth of the Calgary–Cambridge model. Reflecting upon teaching of AP students' consultation and communication skills, there can often be an initial uncertainty about the

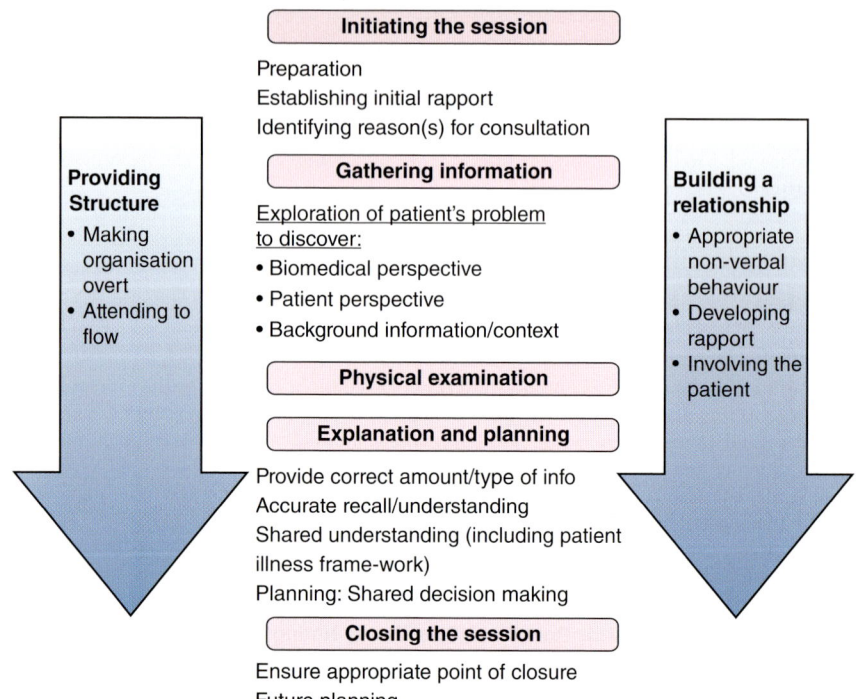

Fig. 4.1 The structure of a patient-centred consultation capturing core elements. *(From Kurtz, S. M., & Silverman, J. D. (1996). The Calgary-Cambridge Referenced Observation Guides: An aid to defining the curriculum and organizing the teaching in communication training programmes. Medical Education, 30, 83–89.)*

application of these communication skills, especially when history taking skills are introduced. Kurtz and Silverman (1996) set out a clear guide to applying communication skills within the challenges of gathering patient data in a history format and supporting a patient-centred approach to the consultation.

In Fig. 4.1, the gathering information stage refers to the biomedical perspective and this would reflect the standard medical approach to undertaking a medical history. Here, like all other stages, communication skills take a central feature, with the identification and exploration of cues, both verbal and nonverbal, and the application of appropriate questioning styles to elicit the information required. It has been suggested that as clinicians, we will conduct between 100,000 and 200,000 patient consultations in our professional lifetime (Nicholas & Mirvis, 1998).

Engel and Morgan's (1973) seminal work about patient consultation reminds us that the consultation is the most 'powerful and sensitive' tool we have at our disposal. In earlier work, Dr William Osler told us to 'Listen to the patient, he is telling you the diagnosis' (Bliss, 1999), as up to 80% of the diagnosis will be derived from a good history (Hampton et al., 1975; Keifenheim et al., 2015; Peterson et al., 1992). History taking and the application of communication skills to a consultation require skill development within practice while working alongside practice supervisors/educators. Denness (2013) recognises that the use of video, recording patient consultations (with patient-informed written consent) and then reviewing these with your practice supervisor/educator is a powerful tool to develop consultation skills and improve the overall consultation.

As we have seen from the various consultation models, decision-making is incorporated into each consultation, and the next part of this chapter focuses on an important element of the clinical pillar, which is clinical decision-making (CDM).

Clinical Decision-Making

WHAT IS CLINICAL DECISION-MAKING?

'Clinical decision making is a contextual, continuous, and evolving process, where data are gathered, interpreted, and evaluated in order to select an evidence-based choice of action.'

(Tiffen et al., 2014)

An interpersonal, holistic assessment requires competency in CDM. Diamond-Fox (2021) identified that advanced practitioners will make a significant difference to those in their care through diagnostic accuracy, patient satisfaction, concordance and healthcare outcomes if they are skilled in consultation and assessment skills. CDM is a core competency for advanced practitioners that needs to be developed (Lawson, 2018). There is a plethora of terms used in the literature that cover CDM, including clinical reasoning, clinical inference, clinical judgement, decision-making, diagnostic reasoning and critical reasoning (Brentnall et al., 2022; Thompson et al., 2004). However, according to Thompson et al. (2004), judgements and decisions are interlinked. Judgements inform clinical decisions, and stem from the critical appraisal of the evidence presented by the patient and other findings. The process of making a judgement comes before decision-making and is almost an unconscious activity. However, be aware that if you have transitioned from a senior role to a trainee or advanced practitioner role, there may be a step back in terms of development of such decision-making skills in relation to Benner's (1984, 1999) framework of novice to expert, and therefore, decision-making in such situations can become a slower and a more conscious activity.

The Benner (1984, 1999) and Benner et al. (1996, 1999) model of skill acquisition based on the work of Dreyfus and Dreyfus (1980) premises that understanding is a skill that develops, knowing 'how' rather than knowing 'that'. The model offers five stages of skill acquisition: novice, advanced beginner, competent, proficient and expert. As you step into the role of an advanced practitioner, there may, as previously mentioned, be an adjustment in the stage of skill acquisition that you occupy within your career, and decision-making may be affected by the role transition. You may therefore move away from 'knowing how' back to 'knowing that' until you develop your experience and abilities, and that your performance becomes less automatic and more reflexive.

Key to the CDM process as an advanced practitioner is that you will be taking responsibility for the decisions you make. This is challenging and can be frightening for advanced practitioners as you may not always make the correct decision.

Problem solving or decision-making ability is dependent upon the amount of knowledge that you have, its specificity and structure and how it is stored, accessed and retrieved (Elstein & Schwartz, 2006). Knowledge alone, however, is not adequate for effective and efficient decision-making, and cognition and metacognition play an essential role in developing expertise.

Cognition is the mental process associated with developing and generating new knowledge and understanding. This occurs through experiences, thought and the senses; it is an activity that gets faster as your practice develops. Metacognition is your understanding and awareness of your thought processes, around decision-making (Church & Carroll, 2023). Metacognition can be described as thinking about your thinking (Elstein, 2009). Metacognition enables you as an advanced practitioner to identify limitations in the quality of information obtained and inconsistencies in the data or unexpected findings. In developing your metacognition, it will enable you to assess and internally observe your decision-making, identifying errors; it will prompt you to recognise when you have limited knowledge and/or insufficient skills to make a decision, and identify when you need to seek advice. Church and Carroll (2023) identified that for healthcare practitioners, metacognition improves decision-making. This occurs through the identification of cognitive bias, and through facilitating a systematic and holistic approach, and in enabling creative thinking.

As an advanced practitioner, you should be aware of the choices and decision-making presented to you, your ability to look inwards at yourself and outward at the situation (Lewenson & Truglio-Londrigan, 2008) and the information/data that will inform your decision-making. This level of self-reflection, cognition and metacognition will enable you to better understand what else you need to know to develop your decision-making skills.

There are a plethora of tools and guidelines you can utilise to help you make a reasoned decision which is defensible should you ever be challenged on your decision.

Trimble and Hamilton (2016) break down CDM into four areas:

1. Information gathering
2. Hypothesis generating
3. Hypothesis testing
4. Reflection

Young et al. (2009) suggest that by gathering and synthesising the information needed to generate a hypothesis, as an advanced practitioner, you can formulate a clinical impression which considers the patient's prognosis, diagnosis, treatment, care and/or management plan. Lawson (2018) recognises that there is little information identifying how advanced practitioners develop CDM skills in clinical reasoning (Lawson, 2018). NHS Scotland (2013) suggests that CDM requires several skills, in addition to experience. The skills they suggest you will need to develop are pattern recognition, critical thinking, communication skills, applying evidence-based practice, developing teamwork and an ethos of sharing and reflection. Your approach will also need to consider the clinical setting you are working within, the resources at hand and your patients' preferences.

These elements enable a healthcare practitioner to select the best course of action which optimises a patient's health and minimises any potential harm. Your role as a clinical decision maker is therefore to be professionally accountable for accurately assessing patients' needs using appropriate sources of information, and planning interventions that address problems and which they are competent to perform (Standing, 2010, 2017).

Decision-Making Process

The factors affecting decision-making processes are:

- Decision maker—this is you as an advanced practitioner.
- Consultation (process)—see later in the chapter how and what affects the process.
- Decision outcome—what this means to your patient.

The decision-making process is influenced by decision-making models and theories. Decision-making theories include hypothetico-deductive theory, pattern recognition, decision analysis and intuition, whereas decision-making models include normative and descriptive models (Khemka, 2021). Both theories and models are interwoven and are dependent on one another.

Normative models, for example, set principles against which individual decision-making behaviours can be compared. Human decision-making is limited and influenced by cognitive capacity and situational constraints. The influences can result in deviation from the normative models. For advanced practitioners in clinical situations, there are regular instances where decision-making occurs with incomplete data sets and knowledge, and where potential outcomes of the decision at hand could be uncertain and obscure. Other factors that influence decision-making include the impact of emotions and individual circumstances (Khemka, 2021).

Decision-making is typified by a limited processing of information, taking cognitive shortcuts (heuristics) to simplify decision-making (Kahneman & Tversky, 1979), and 'satisficing', which is identifying and selecting solutions which meet the least conditions and are 'good enough' (Simon, 1990).

Decision-Making Theories

HYPOTHETICO-DEDUCTIVE DECISION-MAKING

This theory is used frequently by medicine and is rational and based on evidence. It is linked to the normative model of reasoning. Hypothetico-deductive decision-making comprises two types of reasoning: inductive and deductive decision-making. Inductive theory, working from a specific point to a more general point, is where you will collect data, which will lead you to generate hypotheses, and deductive decision works in the opposite direction, from general to specific. You will develop a hypothesis to explain a problem as you collect and search for the presence or absence of data, to confirm or refute the hypothesis/hypotheses (Hughes &

Nimmo, 2017). Literature suggests that more novice individuals use deductive reasoning, while experts will apply inductive reasoning. Nonetheless, in challenging situations, where data are incomplete, where illness patterns are not clear, experts can apply deductive reasoning (Seok Shin, 2019).

PIT STOP!

Read the following paper and the application of hypothetico-deductive reasoning in (nursing) clinical practice. The decision-making process is applicable to all professions:

https://www.cambridge.org/core/journals/british-journal-of-anaesthetic-and-recovery-nursing/article/comparative-theories-in-clinical-decision-making-and-their-application-to-practice-a-reflective-case-study/21AEDD92876160077CBA1FB99BC4B8E9

As advanced practitioners, you will be aware of the incomplete data sets that you work with, as you will likely not obtain all information that you need. Therefore, regardless of the decision-making processes applied, you will never entirely prove or disprove a hypothesis in many cases. You can produce the most likely diagnosis, recognising that you may need to adapt and change the hypothesis should more information be gathered, or the outcome of the treatment decisions/further tests changes the expected outcome.

PIT STOP!

Use a reasoning strategy (deductive versus inductive) to process the information in the clinical context of a patient consultation.

PATTERN RECOGNITION

We have previously identified this theory of decision-making within the reference by NHS Scotland (2013) within the CDM. Pattern recognition is commonly cited in nursing and linked with intuition. When using pattern recognition, you will view the entire situation, as opposed to the reductionist approach of hypothesis generation. It has been noted in the evidence base that practitioners rarely apply pattern recognition and hypothetico-deductive reasoning (Arocha et al., 1993).

Pattern recognition is where you observe patterns or cues, that you then link to previous patient cases who had similar symptoms, without consciously being aware of the process and are therefore given the same diagnosis. This then becomes dependent on your experience and clinical knowledge base (Arocha et al., 1993).

In patients who present with 'nonproblematic' (Offredy, 1998) or 'easy' cases (Elstein & Schwartz, 2002), pattern recognition is useful. However, what this implies is that generating hypotheses and inductively or deductively definitively diagnosing a patient's condition is a completely conscious activity, whereas pattern recognition may be more intuitive (intuition). The language that we use may also infer more intuitive and less conscious decision-making, for example, based on a 'hunch' feeling (Cioffi, 1997) and 'gut feeling' (Melin-Johansson et al., 2017). Intuition, which is principally linked to nursing, is defined as

> *'...something based on an individual's opinion justified by the authority of their experience.'*
>
> (Offredy, 1998)

However, more recent evidence offers insight into how intuition remains valid and amongst a wider community of healthcare practitioners, with medical specialists agreeing that intuition does play a role in the decision-making process (Van den Brink et al., 2019). It is recognised that intuition results from experiential knowledge, and that 'hunches' should be supported by analytical reasoning (Van den Brink et al., 2019) which supports more dated literature that practitioners subconsciously but meaningfully process information (Buckingham & Adams, 2000; Cioffi, 1997; Harbison, 2001).

DECISION ANALYSIS

This refers to a systematic approach to decision-making when there is much uncertainty within the case that you are assessing. The process aims to provide differing options by maximising individual decisions. It is a prescriptive model and breaks down decisions into smaller actions that you can then analyse separately in terms of likelihood and seriousness and reconstruct in a systematic manner to provide you with an option. The prescriptive element should support you in making decisions which can be taken in specific circumstances. It can be seen in practice in the form of decision trees. Harbison (2001) argues that decision analysis theory is not as useful when emergency or urgent decision-making in practice is required; however, recognition of when to use such tools may well be dependent on the clinician's experience.

Dual Process Thinking

Dual process theory sheds light on the intricate interplay between intuitive and analytical processes in human cognition and decision-making. These two modes often interact and mutually influence each other. Let's explore some of the specifics.

INTUITIVE PROCESS (TYPE 1)

The intuitive process operates swiftly and relies on heuristics. It's akin to our gut feeling—quick, automatic, emotional and subconscious. When faced with decisions, we arrive at intuitive answers promptly, often with a sense of confidence. These 'gut' decisions require less working memory and are grounded in instinct (Kahneman, 2011; Sieck, 2011), for instance, swiftly removing an obstacle from a patient's way to prevent a fall.

ANALYTICAL PROCESS (TYPE 2)

The analytical process involves more deliberate thinking. It requires hypothetical considerations and is slower. Type 2 processing engages critical thinking, reflecting on how decisions may impact future events. It's the conscious evaluation of various factors, logical reasoning and weighing options (Kahneman, 2011; Sieck, 2011).

Understanding this dual process framework can enhance our CDM across various spheres of practice. Type 2 thinking is not ideal in an emergency like a cardiac arrest due to the slowness and processing of information. However, for the trainee advanced practitioner, this is an ideal approach as it requires the individual to apply the metacognition ('thinking about thinking') about their decisions. For example, if an advanced practitioner thinks a patient has a suspected urinary tract infection (UTI), type 2 thinking would require processing of the patient's clinical history, examination findings, drawing on current and new knowledge of urinary symptoms and the analysis of relevant clinical guidelines as an example for some type 2 thinking processes. In contrast, type 1 thinking would lead the advanced practitioner to jump to a diagnosis of a UTI based on a limited patient history take and a failure to consider all available information/data, thus not considering other possible causes for the urinary symptoms.

PIT STOP!

Consider the following influences on your decision-making:
- Knowledge (heuristics)
- Experience (heuristics)
- Evidence
- Environment/landscape
- Professional relationship
- Role autonomy
- The patient/client
- Culture
- Legal and ethical issues

To conclude the section, consider a case study from your own practice, and review the decision-making behind each treatment and decision that you made. Consider the following elements:

Describe the case/s using a format familiar to you:
- Presenting complaint.
- History of presenting complaint.
- Past medical history using a format familiar to you and tools such as MJTHREADS and SOCRATES that offer frameworks to guide your questioning (please see Van der Tuijn et al., 2023, for a breakdown of the tools/acronyms).
- Drug history.
- Social/family history.
- What were the decisions that you made?

- Did you use any decision trees?
- What other mechanisms/theories/frameworks did you apply?
- Were there differences in your decision-making and that of other professions/professionals?
- Are there comparisons between other cases that you can think of, and how this affected treatment (did it affect care?)?

DRAWING CONCLUSIONS

Everything isn't always quite as it seems, and conclusions may not always be correct.

"Things are not always what they seem; the first appearance deceives many; the intelligence of a few perceives what has been carefully hidden."

-Phaedrus

The practices and behaviours that you develop as an advanced practitioner are important in decision-making. Poor practices can lead to poor outcomes, in terms of incorrect interpretations based on incorrect use of theories and or models. For example, if, when making a decision, you use pattern recognition without a sufficient experience of knowledge, then this could lead to incorrect diagnosis, treatment, care and poor outcomes and patient satisfaction (Croskerry, 2003).

There are numerous reasons for errors, with five types of diagnostic errors being recognised. They are listed as follows:

- System errors
- Errors related to misinterpretation of data
- Errors related to gaps in knowledge
- Cognitive biases due to the development of too few hypotheses, focusing on a single hypothesis (Elstein & Schwartz, 2002)
- And no-fault errors (Croskerry, 2003)

Others include being influenced by previous, similar patient cases, incorrect interpretation of diagnostic tests, making a decision out of context and not seeking or listening to advice, premature closure of a case/decision and others. Cognitive biases such as anchoring, confirmation bias and framing effect are also common causes for faulty decision-making in practice (Croskerry, 2003; Elstein & Schwartz, 2002).

PIT STOP!

To develop your understanding of errors, take some time to read the following:

Croskerry, P. (2003). The importance of cognitive errors in diagnosis and strategies to minimize them. *Academic Medicine, 78,* 775–780. 10.1097/00001888-200308000-00003

Restrepo, D., Armstrong, K. A., & Metlay, J. P. (2020). Annals clinical decision making: Avoiding cognitive errors in clinical decision making. *Annals of Internal Medicine, 172*(11), 747–751.

Elstein AS, Schwartz A. Clinical problem solving and diagnostic decision making: selective review of the cognitive literature. BMJ. 2002 Mar 23;324(7339):729-32. doi: 10.1136/bmj.324.7339.729. Erratum in: BMJ. 2006 Nov 4;333(7575):944. Schwarz, Alan [corrected to Schwartz, Alan]. PMID: 11909793; PMCID: PMC1122649

As an advanced practitioner, you need to be aware of potential errors in your decision-making, and where these may occur.

Application to Clinical Practice

To conclude this chapter, it would be pertinent to provide a vignette which captures the work of an advanced practitioner working within clinical practice (Box 4.2).

BOX 4.2 ■ Vignette of an Advanced Clinical Practitioner Working in Primary Care

As a registered nurse, I have worked in primary care for almost 25 years as an advanced practitioner and the diversity of patients and the ability to build up relationships with those I care for over time make this a truly rewarding role. Reflecting for this vignette, I am conscious of the many changes primary care has faced and my need to acknowledge that I find it more challenging now in our current health climate. I have less time to spend with each patient and they present with multiple pathologies and complexities which I find stretch me to the edges (not beyond) of my scope of practice. I have less time to develop a rapport and build up the relationships I feel are important in a primary care setting as patients tend to struggle to get appointments with the same clinician. As patients struggle to get an appointment, they often arrive frustrated and have a list of issues which are impossible to safely address in a short consultation. However, I still enjoy the clinical work and feel privileged to be able to care for patients in a holistic way.

Primary care usually comprises of clinicians working two sessions per day with time between for lunch-time home visits and administration work. One practice I worked at had a set break time where all clinicians would have a drink and discuss any concerns they have had with specific patients or presentations. Other practices have a set meeting each week where clinicians can do the same. Several practices I have worked at have practiced in a very different way with no time for clinicians to meet and back-to-back appointments are a normal part of the day with extras added on for emergencies. This way of working can leave advanced practitioners feeling very isolated and unsupported.

My current clinical load is small as my main role is at a university. I have 2 and a half hour surgeries with 15 minutes per patient. My first eight appointments are face-to-face followed by two telephone appointments. I see 'anything and everything' apart from pregnancy-related presentations. Some of my appointments come from the morning triage list, the E-consultation system with others that are pre-booked. There are usually two general practitioners and one advanced practitioner per clinical session which means I am able to seek advice on patients I feel are outside of my scope of practice.

As an example of my work, I will share some patient presentations from a typical clinical session:
Patient one was a 28-year-old man who presented with anxiety and depression symptoms; he had been struggling with these symptoms for 9 months before seeking support. He was using cannabis to try and alleviate his symptoms.
Patient two was a 34-year-old lady with heavy menstrual bleeding; she was tired all the time and was struggling with dysmenorrhoea and passing very large clots.
Patient three was an 18-year-old who had injured his right knee playing football. He was weight bearing but had a significant effusion and was struggling to walk.
Patient four was an 84-year-old lady with end-stage heart failure, mobility issues and multiple falls. She had injured her left leg falling last night.
Patient five was a 5-year-old boy who had upper respiratory symptoms of nasal congestion, temperature and cough. Mum brought him today as she was worried as he was now wheezing at night.
Patient six was a 26-year-old lady who had recently moved to the United Kingdom from Nigeria. She had been treated for a psychotic episode in Nigeria but had now run out of her medication. She had a handwritten letter from a psychiatrist and was on multiple high-dose antipsychotics.
Patient seven was a 64-year-old man with left-sided chest pain and shortness of breath.

> **BOX 4.2 ■ Vignette of an Advanced Clinical Practitioner Working in Primary Care—cont'd**
>
> Patient eight was a 42-year-old lady who was struggling with long COVID. She had multiple joint pains, exhaustion, headaches and low mood. She had been referred to the long COVID clinic but had not heard from them and felt she could not continue with the symptoms she was experiencing, and had thoughts of self-harm.
>
> The final two telephone appointments were to discuss bloods results; one patient needed referral for a liver ultrasound and one patient needed to start on ferrous sulphate for iron deficiency anaemia.
>
> As you can see from the patients seen, there was a large diversity of presentations which necessitated a range of clinical skills. History taking within a holistic consultation approach was utilised with every patient. This took between 8–15 minutes per patient depending on the complexity. All three patients with mental health symptoms took longer to assess; these required risk assessments in addition to their histories. Clinical examinations skills included many of the systems: gynaecological, abdominal, knee, neurological, ear, nose and throat, respiratory and cardiovascular. Referral was needed for five of my patients to secondary care, one to our in-house mental health nurse and one to musculoskeletal physiotherapy. Two patients were referred for blood tests and one for a pelvic ultrasound.
>
> I was particularly concerned about three of my patients, but all my patients had presentations which could be serious and required safety netting. Patient seven was sent directly to emergency care after receiving aspirin, glyceryl trinitrate and oxygen. Patient six was discussed with the on-call psychiatric team who agreed to see her the next day. Patient eight was referred to the hospital at home team who arranged a falls assessment later that day.

Conclusion

This chapter has covered some of the main elements of the clinical pillar, related to communication, consultation and decision-making. Decision-making will impact your practice as an advanced practitioner across the other three pillars, offering you an opportunity to develop your thinking and expertise within your practice.

References

Arocha, J. F., Patel, V. L., & Patel, Y. C. (1993). Hypothesis generation and the coordination of theory and evidence in novice diagnostic reasoning. *Medical Decision Making, 13*(3), 198–211. https://pubmed.ncbi.nlm.nih.gov/8412548/. Accessed April 20, 2024.

Benner, P. (1984). From novice to expert: Excellence and power in clinical nursing practice. *American Journal of Nursing, 84*(12), 1480. doi:10.1097/00000446-198412000-00025

Benner, P. (1999). Nursing leadership for the new millennium. Claiming the wisdom & worth of clinical practice. *Nursing and Health Care Perspectives, 20*(6), 312–319.

Benner, P., Hooper-Kyriakidis, P., & Stannard, D. (1999). *Clinical wisdom and interventions in critical care: A thinking in action approach.* London: W.B. Saunders.

Benner, P., Tanner, C., & Chesla, C. (1996). *Expertise in nursing practice: Caring, clinical judgment, and ethics.* New York: Springer Publishing

Bliss, M. (1999). *William Osler: A life in medicine.* Oxford University Press.

Bodegard, H. (2019). Challenges to patient centredness – a comparison of patient and doctor experiences from primary care. *BMC Family Practice, 20*, 83. https://doi.org/10.1186/s12875-019-0959-y

Brentnall, J., Thackray, D., & Judd, B. (2022). Evaluating the clinical reasoning of student health professionals in placement and simulation settings: A systematic review. *International Journal of Environmental Research and Public Health, 19*(2), 936. doi:10.3390/ijerph19020936

Buckingham, C., & Adams, A. (2000). Classifying clinical decision making: Interpreting nursing intuition, heuristics and medical diagnosis. *Journal of Advanced Nursing, 32*(4), 990–998.

Byrne, P. S., & Long, B. E. L. (1976). *Doctors talking to patients*. London: HMSO.

Church, D., & Carroll, M. (2023). How does metacognition improve decision-making in healthcare practitioners? *Journal of Paramedic Practice*, *15*(3). https://doi.org/10.12968/jpar.2023.15.3.113. Accessed April 20, 2024.

Cioffi, J. (1997). Heuristic, servants to intuition in clinical decision making. *Journal of Advanced Nursing*, *26*, 203–208.

Craske J., Carter, B., Jarman I. H., Tume, L. N. (2017). Nursing judgement and decision-making using the Sedation Withdrawal Score (SWS) in children. *Journal of Advanced Nursing*, *73*, 2327–2338.

Croskerry, P. (2003). The importance of cognitive errors in diagnosis and strategies to minimize them. *Academic Medicine: Journal of the Association of American Medical Colleges*, *78*, 775–780. doi:10.1097/00001888-200308000-00003

Dart, M. (2010). Making the pieces fit: Therapeutic communication and the nursing process. In M. Dart (Ed.), *Motivational interviewing in nursing practice: Empowering the patient*. MA: Jones and Bartlett Publishers.

Denness, C. (2013). What are consultation models for? *InnovAiT*, *6*(9), 592–599. doi:10.1177/1755738013475436

Diamond-Fox, S. (2021). Undertaking consultations and clinical assessments at advanced level. *British Journal of Nursing*, *30*(4), 238–243. https://doi.org/10.12968/bjon/2021.30.4.238

Dreyfus, S. E., & Dreyfus, H. L. (1980). *A five-stage model of the mental activities involved in directed skill acquisition*. Berkeley: University of California.

Dunn, N. (2003). Practical issues around putting the patient at the centre of care. *Journal of the Royal Society of Medicine*, *96*(7), 325–327.

Edwards, M., Davies, M. M., & Edwards, A. G. (2009). What are the external influences on information exchange and shared decision-making in healthcare consultations: A meta-synthesis of the literature. *Patient Education and Counselling*, *75*(1), 37–52. doi:10.1016/j.pec.2008.09.025

Elstein, A. (2009). Thinking about diagnostic thinking: A 30-year perspective. *Advances in Health Sciences Education: Theory and Practice*, *14*(Suppl. 1), 7–18. https://pubmed.ncbi.nlm.nih.gov/19669916/. Accessed April 22, 2024.

Elstein, A. S., & Schwartz, A. (2002). Clinical problem solving and diagnostic decision making: Selective review of the cognitive literature. *BMJ*, *324*, 729–732.

Elstein, A., & Schwartz, A. (2006). Clinical problem solving and diagnostic decision making: Selective review of the cognitive literature. *BMJ*, *333*, 944. https://doi.org/10.1136/bmj.333.7575.944-c

Engel, G., & Morgan, W. (1973). *Interviewing the patient*. London: Saunders.

Frain, J. (2017). Why clinical communication matters. In N. Cooper & J. Frain (Eds.), *ABC of clinical communication*, 1–6 Sussex: Wiley & Sons Ltd.

Hampton, J. R., Harrison M. J., Mitchell J. R., Prichard, J. S., & Seymour, C. (1975). Relative contributions of history-taking, physical examination, and laboratory investigation to diagnosis and management of medical outpatients. *BMJ*, *2*, 486–489.

Harbison, J. (2001). Clinical decision making in nursing: Theoretical perspectives and their relevance to practice. *Journal of Advanced Nursing*, *35*(1), 126–133.

Health Education and Improvement Wales (HEIW). (2023). *Professional framework for enhanced, advanced and consultant clinical practice*. https://heiw.nhs.wales/files/enhanced-advanced-and-consultant-framework/. Accessed April 7, 2024.

Helman, C. G. (1981). Disease versus illness in general practice. *Journal of the Royal College of General Practitioners*, *31*(230), 548–552.

Kahneman, D. (2011). *Thinking, fast and slow*. Farrar, Straus and Giroux.

Kahneman, D., & Tversky, A. (1979). Prospect theory: An analysis of decision under risk. *Econometrica*, *47*(2), 263–291. https://doi.org/10.2307/1914185

Hughes, M., & Nimmo, G. (2017). Models of clinical reasoning. In N. Cooper & J. Frain (Eds.), *ABC of clinical reasoning*, 17–21. Sussex: Wiley & Sons Ltd.

Keifenheim, K., Teufel, M., Speiser, N., Leehr, E., Zipfel, S., & Herrman-Werner, A (2015). Teaching history taking to medical students: A systematic review. *BMC Medical Education*, *15*, 159. doi:10.1.1186/s12909-015-0443-x

Khemka, I. (2021). Theoretical perspectives on decision making. In I. Khemka & L. Hickson (Eds.), *Decision making by individuals with intellectual and developmental disabilities*. Positive Psychology and Disability Series. Springer, Cham. https://doi.org/10.1007/978-3-030-74675-9_6

Kumar, P. M., Nagate, R. R., Alqahtani, S. M., Sarma, G. S. N., & Supraja, S. (2023). Role of jargon in the patient–doctor communication in the dental healthcare sector—A systematic review and meta-analysis. *Journal of Education and Health promotion*, *12*(198). doi:10.4103/jehp.jehp_1442_22

Kurtz, S., Silverman, J., Benson, J., & Draper, J. (2003). Marrying content and process in clinical method teaching: Enhancing the Calgary-Cambridge guides. *Academic Medicine*, *78*(8), 802–809. doi:10.1097/00001888-200308000-00011

Kurtz, S. M., & Silverman, J. D. (1996). The Calgary-Cambridge Referenced Observation Guides: An aid to defining the curriculum and organizing the teaching in communication training programmes. *Medical Education*, *30*(2), 83–89. https://doi.org/10.1111/j.1365-2923.1996.tb00724.x

Lawson, T. N. (2018). Diagnostic reasoning and cognitive biases of nurse practitioners. *Journal of Nursing Education*, *57*(4), 203–208. doi:10.3928/01484834-20180322-03.

Lewenson, S., & Truglio-Londrigan, M. (2008). *Decision making in nursing*. Sudbury: Jones and Bartlett.

Mahendran, A. (2014). Improving your communication skills. *BMJ Careers*. https://www.bmj.com/careers/article/improving-your-communication-skills. Accessed January 10, 2024.

Melin-Johansson, C., Palmqvist R., & Rnnberg., L. (2017). Clinical intuition in the nursing process and decision-making—A mixed-studies review. *Journal Clinical Nursing*, *26*, 3936–3949.

Moulton, L. (2007). *The naked consultation – A practical guide to primary care consultation skills*. Oxford: Radcliffe Medical Press.

Neighbour, R. (1987). *The inner consultation: How to develop an effective and intuitive consulting style*. MTP Press.

Neighbour, R. H. (2004). *The Inner Consultation: How to develop an effective and intuitive consulting style* (2nd ed). London: Radcliffe Publishing.

NHS England. (2025). *Multi-professional framework for advanced Practice in England*. Birmingham: Centre for Advancing Practice.

NHS Scotland. (2013). *Clinical decision making*. https://www.effectivepractitioner.nes.scot.nhs.uk/media/254840/clinical%20decision%20making.pdf. Accessed 20.04.2024.

Nicholas, L., & Mirvis, D. (1998). Physician-patient communication: Does it matter? *Tennessee Medicine—Journal of the Tennessee Medical Association*, *91*(3), 94–96.

Nursing and Midwifery Board Australia. (2021). *Nurse practitioner standards for practice – Effective from 1 March 2021*. https://www.nursingmidwiferyboard.gov.au/Codes-Guidelines-Statements/Professional-standards/nurse-practitioner-standards-of-practice.aspx. Accessed March 2, 2024.

Nursing Council of New Zealand. (2017). *Education programme standards for the mātanga tapuhi nurse practitioner scope of practice*. https://nursingcouncil.org.nz/Public/NCNZ/nursing-section/Nurse_practitioner.aspx. Accessed March 2, 2024.

Offredy, M. (1998). The application of decision-making concepts by nurse practitioners in general practice. *Journal of Advanced Nursing*, *28*(5), 988–1000. doi:10.1046/j.1365-2648.1998.00823.x.

Peart, P. (2022). Clinical history taking. *Clinics in Integrated Care*, *10*, 100088. https://doi.org/10.1016/j.intcar.2021.100088

Pendleton, D. (1984). *The Consultation: An approach to learning and teaching*. Oxford: Oxford University Press. Accessed 02.04.2013.

Peterson, M., Holbrook, J., Hales, D., Smith, N., & Staker, L. (1992). Contributions of the history, physical examination and laboratory investigations in making medical diagnoses. *Western Journal of Medicine*, *156*(2), 163.

Restrepo, D., Armstrong, K. A., Metlay, J. P. (2020). Annals clinical decision making: Avoiding cognitive errors in clinical decision-making. *Annals of Internal Medicine*, *172*(11), 747–751.

Rushforth, H. (2008). Reflections on a study tour to explore history taking and physical assessment education. *Nurse Education in Practice*, *8*(1), 31–40.

Sieck, W. (2011). *Dual process theory: Two ways to think and decide*. https://www.globalcognition.org/dual-process-theory/. Accessed April 22, 2024.

Seok Shin, H. (2019). Reasoning processes in clinical reasoning: From the perspective of cognitive psychology. *Korean Journal of Medical Education*, *31*(4), 299–308. https://www.ncbi.nlm.nih.gov/pmc/articles/PMC6900348/. doi:10.3946/kjme.2019.140. Accessed April 20, 2024.

Silverman, J. (2017). The Consultation. In Cooper, N., & Frain, J (Eds.), *ABC of clinical communication*, 7–12 Sussex: Wiley & Sons Ltd.

Silverman, J., Kurtz, S., & Draper, J. (2008). *Skills for communicating with patients*. Oxford: Radcliffe Medical Press.

Simon, H. (1990). *Reason in human affairs.* Stanford University Press.

Slater, N. (2014). *Appetite.* London: Fourth Estate.

Standing, M. (2010). Cognitive continuum theory – Nine modes of practice. In Standing, M. (Ed.), *Clinical judgement and decision-making in nursing and interprofessional healthcare.* Maidenhead Open University Press.

Standing, M. (Ed.). (2017). *Clinical judgement and decision making in nursing* (3rd ed.). London: Learning Matters.

Stoeckle, J. D., & Billings, A. J. (1987). A history of history-taking. *Journal of General Internal Medicine, 2,* 119–127.

Stott, N. C. H., & Davis, R. H. (1979). The exceptional potential in each primary care consultation. *Journal of the Royal College of General Practitioners, 29,* 201–205.

The Health Foundation. (2012). *When doctors and patients talk: Making sense of the consultation.* https://www.health.org.uk/publications/when-doctors-and-patients-talk-making-sense-of-the-consultation. Accessed March 13, 2024.

Thompson, T., Dowding, D., & McCaughan, D. (2004). Strategies for avoiding pitfalls in clinical decision-making *Nursing Times, 100*(20), 40–42.

Tiffen J., Corbridge S. J., and Slimmer L. (2014). Enhancing clinical decision making: development of a contiguous definition and conceptual framework. *Journal of Professional Nursing.* (5):399–405. DOI: 10.1016/j.profnurs.2014.01.006.

Trimble, M., & Hamilton, P. (2016). The thinking doctor: Clinical decision making in contemporary medicine. *Clinical Medicine, 16*(4), 343–346.

Van den Brink, N., Holbrechts, B., Brand, P. L. P., Stolper, E. C. F., & Van Royen, P. (2019). Role of intuitive knowledge in the diagnostic reasoning of hospital specialists: A focus group study. *BMJ Open, 9,* e022724. doi:10.1136/bmjopen-2018-022724

Van der Tuijn, K., Kavanagh, S., & Bain, A. (2023). *Principles of effective history taking when prescribing.* https://pharmaceutical-journal.com/article/ld/principles-of-effective-history-taking-when-prescribing. Accessed April 22, 2024.

Young, K., Duggan, L., & Franklin, P. (2009). Effective consulting and history–taking skills for prescribing practice. *British Journal of Nursing, 18*(17), 1056–1061.

CHAPTER 5

Four Pillars of Advanced Practice—Leadership

Jonathan Thomas ■ Melanie Rogers ■ Colette Henderson

CHAPTER OUTLINE

This chapter compliments Chapters 3, 4 and 6, which are dedicated to exploring each of the four pillars. It is beyond the scope of this chapter to discuss and analyse each leadership theory and style; however, it introduces the foundations of some of these theories. This chapter will explore what leadership is and how this differs from management and why leadership is important in health and social care. It explores the qualities that make a good leader and then concludes with two stories from leaders about their leadership.

Introduction

Across the UK, each advanced practice (AP) framework has leadership as a specific pillar for practice, thus highlighting the importance of this within the AP role. Embarking upon your AP journey, education programmes will encapsulate leadership, whether this be in a distinct module or integrated throughout the programme of study.

Leadership can often be confused with management but both concepts are completely different; however, these terms will often be used interchangeably in practice. Jonas et al. (2017) recognise that both management and leadership have an integrated part to play with supporting effective organisational change, with leadership setting the vision and direction, whilst management focuses upon the direction of resources to achieve organisation goals and targets. The aim of this chapter will be to explore the theory of leadership and how this can be applied to clinical practice which will draw upon personal stories of own leadership journeys.

What Is Leadership Versus Management?

PIT STOP!

What does leadership mean to you? Does this differ from management? Or do you see both being the same?

Leadership appears to have many definitions and associated theories; however, Bennis (2009) argues that it remains poorly understood despite being well researched. Kotter (1999) highlights that leadership is around setting direction and the vision to bring about change, with a leader being able to motivate and inspire others to follow. There are many factors that underpin being a good leader, such as the behaviours adopted and displayed, the relationships developed with others and the leadership style (Northouse, 2007). There might be some clear similarities with management; however, Bass (1990) provides a well-defined explanation of both leaders and managers:

> 'Leaders manage and managers lead, but the two activities are not synonymous. Management functions can potentially provide leadership; leadership activities can contribute to managing. Nevertheless, some managers do not lead, and some leaders do not manage.'

(Bass, 1990, p. 383)

Uhl-Bien and Arena (2017) and Azad et al. (2017) indicate that there is overlap between the concepts of management and leadership. In fact, at times the two concepts appear to be used interchangeably (Azad et al., 2017; Christensen et al., 2018). Azad et al. (2017) argue that attempting to differentiate may lead to an oversimplification of a complex concept that is not reflective of contemporary practice where adaptability is a core skill (Uhl-Bien & Arena, 2017). Whilst arguably overlap between these two concepts occurs, there is agreement between authors that there are key attributes of leaders such as adaptability (Azad et al., 2017; Uhl-Bien & Arena, 2017), shared vision, authenticity, self-awareness and personal integrity (Giordano-Mulligan & Eckardt, 2019; Leithwood et al., 2020). The Center for Creative Leadership (2023) identified 12 qualities that make a good leader, and Wong (2023) identifies 12 qualities to be a good manager, as highlighted in Box 5.1.

As we can note from Box 5.1, there are some qualities that cross over between leadership and management such as communication and the supportive role. Clearly, there is scope to be both a leader and a manager and these can occur in

---

BOX 5.1 ■ Leadership Versus Management Qualities

The 12 Essential Qualities of Being a Good Leader (Center for Creative Leadership, 2023)

1. Self-awareness
2. Respect
3. Compassion
4. Vision
5. Communication
6. Learning agility
7. Collaboration
8. Influence
9. Integrity
10. Courage
11. Gratitude
12. Resilience

The 12 Qualities for a Manager (Wong, 2023)

1. Build trust
2. Focus of employee strengths
3. Do not micromanage
4. Assertive
5. Develop employees' careers
6. Manage pressure
7. Effective communicators
8. Open to ideas
9. Analytical
10. Recognise and reward hard work
11. Role model
12. Demonstrate appreciation

various formats such as leading and managing change, leading and managing a team or leading and managing an organisation.

Clinical Leadership

In relation to clinical leadership, this applies to healthcare staff and their ability to act as leaders within the practice setting (Jonas et al., 2017). All clinicians can act as leaders no matter what stage of their career they are at. Within the UK, clinical leadership has a high agenda; however, Mrayyan et al. (2023) imply that clinical leadership is not fully understood by many clinicians. Poor leadership can have a significant impact upon healthcare practice, and this was tragically witnessed at the Mid Staffordshire NHS Foundation Trust which led to the Francis Inquiry (Francis, 2013). Poor clinical leadership emerged as an underlying theme at the failings of a Welsh health board where the standards of care for elderly people led to an independent review which was led by Dame June Andrews (Trusted to Care; Andrews Report, 2014). There are many more failures within health and social care that can be attributed to both poor leadership and management which have escaped public attention. Within the recommendations from both the Francis Inquiry (Francis, 2013) and Trusted to Care (Andrews Report, 2014), leadership was an embedded theme to develop collaborative working to change failures identified in the system.

Across the UK, health bodies have developed a wealth of leadership resources for clinicians, with some examples and links in the Pit Stop.

PIT STOP!

Take time to look at some of the UK's online leadership resources

Scotland—https://learn.nes.nhs.scot/506/leadership-and-management-zone
Wales—https://heiw.nhs.wales/our-work/leadership/
England—https://www.leadershipacademy.nhs.uk/
Northern Ireland—https://leadership.hscni.net/

The importance of leadership is also being captured at preregistration education level. The Council of Deans of Health, an organisation that represents educators and researchers that delivers university health-based education, has developed the student leadership programme (see Pit Stop for web link). The aim of this programme is to develop leadership skills into the future healthcare workforce.

PIT STOP!

Review the Student Leadership Programme website:
https://www.councilofdeans.org.uk/studentleadership/

Leadership Theory Versus Style

Embarking upon a leadership journey, the terms of leadership theory and style will be well discussed within any leadership literature; however, it is important to understand what these both mean. Leadership theories and styles are related but are not the same. A leadership theory helps inform understanding of the ideas or principles that makes someone a successful leader in comparison to a leadership style, which relates to a set of behaviours within these theories. Table 5.1 provides a summary of some of the common leadership theories.

There are many more leadership theories, too many to capture within one book chapter. Leadership theories are not static and have continued to develop and evolve over time. Having an understanding and being able to apply these theories to practice will have clear benefits to you as a practitioner, our patients, colleagues and the organisation. As advanced practitioners, leadership skills are required throughout the role, from leading self to others and then to leading change and through to leading services and complex episodes of patient care (Bailey & West, 2022). The compassionate leader has been given greater focus with the current health service, recognising the need to develop more compassionate leaders as this has improved patient and staff outcomes (Bailey & West, 2022).

TABLE 5.1 ■ **Summary of Leadership Theories**

Theory	Explanation
Trait theory/ Great man theory	The great man theory emerged in the 19th century when it was proposed that leaders are born and are not made. These leaders have inherent qualities that make them good leaders. However, this theory is rather simplistic and has come under great scrutiny. The trait theory builds upon the great man theory and will often be used interchangeably in the literature. Within the trait theory, it is theorising that leaders have a set of traits that make them an effective leader. There are many criticisms to this theory, including too many identifiable traits and unreliable research data (Northouse, 2007).
Behavioural theory	The behavioural theory has developed from the trait theory, in which the idea that leaders are made through the development of learnt behaviours was introduced. This supports the principle that leadership can be learnt especially from role modelling key sets of behaviours. However, criticism of this this theory relates to situational factors (Harrison, 2018) which relate to what sets of behaviours are required for different situations.
Contingency and Situational theories	Building upon the trait and behavioural theories, situational theory focusses on the leadership within a particular situation (Graeff, 1997). Here, the leader is assessing the situation and applying which leadership style best fits the situation they are placed within (Contingency Theory). This theory suggests that no one set best of styles or behaviours and that these must change pending the situation.
Transformational theory	Transformational theory is centred around making change happen (Bass & Avolio, 1994). The leadership within this theory is based on challenging the norms to set about change based upon a vision. Achieving this vision requires followers, and these followers need to be motivated and empowered to share and achieve that vision (Swanwick, 2017). Lee (2014) argues that this most researched theory has many advantages, such as accumulated evidence of benefit in terms of profit, satisfaction from stakeholders and staff, sense of identity and transformation.
Transactional theory	The transactional theory is based on the notion of control and order, with the leader rewarding those followers who achieve their set goals but will also punish those who fail to achieve their goals (Burns, 1978). This theory has been aligned to the operational functions of an organisation in that a set task needs to be achieved. Like all leadership theories, this has many criticisms, yet it can be argued that this does have a place to ensure tasks/targets are met.

TABLE 5.1 ■ Summary of Leadership Theories—cont'd

Theory	Explanation
Authentic leadership	Authentic leadership is regarded as a modern leadership theory. This theory is based on the principles that the leader is true to their own beliefs and values. They have self-integrity and have great respect for others. The authentic leader is often seen as a role model to others (Bhindi & Duignan, 1997). Nursing leadership literature aligns authentic leadership with nursing core values (Doherty & Hunter-Revell, 2020; Giordano-Mulligan & Eckardt, 2019) and recognises the effect of individual values on the development of authentic leaders.
Servant leadership	Servant leadership was theorised by Greenleaf (1997) and the leader has greater investment within their followers to ensure growth. The leader is seen to serve their followers. Ten key principles are associated with servant leadership (Spears, 1995), which include empathy, healing, awareness, persuasion, foresight, stewardship, commitment to growth of people and building a community.
Compassionate leadership	Compassionate leadership (De Zulueta, 2016) has a significant drive within the UK health service based on the principles that can have positive impact upon outcomes (Bailey & West, 2022). The notion of compassionate leadership is that listening, valuing and supporting improve new ways of working as staff feel appreciated (Stanley, 2022). Compassionate leadership has four underlying sets of behaviours, which are (1) attending, (2) understanding, (3) empathising and (4) helping (Atkins & Parker, 2012).
Collaborative leadership	Collective leadership is the working together to share the leadership responsibility (Archer & Cameron, 2013). With this approach, people involved will have shared leadership so might feel a greater sense of ownership for the project, service or task being led. However, like all the leadership theories, this also does have some drawbacks, for example, if someone within the team does not want to share.

PIT STOP!

To learn more about compassionate leadership, the King's Fund has a free online course which can be accessed here:

https://www.kingsfund.org.uk/leadership-development/courses/leading-kindness-compassion-health-social-care

Leadership Styles

The leadership style relates to the behaviours and approaches towards leadership, with many being cited within the literature. The style will underpin the theory; for example, a coaching style (see next paragraph) could support the situational leader through their ability to support a collaborative input for a particular situation. Common styles include:

Coaching: Coaching enables development; therefore, the principle of this style is around providing guidance, support and feedback to help individuals develop their skills and achieve their goals. The coaching leader identifies the strengths and weaknesses of their team or individuals and works to develop these (Layton & Pearson-Shaver, 2021). Leadership coaching is recognised as an important style within healthcare to ensure long-term success of objectives (Hu et al., 2022); however, Layton and Pearson-Shaver (2021) suggest that this is the least used as it is time consuming.

Visionary: A visionary leader inspires and motivates others by communicating a compelling vision for the future and instilling confidence in the team's ability to achieve it. This style is effective for fostering innovation, aligning the team's efforts and driving organisational change.

Servant: A servant leader puts the needs of their team members first and focuses on empowering them to succeed. Servant leadership is both a theory and style.

Autocratic or authoritarian: An autocratic leadership style is centred around control. This style observes the leader making all the decisions based on their own ideas and seeking no input from others. This style can be useful when immediate decisions are needed such as a clinician leading a trauma call. However, long-term use of this style has the potential to disengage people, leading to resentment which will result in a breakdown of the leader's ability to lead (Cherry, 2023).

Laissez-faire or hands-off: This 'hands-off' approach allows for the delegation of tasks and responsibilities to team members with minimal supervision. Decisions are made within the team. Whilst this approach can foster autonomy, creativity and personal growth, it may also result in confusion or lack of direction, lack of role clarity and the avoidance of leadership by the leader (Cherry, 2022).

Democratic: Or participative leadership, values the views of others in decision-making. With this style, decisions made are often well balanced because the leader has listened to and involved others through a collaborative style. Clearly, this will lead to colleagues feeling appreciated which impacts upon team dynamics and the overall organisation (National Society of Leadership and Success, 2022).

Pacesetter: A pacesetter leader sets high standards of performance, high pace and quality and leads by example. The leadership is about doing things faster and better, fostering a culture of excellence. However, this style could be destructive as it may lead to burnout or frustration among team members if expectations are unrealistic or if the leader fails to provide adequate support (Layton & Pearson-Shaver, 2021).

Bureaucratic: A bureaucratic leader likes to adhere to authority (Fata, 2020) such as sticking to and following rules, protocols, guidance and procedures. The expectation is that the followers adhere to this authority. Whilst this approach can ensure consistency and order, the bureaucratic leader can struggle with change and can lack creativity and innovation (The Economic Times, 2023).

It should be noted that some leadership theories and styles are the same, for example, the servant leader and the transformational leader. Price-Dowd (2020) recognises that we need to move between different styles depending on the situation. However, Goleman (2000) notes that leaders tend to follow a style that they are familiar and comfortable with, regardless of the situation. This clearly has significant concerns as a laissez-faire leadership approach would not be ideal in an emergency. Price-Dowd (2020) suggests that leaders will often use an inappropriate or wrong style to lead people. Hence, the importance is to recognise that styles are 'fluid' and

> **BOX 5.2 ■ Example of Poor Leadership**
>
> A hospital admission avoidance team based within the community has appointed a new team leader to lead the team. The newly appointed team leader is new to the line management role and has never had formal support/training to develop their leadership skills. Their exposure to leadership has been role modelled on former managers who have been transactional and authoritarian. With no exposure or understanding of leadership, the newly appointed team leader adopts these two approaches that they have been exposed to. This has a detrimental impact upon the wider team, which results in team members feeling undervalued and demoralised. This led to increased staff sickness levels and high staff turnover resulting in staff retention and recruitment issues. With these human resources issues, the service delivery is impacted which results in poor care for the patients.
>
> What should have happened here to prevent this escalation and damage to this team?

not one can 'fit all'. Inappropriate leadership styles can lead to negative impacts upon individuals, teams and organisations; an example is provided in Box 5.2.

> **PIT STOP!**
>
> In relation to the different leadership styles, reflect upon a situation you were involved in and where a leadership style was displayed by a colleague; consider if this was appropriate or not for that situation.

Knowing Yourself as a Leader

As a leader, you need to understand yourself as this understanding will help inform the strengths and limitations to your leadership skills; it is a case of being able to lead ourselves before leading others (Price-Dowd, 2020). However, this understanding has multiple facets, including the understanding of your personality, emotions, beliefs and values (Bean, 2020). For example, personality will impact upon emotions and the way you respond to individuals. So, if a leader is very emotional and prone to inappropriate outbursts, then that will have an impact upon their ability to lead as colleagues might be afraid of the leader or lose trust. Likewise, if a leader has poor values like negativity to their work, then this will filter through to those who are being led. A good leader needs to both recognise themselves and also be able to challenge others in relation to their behaviours, values and beliefs.

There are many tools that can help you understand yourself as a leader; however, Bean (2020) recognises that there is no gold standard tool. Multisource feedback, performance annual reviews, personal reflections and 360 reviews are all helpful means to help an individual understand themselves as a leader.

> **PIT STOP!**
>
> How do you respond to feedback? Do you embrace it to aid your growth and development or are you resistant to feedback?
>
> As a leader, you need to be able to embrace all feedback as this will help you further develop your understanding of yourself!

Emotional Intelligence

The theory of emotional intelligence (EI) focusses on the individual's ability to recognise their own emotions and how these can impact upon others. EI requires you to understand your own emotions and to manage these to develop effective relationships with others. However, with EI, there needs to be an understanding of how others emotionally respond and act which influences our communication and relationship at that specific time (Goleman, 1995). EI has been linked to both situational and compassionate leadership (James & Bennett, 2020), because the EI leader will be able to recognise and respond to the different emotions that they are faced with at any particular situation.

EI has five recognised characteristics (Goleman, 1995), which are listed in Table 5.2. Imagine a leader lacking EI and these key characteristics when faced with a daily challenge; this would convey an image of a leader who is potentially stressed and volatile who makes bad decisions and does not inspire, motivate or communicate with others. Clearly, this would have a negative impact upon any team; however, Lambert (2021) recognises that healthcare workers need the time and training to be able to develop their EI skills in practice.

Developing as a Leader

With clinical leadership, all healthcare professionals can become leaders in practice, and this means that you do not have to be working at a senior role. As highlighted earlier, the development of leadership skills will start within preregistration education programmes, and this has been supported with the Student Leadership Programme (Council of Deans, 2019). Leadership in practice is important as it can help identify and set about making change; it can create a healthy workplace environment and improve and develop working practices. The NHS Healthcare Leadership Model has been developed to help develop leadership in practice for those new to leadership and is for those in both clinical and nonclinical roles. This model has nine dimensions which set about to challenge and explore behaviours and motivators. The nine dimensions are:

1. Inspiring share purpose
2. Leading with care
3. Evaluating information
4. Connecting our service
5. Sharing a vision
6. Engaging the team
7. Holding to account
8. Developing capability
9. Influencing for results

PIT STOP!

You can review the NHS Healthcare Leadership Model website here:
https://www.leadershipacademy.nhs.uk/healthcare-leadership-model/

TABLE 5.2 ■ EI Characteristics

EI Characteristics	Description and Discussion
Self-awareness	You need to be able to know yourself in terms of emotions, your mood and reactions. For example, you may not have an awareness that a certain mood might have on both you and others, such as being stressed. Self-reflection on incidents and daily events can help develop greater self-awareness.
Self-regulation	This concerns the ability to stay calm and control your mood, behaviour and impulses. For example, you might be prone to shouting at people when a task has not been achieved or when feeling stressed, yet you do not recognise this as a bad emotional response, nor do you recognise the impact this has upon others. Self-regulation is important as leaders need to stay calm at stressful times since they would need to make rational decisions. To develop self-regulation skills, self-reflection upon events and situations might be a starting point; however, calming techniques such as breathing exercises to aid calmness might help. An important feature here is the recognition and trying to manage the internal responses.
Motivation	The drive to motivate others with the ability to identify and support the achievement of individual's full potentials. Those motivational skills are key here, such as passion, empowerment, inspirational and visionary. An example of motivational skills within EI relates to the leader recognising the team's self-doubt and being able to draw on each member's strengths to inspire and empower to achieve a set goal. To develop motivational skills, you should be able to self-reflect upon what motivates you as a leader, adopting the notion of being a 'half glass full' type of leader as opposed to being a 'half glass empty' type of leader.
Empathy	Empathy is putting yourself in someone else's position to understand their emotions, thoughts and feelings. Being empathetic is an essential requirement of working within healthcare and something we should all have awareness of and apply to one's own practice. Unfortunately, this is not often the case, and you might be able to reflect upon a situation when there was no empathy demonstrated to you by someone.
Social skills	Social skills focus on relationship development with others, being able to draw on the key communication skills needs to develop and maintain their relationships. Developing relationships with others is key to support both personal and organisation growth. A leader with good social skills would be better at providing bad news as they would have well-defined social skills to communicate this to others. Social skills will also relate to those nonverbal skills such as posture and facial expression, so there is an awareness needed of how you portray yourself amongst others.

EI, Emotional intelligence.
Modified from Goleman, D. (1995). Emotional intelligence. New York: Bantam Books, Inc.

The NHS Healthcare Leadership Model might be a starting point for those looking to develop as a leader; however, there are many opportunities to develop leadership skills for practice. Within many MSc AP programmes, there might be specific leadership modules. Alternatively, the graduate advanced practitioner might wish to undertake an accredited leadership module as part of their continuing professional development. Other opportunities to develop leadership skills can include coaching and mentoring, gaining feedback, shadowing colleagues and clinical supervision. As highlighted at the start of the chapter, each country in the UK has a wealth of leadership resources available which have been captured within the Pit Stops.

Storytelling in Leadership

The final part of this chapter will be dedicated to storytelling by some senior AP clinicians and educators. Storytelling in leadership is a powerful tool that leaders can use to narrate their leadership journey (Kouzes & Posner, 2012) and through doing this demonstrate their own values and beliefs that are core to them as leaders. The aim of personal stories is to narrate the passion for AP and how leadership has helped develop the person, their practice and others around them.

MELANIE ROGERS—LEADERSHIP STORY

Mindset versus Skills Set: Leadership Vignette—Professor Melanie Rogers, whose background is an advanced nurse practitioner primary care, AP educator, professor of AP and Inaugral Director ICN Nurse Practitioner/Advanced Practice Nurse Network Global Academy of Research and Enterprise.

I, Melanie, have had the opportunity to develop my leadership skills in every area of my professional practice. It has been developmental, and at times, I have had to encourage myself to have confidence in my own leadership skills. Wherever you work and at whatever level you are, you can lead. This may be leading an aspect of service development to improve patient care; it may be leading meetings, developing networks regionally, nationally or internationally. It may be leading a ward round or a mortality and morbidity meeting. Try not to think of leadership as something someone else will do. As an advanced practitioner, part of your role is to lead.

I want to share with you a leadership skill which has helped me. This is understanding the difference between a skill set and a mindset. Our mindset is often thought of as a key aspect of our personality that can influence our success or failure in all aspects of our lives. Mindset is often aligned to how we see ourselves and approach the world we live in (Dunn, 2015). In leadership, a mindset develops through the experiences that shape our behaviours (Britto, 2019).

> **PIT STOP!**
>
> Take a few minutes now to think about how your personal and professional experiences have shaped your own behaviour.

Britto (2019) suggests that a mindset is a nebulous concept unless understood within a roadmap. He suggests six attributes which are needed: mindfulness, genuine curiosity, a flexible mind, resilience, an ability to create leaders and an enterprise thinking style. These attributes he suggests are a way of thinking rather than a skill.

Carol Dweck (2016) has been identified as one of the pioneers of the fixed versus growth mindset theory. She states that a growth mindset is an individual who through having good strategies and hard work develops their talents with the input of others (Dweck, 2016). Her work connects closely with that of Britto (2019). Those who lean towards a growth mindset tend to have a desire to develop themselves personally and professionally through hard work. They believe their talents can improve and attributes are not fixed but are changeable. Challenges and setbacks are often viewed as a motivator to succeed even when it is difficult. It is usual for those with a growth mindset to be willing to react constructively to feedback and see mistakes made as an opportunity to learn.

In contrast, those with a fixed mindset believe that their talents are innate so put less energy into hard work and personal development (Dweck, 2016). They tend to believe their talents and attributes cannot change and often approach projects and tasks with pessimism. Those with a fixed mindset can be hypercritical of themselves, seek validation from others and avoid challenges because they fear failing. They often do not learn from their mistakes and do not take criticism well, turning any criticism into proof of their own inadequacy.

PIT STOP!

Do you have a fixed or a growth mindset? How do you receive feedback?

Dweck's earlier work considered the helpless response vs the mastery orientated response (Dweck & Leggett, 1988) which correlate to the fixed and growth mindsets. This early work led onto further theories about the malleability of attributes including the fixed and growth mindset theories. McGrath and MacMillan (2000) have posited that mindset can be changed through prescriptive techniques; others suggest that the mindset development is more nuanced, needing persuasion to change (Limeri et al., 2020).

When I learned about this new theory, I began to understand how my personality and achievements have been moulded by more of a growth mindset. I would argue that all of us have times when both growth and fixed attributes can be more recognisable at various times in our lives. One possible reason for my development of a leaning towards a growth mindset comes from my early childhood where I faced many challenges whilst growing up with a parent with a mental health problem. I learned to navigate challenges and have a 'can do' attitude. This continued through my adolescence when I sought out challenges to learn more about team working and overcoming adversities. These challenges included applying to participate in various adventures from an expedition to the Himalayas to being a volunteer crew on a three-masted schooner. I was often told I would not be selected to take part in these challenges as I was not particularly sporty. However, I believed I could rise to the challenges and was selected to participate in both expeditions out of hundreds of young people in the region who applied to take part. This approach followed through into my work as a nurse and then as an advanced nurse practitioner. I continue to believe that challenges are something we can navigate and by building networks of colleagues who can support us and encourage us, we can navigate most things!

In contrast to mindset, a skill set is more about the capabilities we each possess. Maxwell (2021) identifies the need for both sets to reach your full potential. He states that if you do not have a 'proper mindset', no matter how good your skill set is, you will never reach your full potential. Skills are innate or developed abilities and can be soft, related to our behaviours, or hard, related to functional or technical abilities. Cheary (n.d.) identified in a survey that 96% of 800 employers valued mindset over skill set, stating that mindset stays constant. Both mindset and skills set are important for leaders to develop professionally and personally. For me, key is humility and self-awareness. Capozzi (2017) suggests that leaders who have humility are much more likely to want to develop their mindset and skills set.

Finally, whilst researching mindset and skill set, I came across the following quote from John Timpson which reminds me of the importance of mindset, here talked about as character:

> 'We can teach a guy with character how to repair shoes, but you can't put personality into a grumpy cobbler.'
>
> (Timpson, 2014)

LEADERSHIP STORY—MICHELLE ACORN

My nursing leadership path consisted of a combination of both informal and formal leadership roles as a clinician, educator and in executive practice roles. My bedside, classroom, boardroom and bureaucrat lens will be embedded across my local to global career trajectory to illuminate impactful influences, opportunities and personal and professional challenges.

Registered Nurse (RN)—Clinician and Education Leader

I was barely 20 when I graduated as an RN from a 3-year nursing diploma programme. It prepared me clinically to be entry-level competent as I hit the floor running to provide emergency care. I was knocked down hard when I was laid off within 6 months of entering the nursing profession. I relocated for full-time hospital employment at a community hospital and never looked back. My emergency department (ED) role was sentinel and remains my pulse check. It shaped my prioritisation and critical assessment that hold true today. Is the situation stable, nonurgent, urgent or life threatening? Context, prioritisation and your moral and ethical compass will steer your leadership immersion. They help inform and guide you. Is this the mountain you wish to die on? What is the cost or outcome of the decision, action or inaction? There will be formal and informal decisions among your career path that shape the future for both you and others. My advice is do not say no to career opportunities. They are a gift that keeps giving and revealing.

Over the next few years, I moved from novice to expert as a clinician delivering care at the bedside and became specialised and emergency certified. The shift to leadership was not as easy. I tracked quickly into clinical leadership roles as a young team lead, next to a charge nurse and then clinical education leader. My peers who were older and more experienced were not always as supportive as they could have been. Balancing imposter syndrome and building your competence in initial leadership roles is hard enough without peer support and mentoring.

Bullying and unsolicited judgement in nursing are very real—horizontally and vertically. I remained professional, and balanced my emotional and professional intelligence while building my credibility.

I worked full-time while raising a family, and part-time continuing my professional development to become the first nurse practitioner (NP) in the ED. My peers recognised my drive and determination and witnessed me immersed in my homework on breaks together. A few colleagues questioned and counselled on my ability to be both a 'good mom' and my pursuit of my 'NP' career choice.

As I transitioned from RN to NP to implement the value-added role that embeds all the domains of practice including leadership through capacity building, I developed dozens of medical directives that would support my RN colleagues to work to the top of their knowledge and scope as well which was very well received. I became actively involved in organisational councils and quality improvement opportunities.

Over time, a few of those colleagues who were less supportive over the years continued their professional development, obtaining their baccalaureate to graduate education and I became been their instructor. They apologised to me. I congratulated them and gave them my best professional support to optimise their success. I also challenged them to pay it forward in teaching, precepting and mentoring.

Nurse Practitioner: Clinician, Leader and Political Advocacy

I will never regret becoming an NP, nor the diverse opportunities it has afforded me. I was always a disruptive innovator, creating the first NP role in the ED. Weaving into the Professional Practice Leader with dedicated protected time, I aimed to target impact, by enabling and empowering AP nurses (APNs) to showcase their contributions across all the domains of practice, not just clinically, in an effort to build capacity for full scope of practice for NPs and clinical nurse specialists (CNSs) to contribute to patient and organisational outcomes.

I wanted to catapult my leadership experience, advocacy and political acumen externally to my employment. I was a member of my provincial nursing association, but not actively engaged until I became a board member and eventually president of the Nurse Practitioner Association. As part of the executive, I learned the power and passion that drive leadership volunteerism. The governance and leadership experience, learning how decisions are made, building relationships with stakeholders, fostering a community of practice network and forming friendships with nurse leaders across health systems that leverage nursing are far reaching and cherished. During my term, we worked closely with the government to modernise the Nursing Act to authorise open prescribing and hospital admission, treatment and discharge by NPs. We led the first ever adoption of the NP role as the most responsible provider caring for geriatric and rehabilitation patients' model for care to drive quality care.

My transition into executive leadership practice began as the provincial government chief nursing officer (CNO). I provided nursing strategic, clinical and technical advice to the Ministry as a bureaucrat that aligned with government mandates. I learned how to navigate interministerial and cross-functional intersections with regulation, education and scope of practice policy. I also experienced the challenges of leading if your positional authority and resources are misaligned.

I am now into my second year as the inaugural chief nurse of the International Council of Nurses representing over 28 million nurses around the world in a non-governmental organisation to enable advocacy and amplification of nurses' voices as experienced thought leaders. I continue my intent to lead through transformational leadership efforts collectively. We must advance universal health coverage, primary healthcare and sustainable development goals to leave no one behind. The populations we target are health equity and nursing professional equity. Let's lead together!

Conclusion

This chapter has set out to define the differences between leadership and management, recognising that these can both compliment and share some individual qualities. There has been a recognition of the importance of good clinical leadership in practice, and when this is absent along with poor management, the consequences can be devastating (Andrews Report, 2014; Francis, 2013). An overview of both leadership styles and theories has been presented and aims to provide a foundation of understanding for the need for both in practice, recognising that leaders will adopt many pending on the situation they face. Developing as a leader and the importance of EI in supporting this development have been recognised. With the use of storytelling, two AP leaders have been invited to share their leadership journey.

References

Andrews Report. (2014). *Trusted to care: An independent review of the Princess of Wales Hospital and Neath Port Talbot Hospital at ABMU Health Board.* Cardiff: Dementia Services Development Centre.

Archer, A., & Cameron, A. (2013). *Collaborative leadership building relationships, handling conflict and sharing control.* London: Routledge.

Atkins, P. W. B., & Parker, S. K. (2012). Understanding individual compassion in organizations: The role of appraisals and psychological flexibility. *Academy of Management Review, 37*(4), 524–546.

Azad, N., Anderson, H. G., Jr, Brooks, A., Garza, O., O'Neil, C., Stutz, M. M., & Sobotka, J. L. (2017). Leadership and management are one and the same. *American Journal of Pharmaceutical Education, 81*(6), 102–107.

Bailey, S., & West, M. (2022). *What is compassionate leadership?* https://www.kingsfund.org.uk/insight-and-analysis/long-reads/what-is-compassionate-leadership. Accessed March 3, 2024

Bass, B. M. (1990). From transactional to transformational leadership: Learning to share the vision. *Organizational Dynamics, 18*(3), 19–31.

Bass, B. M., & Avolio, B. J. (Eds.). (1994). *Improving organizational effectiveness through transformational leadership.* London: Sage Publications, Inc.

Bean, A. (2020). Understanding yourself as a leader: Diagnostics and tools. *BMJ Leader, 4,* 168–170.

Bennis, W. (2009). *On becoming a leader* (revised ed.). New York: Addison-Wesley Publishing.

Bhindi, N. L., & Duignan, P. (1997). Leadership for a new century: Authenticity, intentionality, spirituality and sensibility. *Educational Management Journal, 25*(2), 117–132.

Britto, J. (2019). *Six attributes of a leadership mindset: Flexibility of mind, mindfulness, resilience, genuine curiosity, creating leaders, enterprise thinking.* Crown House Publishing.

Burns, J. M. (1978). *Leadership.* New York: Harper & Row.

Capozzi, R. (2017). *The growth mindset: Leadership makes a difference in wealth management.* New York: Wiley & Sons.

Center for Creative Leadership. (2023). *12 Characteristics of a good leader.* https://www.ccl.org/articles/leading-effectively-articles/characteristics-good-leader/

Cheary, M. (n.d.). *Five characteristics of successful jobseekers.* https://www.reed.co.uk/career-advice/five-characteristics-of-successful-jobseekers/. Accessed March 3, 2024

Cherry, K. (2024). *The Pros and Cons Laissez-Faire Leadership? When hands-off leadership may be best…and worst.* https://www.verywellmind.com/what-is-laissez-faire-leadership-2795316#:~:text=Laissez%2Dfaire%20leadership%2C%20also%20known,1. Accessed April 5, 2024.

Cherry, K. (2023). *What is autocratic leadership?* https://www.verywellmind.com/what-is-autocratic-leadership-2795314#:~:text=Autocratic%20leadership%2C%20also%20known%20as,rarely%20accept%20advice%20from%20followers. Accessed April 5, 2024.

Christensen, S. S., Wilson, B. L., & Edelman, L. S. (2018). Can I relate? A review and guide for nurse managers in leading generations. *Journal of Nursing Management, 26*(6), 689–695.

Council of Deans. (2019). *Student leadership programme.* https://www.councilofdeans.org.uk/studentleadership/. Accessed March 18, 2024

De Zulueta, P. C. (2016). *Developing compassionate leadership in health care: An integrative review. Journal of Healthcare Leadership, 18*(8), 1–10.

Doherty, D. P., & Hunter-Revell, S. M. (2020). Developing nurse leaders: Toward a theory of authentic leadership empowerment. *Nursing Forum, 55*(3), 416–424.

Dunn, J. (2015). *The difference between fixed and growth mindsets.* https://dailygenius.com/the-difference-between-fixed-and-growth-mindsets/. Accessed March 16, 2024.

Dweck, C. (2016). *What having a "growth mindset" actually means.* Harvard Business Review. https://hbr.org/2016/01/what-having-a-growth-mindset-actually-means. Accessed January 10, 2024

Dweck, C. S., & Leggett, E. L. (1988). A social-cognitive approach to motivation and personality. *Psychological Review, 25*(2), 109–116. doi:10.1037/0033-295X.95.2.256G

Fata, E. (2020). *5 Examples of bureaucratic leadership in action.* https://www.startingbusiness.com/blog/bureaucratic-examples. Accessed April 2, 2024.

Francis, R. (2013). *Report of the Mid Staffordshire NHS Trust Public Inquiry—Executive summary.* https://commonslibrary.parliament.uk/research-briefings/sn06690/

Giordano-Mulligan, M., & Eckardt, S. (2019). Authentic nurse leadership conceptual framework: Nurses' perception of authentic nurse leader attributes. *Nursing Administration Quarterly, 43*(2), 164–174.

Goleman, D. (1995). *Emotional intelligence.* New York: Bantam Books, Inc.

Goleman, D. (2000). Leadership that gets results. *Harvard Business Review, 78*, 78–90.

Graeff, C. L. (1997). Evolution of situational leadership theory: A critical review. *The Leadership Quarterly, 8*(2), 153–170.

Greenleaf, R. K. (1997). The servant as leader. In R. P. Vecchio (Ed.), *Leadership: Understanding the dynamics of power and influence in organizations* (pp. 429–438). Indiana: University of Notre Dame Press.

Harrison, C. (2018). *Leadership theory and research: A critical approach to new and existing paradigms.* New York: Springer Link.

Hu, S., Chen, W., Hu, H., Huang, W., Chen J., and Hu J. (2022). Coaching to develop leadership for healthcare managers: A mixed-method systematic review protocol. *BMC, 11*, 676. doi:10.1186/s13643-022-01946-z

James, A., & Bennett, C. (2020). Effective nurse leadership in times of crisis. *Nursing Management, 27*(4), 32–40.

Jonas, S., McCay, L., & Keogh, B. (2017). The importance of clinical leadership. In T. Swanwick & J. McKimm (Eds.), *ABC of clinical leadership* (2nd ed., pp. 1–4). Wiley-Blackwell.

Kotter, J. P. (1999). *What leaders really do.* Boston; Harvard Business School Press.

Kouzes, J. M., & Posner, B. Z. (2012). *The leadership challenge: How to make extraordinary things happen in organizations.* New York: Wiley & Sons.

Lambert, S. (2021). Role of emotional intelligence in effective nurse leadership. *Nursing Standard, 36*(12), 45–49.

Layton, E., & Pearson-Shaver, A. (2021). Leadership. *HCA Healthcare Journal of Medicine, 2*(1), 9–15.

Lee, M. (2014). Transformational leadership: Is it time for a recall? *International Journal of Management and Applied Research, 1*(1), 17–29.

Leithwood, K., Harris, A., & Hopkins, D. (2020). Seven strong claims about successful school leadership revisited. *School Leadership & Management, 40*(1), 5–22.

Limeri, L. B., Carter, N. T., Choe, J., Harper, H. G., Martin, H. R., Benton, A., & Dolan, E. L. (2020). Growing a growth mindset: Characterizing how and why undergraduate students' mindsets change. *International Journal of STEM Education, 7,* 35. https://doi.org/10.1186/s40594-020-00227-2

Maxwell, J. (2021). *Which is more important – Your skill set or your mindset?* https://www.maxwellleadership.com/blog/which-is-more-important-your-skill-set-or-your-mindset/. Accessed March, 3, 2024.

McGrath, R., & MacMillan, I. (2000). *The entrepreneurial mindset: Strategies for continuously creating opportunity in an age of uncertainty.* Harvard Business School Press.

Mrayyan, M. T., Algunmeeyn, A., Abunab, H. Y., Kutah, O. A., Alfayoumi, I., and Abdallah, A. K. (2023). Attributes, skills and actions of clinical leadership in nursing as reported by hospital nurses: A cross-sectional study. *British Medical Journal, 7,* 203–211.

National Society of Leadership and Success. (2022). *Key characteristics of democratic leadership.* https://www.nsls.org/blog/key-characteristics-of-democratic-leadership. Accessed March 5, 2024

Northouse, P. G. (2007). *Leadership theory and practice* (4th ed.). California: Sage Publications, Inc.

Price-Dowd, C. F. J. (2020). Your leadership style: Why understanding yourself matters. *BMJ Leader, 4*(4). https://doi.org/10.1136/leader-2020-000218

Spears, L. C. (1995). *Reflections on leadership.* New York: John Wiley & Sons

Swanwick, T. (2017). Leadership theories and concepts. In T. Swanwick & J. McKimm (Eds.), *ABC of clinical leadership* (2nd ed., pp. 8–13). Wiley-Blackwell.

Stanley, D. (2019). Values-Based Leadership in Healthcare Congruent Leadership Explored. SAGE Publications Ltd.

The Economic Times. (2023). *The 10 Most Common Leadership Styles.* https://economictimes.indiatimes.com/jobs/c-suite/the-10-most-common-leadership-styles/articleshow/102808003.cms?from=mdr. Accessed Jan 20, 2025

Timpson, J. (2014). *Acceptance speech when receiving the Lifetime Achievement Award at the SFEDI and IOEE Celebrating Enterprise Awards.* https://campus.ioee.uk/acceptance-speech-by-john-timpson-cbe/

Uhl-Bien, M., & Arena, M. (2017). Complexity leadership: Enabling people and organizations for adaptability. *Organizational Dynamics 46*(1), 9–20.

Wong, K. (2023). *12 must-have qualities of a manager and 20 other good traits.* https://www.achievers.com/blog/12-traits-make-great-manager/. Accessed April 3, 2024

CHAPTER 6

Four Pillars of Advanced Practice: Research

Anna Jones ■ Melanie Rogers

CHAPTER OUTLINE

The aim of this chapter is to consider the origins of evidence-based practice and what is meant by research. Research is one of the four pillars of advanced practice. However, it is frequently acknowledged as being one of the most difficult to achieve, to get involved with and to maintain.

We will therefore consider how as an advanced practitioner you can integrate the research pillar into your own work. We finish the chapter describing a personal journey that we hope will inspire you.

Introduction

Research is one of the four pillars of advanced practice (AP); it is frequently acknowledged by our students as being one of the most difficult to achieve, to get involved with, and to maintain.

'(I have an)...interest in research...not sure how to get involved in current role (and)...fulfilling research pillar'

(First year AP student)

'Research is important for making sure I'm evidence based but where I work we are so busy it is never something I have time for'

(Third year AP student)

Research is key to providing care at an advanced level as it helps to maintain patient safety and lower healthcare costs and clinical risk through limiting variations in practice (National Institute for Health and Care Excellence (NICE), 2018). Understanding and knowing the evidence base in order to make changes in practice are underpinned by leadership, sharing of good practice and lessons learned (NHS Education Scotland (NES), 2024; NICE, 2018) and integration of the research pillar with the other three AP pillars. This chapter highlights some of the key areas related to the research pillar and gives you suggestions on how you can begin to integrate research into all aspects of your AP work.

Evidence-Based Practice

As part of the competence and capabilities that you are building and consolidating as an advanced practitioner, be it as a trainee or if you have been in practice for some time, you will need to learn and maintain your skills in searching for, critical appraisal of, synthesis and evaluating the evidence base available (Fielding et al., 2022). With the breadth of methodologies that are currently used, across primary research and quality improvement (QI), it is indeed a challenge. However, developing strategies to maintain currency within your specialist areas of practise and expertise is essential in improving the quality of care. This links with the development of study skills (see Chapter 9). It also ensures you can challenge outdated practice by being able to identify the current evidence. You should also develop an awareness of the evidence base of other professions and specialities to ensure that your decision-making is not based on a limited or a professionally biased evidence base (see Chapter 4).

What Is Evidence-Based Practice?

Evidence-based practice's foundations were born in evidence-based medicine (EBM) and have reflected the impact that EBM has had in changing medical practice (Carrier & Jones, 2023). EBM has been described as a paradigm shift because of the integration of clinical research into practice (EBM Working Group, 1992; Hallas & Melnyk, 2003). Evidence-based practice was established by a group of practitioners in the 1980s by the Department of Clinical Epidemiology and Biostatistics at McMasters University, Canada. The practitioners sought to discover new methods of sourcing, critically appraising and applying research, using the best evidence/data to advance scientific standards and principles that would support and aid clinicians in decision-making (Carrier & Jones, 2023; Faubion, 2024).

The term EBM was initially proposed by Dr Gordon Guyatt in the 1990s, influencing bedside decision-making, and was initially published by the EBM Working Group in 1992 (p. 2420, original emphasis) as:

> *'A NEW paradigm for medical practice is emerging. Evidence-based medicine de-emphasizes intuition, unsystematic clinical experience, and pathophysiologic rationale as sufficient grounds for clinical decision making and stresses the examination of evidence from clinical research.'*

NICE (2018) suggests the following key principles and strategies for putting the evidence base into practice. The guide includes a commitment to QI, effective leadership, the right culture and working together.

PIT STOP!

Examples of evidence-based interventions can be found in the following links:
https://www.ncbi.nlm.nih.gov/pmc/articles/PMC8396772/
https://www.nursingprocess.org/evidence-based-practice-in-nursing-examples.html

Quality in Healthcare

Differing definitions of quality abound, with an early definition being set by the Institute of Medicine (IOM) (1990, p. 21) as:

'Quality of care is the degree to which health services for individuals and populations increase the likelihood of desired health outcomes and are consistent with current professional knowledge.'

Six dimensions of quality in healthcare identified by the IOM and adapted by the Institute of Healthcare Improvement were widened by The Health Foundation in 2021 (p6) to:

"care that is effective, safe and provides as positive an experience as possible by being caring, responsive and personalised. This definition also states that care should also be well-led, sustainable and equitable, achieved through providers and commissioners working together and in partnership with, and for, local people and communities"

PIT STOP!

Consider how you as a trainee or qualified advanced practitioner could improve quality in healthcare.

The Health Foundation (2021) makes several suggestions about how you might improve quality in healthcare. These have been slightly adapted here. It is important to reflect and consider how you might apply the following points to your practice areas when you notice an area where quality is being compromised:

- What is the issue or problem that you have identified in practice?
- What impact does this have on the different stakeholders, for example, patients/service users, clinicians, managers?
- What solutions could you develop to resolve the issue, or reduce the problem?
- What data would you need to collect to measure the impact of any changes to improve?

Once you have implemented the solution/s, how would you sustain this practice, to ensure that standards and the quality of the service are ensured? (Adapted from The Health Foundation, 2021)

QI methodologies can be utilised in all practice settings to improve patient safety, reduce clinical risk concerns and ensure services' safety and clinical effectiveness. This is where QI and research (evidence-based practice) further align, with the use of clearly defined methods, tools and systematic and coordinated approaches.

Commitment to Quality Improvement

To further help you consider how to implement QI, consider the following:
- Set clear directions and priorities based on evidence.

- Utilise NICE quality standards to specify what high-quality care looks like (NICE, 2018).
- Measure and publish quality data to track progress.
- Recognise and celebrate outstanding care.
- Build capability through leadership development and continuous QI (Faubion, 2024).

EFFECTIVE LEADERSHIP AND CULTURE

As you consider QI, you also need to think about the impact of leadership and the organisation culture. Many times, QIs do not happen because of inadequate leadership or a culture which does not support QI and change. As an advanced practitioner, you need to develop your leadership skills and also be willing to challenge cultures which do not foster change. You can consider the following suggestions to help you:

- Foster an organisational culture that encourages innovation and continuous improvement.
- Encourage professional curiosity within a robust governance framework.
- Prioritise interventions that have a real impact on patient safety, such as those targeting delirium prevention, cardiopulmonary arrest, adverse drug events, infections and falls (NHS England, 2024a).

In Chapter 5, we explored leadership theories and styles and how you can develop as a leader.

> **PIT STOP!**
>
> Revisit Chapter 5 and consider the content again, refreshing your understanding as you consider leadership from a research angle.

Research and Advanced Practice

LACK OF REGULATION AND ITS IMPACT ON RESEARCH

Mackavey et al. (2024a) stated that since the inception of AP and its integration into healthcare on a much larger scale, there has been a proliferation of roles and titles associated with AP. The Health and Care Professions Council (HCPC) (2021) in their review of AP regulation recognised that there was no indication for additional regulation of allied health practitioners who practiced at an advanced level. In 2024 the Nursing and Midwifery Council (NMC) reviewed AP regulation (NMC, 2024a). A decision was made by the NMC Council to proceed to additional regulation, to ensure protection of the public and individuals who use health and care services. This will support the AP research pillar for nurses through providing education standards and proficiencies related to research.

The NMC (2024a) have agreed to the following:

- 'Develop standards of proficiency for advanced level practice (and associated programme standards).

- adopt a collaborative approach to develop a UK-wide AP principles framework incorporating a shared position or definition of advanced level practice.
- ensure that advanced level practice requirements are included in the wider reviews of revalidation and the Code scheduled for 2025/26' (NMC, 2024b).

The setting of regulatory standards for nurses and midwives should result in a greater level of standardisation of education and consequentially practice, across the four pillars including impacting the research pillar. Educational standards and proficiencies directly related to research will promote the knowledge and understanding of (trainee) advanced practitioners. This may enable more research by advanced practitioners and more consistent research about AP in general which will lead onto ensuring advanced practitioners are able to deliver the best quality care (NMC, 2024a). It may also provide more impetus for all professions to consider regulation of AP.

THE RESEARCH-TO-PRACTICE LAG

Research as a pillar is acknowledged as being essential because current and contemporaneous knowledge introduction and integration into clinical practice will reduce risk (Dean, 2023). The inclusion of the research pillar in all four UK country AP frameworks underpins its importance (Department of Health, Social Service and Public Safety Northern Ireland (DHSS), 2023; Health Education and Improvement Wales (HEIW), 2023; National Health Service England (NHSE) 2025; NES, 2024).

Nevertheless, it is worth noting that there is a notable lag in turning research into a clinical reality (Kristensen et al., 2015). It is recognised that there can be a 17-year lag between the publication of results and the implementation of the research in practice (Morris et al., 2011; Robinson et al., 2020). To bridge this gap, and to ensure that local practice is delivered safely and meets quality standards, the answer may lie in the use of QI methodologies.

Quality Improvement

In addition to the length of time that research takes to be implemented into practice, it has been noted that clinical guidelines can also be restrictive, in that they overlook the clinical autonomy and wealth of knowledge and experience of clinicians (Gabbay, 2016; Gabbay & Le May, 2011). As an advanced practitioner or student, you will bring with you accumulated experience and knowledge. Advanced practitioners play a key role in the use of QI and service improvement, to measure current practice against best practice, and monitoring (British Medical Journal, 2020). As such, the use of health improvement or QI methodologies can offer different and faster methods of changing practice, when faced with small-scale local issues and complications. The goal of quality/service improvements is to result in small-scale changes, which is where research and QI deviate from one another (University of Tennessee, 2018).

Research focuses on developing new knowledge, whilst QI could be a mechanism with which to apply your research into practice, on a small scale. Effective and elevated impact, outcomes and improvement are based on thoughtful, data-driven approaches, which are coupled with continuous learning. Procuring time to objectively view and consider what changes are required is a challenging 'ask' in the current health and social care climate, with constrained resources and time (Healthcare Quality Improvement Partnership (HQIP), 2024a). Other key differences between research and QI is that research can be based on one study, test or trial, whilst QI projects often run several sequential tests (or cycles) to generate data that can be used to improve practice. Whereas research attempts to control as many biases as possible, QI does not. QI instead aims to stabilise these biases from each sequential test to the next test. Research is about gathering as much information/data as possible, whereas QI aims to collect 'just enough' data between each cycle to influence the next cycle (Institute for Healthcare Improvement, 2022). To clarify whether your project ideas are classed as research or not, the Health Research Authority (HRA, 2023) offers an online tool which helps you determine whether your study is classed as empirical research, which requires ethical approval, or QI, which does not. Please visit the HRA website for details.

> **PIT STOP!**
>
> The differences between research and QI can be found at the following link:
>   Table 1: The HRA decision-making tool is available at: Is my study research? https://hra-decisiontools.org.uk/ethics/

Quality and Service Improvement

Service improvement and QI are related concepts in healthcare, but they have distinct foci.

SERVICE IMPROVEMENT

Service improvement encompasses a broader range of activities aimed at enhancing various aspects of healthcare services. Its scope goes beyond solving problems in failing parts of an organisation. Instead, it aims to expand improvement across organisational and functional boundaries, impacting the entire health and social care system.

Key aspects include:
- Empowering staff to take on a wider range of clinical tasks
- Encouraging continuous QI
- Being a change agent
- Sharing learning and knowledge with other organisations

QUALITY IMPROVEMENT

QI is a systematic approach to enhancing service quality, efficiency and morale. Improvement Cymru (2024) offer a series of questions to help you to think about what areas you could review and apply QI methodologies.

PIT STOP!

Please visit this link, and think about how you would consider improvements in your clinical practice:

https://phw.nhs.wales/services-and-teams/improvement-cymru/improvement/

QI focuses on, and specifically targets, improving the quality of care, reducing patient harm, enhancing operational performance and achieving financial savings. Benefits from service improvement projects can include, for example, a reduction in patient harm, improved operational performance, increased staff satisfaction and reduced staff sickness and absence (Healthcare Improvement Scotland, 2023; The Health Foundation, 2023).

Quality Improvement Approaches

Approaching changes in clinical practice and to services can be challenging, and whilst there is no one single approach to QI, each of the approaches does offer an alternative method of undertaking change. The Institute for Healthcare Improvement (2024) suggests some of the issues include the constant evolution and complexity of healthcare delivery, which means that QI (and research in general) is about an ongoing journey rather than a destination. Having identified an issue in practice as a trainee or qualified advanced practitioner, think broadly when deciding on a 'thoughtful and tailored' approach to QI (HQIP, 2024b). The issue or problem you identify will influence the choice of QI methodology to use. This may include a combination of approaches, models and tools. The Health Foundation (2021) recognises that QI approaches have comparable core elements. Approaches that you may want to review include the Model for Improvement and Plan, Do, Study, Act (PDSA) cycles (Langley et al., 2009) and total quality management (TQM), which is aligned to Lean system/Six Sigma (NHS England, n.d.). However, you should read more widely, as this is not an exhaustive list. To support you in exploring QI, the Model for Improvement will be discussed next.

Model for Improvement

To enable you to make small-scale changes in practice, the Model for Improvement, which was developed by Langley et al. in 1992 (Langley et al., 2009), offers you a framework to develop your ideas, test them and then implement any small-scale changes. Tools that are used include the PDSA cycles (NHS England, 2022).

The Model for Improvement will take you through the steps towards improving practice and/or services and asks, firstly, a series of questions that you may want to take some time to consider, prior to moving on to the second section, which is where the 'actions' are realised. The questions asked in the first part are:

1. **What are we trying to accomplish?** This is where you consider and develop the aim of your service improvement project.

2. **How will we know whether the change is an improvement?** Consider the following points: What and how will you measure your improvement? What measures do you need, for example, do you need to measure the length of stay of patients, or to gather their feedback on the service that you are providing? How will you do this? Consider the tools that you need to measure. Measuring in this way enables you to learn as the process unfolds. Establishing a baseline to compare new data with is key, as you measure little and often, to offer means of measuring success. When considering what data you need to collect, think about how you will record your data, and the tools that can be used for this, such as Run charts, Control charts or Pareto charts.

3. **What changes can we make that will result in improvement?** What changes can you put in place to test your ideas?

The PDSA cycle (The Deming Institute, 2022) is a tool that enables small-scale testing, which will result in establishing data on how effective your change is, and can be broken down as follows:

Plan: What is your objective now that you have identified the issue in practice? What data do you think that you will need to collect? What might happen when the change is implemented?

Do: This is where you implement your plan. It is important that you ensure that any observations and data that you collect are recorded accurately.

Study: You will need to reflect on how the cycle went and analyse the data thoroughly. What have you learned? What did the data demonstrate? Did this tally with your forecasts and estimations from the planning phase?

Act: Will you need to make any changes to the process/data collection tools before you undertake the next cycle? Is there a need to collect any more evidence/data?

Process Mapping

To help you to understand the process, you may want to use a process mapping tool. The use of a process mapping tool helps you to identify issues and problems and reduces the risk of waste and inefficiency (Improvement Cymru Academy, 2024).

Stakeholders

To increase the success of the improvement project, ensure that you involve all stakeholders from the start of the project; stakeholders vary, depending on the scope and context of your improvement project, but may include patients/service users and carers, and clinical staff, for example. It is important to recognise patient/service user perspectives as their views can differ from yours as an advanced practitioner/trainee and health and care staff generally, offering different perspectives that will make the service improvement more robust and inclusive (HQIP, 2015).

Currently, Scotland has identified a need for trainee and qualified advanced practitioners to demonstrate an ability to implement and use a breadth of QI, audit, research skills and tools and to improve practice (NES, 2024). Having a breadth of ability like this provides greater leeway in demonstrating your skill set, rather than having to only focus on empirical research.

> **PIT STOP!**
>
> Consider how you could evidence the research pillar, thinking more widely about how QI, audit and participation in, and implementation of, empirical research are present in your everyday clinical role.

Audit

Audits are an important tool to support and ensure that quality care is delivered in practice. Clinical audits in the context of the National Health Service (NHS) are a systematic process that assesses whether healthcare services are provided in line with established standards. Their purpose is to inform those working in AP about areas where services excel, and where improvements are needed. Audits can be conducted nationwide, with over 30 national audits existing in England, focusing on specific conditions. Additionally, local clinical audits are conducted within health boards, trusts, hospitals or general practice, and across social care and third sector institutions; these audits identify areas for improvement at a local level (NHS England, 2024b).

> **PIT STOP!**
>
> For further information on clinical audits, visit the website commissioned and maintained for NHS England by HQIP.
>
> https://www.hqip.org.uk/a-z-of-nca/
> https://www.hqip.org.uk/
> Other resources that you may wish to explore include:
> Clinical Outcome Review Programmes (CORP). https://www.hqip.org.uk/clinical-outcome-review-programmes/
> National Quality Improvement and Clinical Audit Network (NQICAN). nqican.org.uk/our-work/

The resources identified in the earlier Pitstop provide support, training and resources for you and health and social care colleagues. They also are places where you can get involved and have your voice heard at a national level. The organisations listed previously collaborate and corroborate with NHS England, NICE and HQIP. For practical resources, a search of your local intranet should provide you with audit proposal forms and templates.

Remember, clinical audits contribute to better patient outcomes and continuous QI in healthcare.

Sustainability

Embedding changes into practice is challenging and is an important part of improving care and services. It will require you as an advanced practitioner to consider more widespread support. By recognising the stakeholders and involving individuals from across services and systems (including service users and carers), you could enable a more effective change to practice. It is important that you recognise concepts such as compassionate and effective leadership, to advocate for QI, and how a positive organisational culture influences the success of the project (The Health Foundation, 2021).

PIT STOP!

Further Reading
- Public Health Wales (2024). Improvement Cymru. Available at: https://phw.nhs.wales/services-and-teams/improvement-cymru/
- NHS Education for Scotland. Quality improvement. Available at: https://www.nes.scot.nhs.uk/our-work/quality-improvement/
- NHS England. Available at: https://www.england.nhs.uk/nhsimpact/

Research and Advanced Practice

There are two ways to view AP research—research by advanced practitioners and research about AP. A recent umbrella review undertaken by the International Council of Nurses (ICN) Nurse Practitioner/Advanced Practice Nurse Network highlighted some of the challenges with identifying research undertaken by advanced practice nurses (APN) (Kilpatrick et al., 2023). As a trainee or qualified advanced practitioner, you might be interested in reviewing this work which identifies gaps in the global research evidence specific to APNs. This may give you some ideas about areas that are under-researched and that you are interested in.

Enablers and Barriers to Research

There is an increasing volume of literature available on AP research (Kilpatrick et al., 2023; Mackavey et al., 2024a, 2024b; Ndirangu-Mugo et al., 2024). Additionally, research about AP by advanced practitioners and across professions is increasing (Hooks & Walker, 2020; Mann et al., 2023).

Some notable challenges to partaking in research include difficulty in accessing continuing education to upskill and maintain research and QI skills, organisational barriers such as lack of time allocated to the pillar, a lack of role modelling and experience in those supervising trainee advanced practitioners (Dugani et al., 2020; Hooks & Walker, 2020; Mackey et al., 2016). Support by line managers who understand and appreciate the complexity of the AP role is crucial in enabling development of the research pillar (Mann et al., 2023); this will also level the playing field in terms of equity of research education and training that other professions are afforded.

PIT STOP!

The literature, where available, focuses on the barriers to research; however, take a moment to consider what could, or does, enable you to partake in and maintain competence and capability about the research pillar.
- Are there individuals who encourage you to participate and to engage? Does this merge with the Leadership pillar, and the Education pillar?
- Does QI offer an alternative approach, and does thinking about research on a smaller scale, such as evaluative research, offer you alternative options?

Kelley et al. (2015) state several potential actions to enable practitioners to partake in research within clinical practice, such as:

- Identifying times and arranging face-to-face meetings with research supervisors, researchers and collaborators. Ensure that all of your stakeholders are included and provided with sufficient and timely information; for example, contact your research and development teams in good time and use their expertise to shape your project. Time management is key, with an awareness of the requirements of the other three pillars, other work commitments and those of your personal life. Holistic care extends to you too; if you are too busy to be able to engage in research, then you will be at risk of burnout (Stallter & Gustin, 2021). However, if you view research not as an additional chore but as a way of improving patient care where you can make a difference, you will begin to enjoy the research pillar more.

- Applying reliable and economic data collection methods that can be manageable within the business and demands of practice is important. You can collaborate with colleagues to help support data collection and help each other to increase research knowledge and ability. Ethics, development of protocols, proposals and processes should be given sufficient consideration. Whether or not you are conducting empirical research or a QI project, you must follow ethical guidelines and principles, such as beneficence, nonmaleficence and justice (see Chapter 10), and adhere to your local institution's requirements (UK Research and Innovation, 2021). If you are carrying out empirical research, you will need ethical approval and will have to seek and obtain informed consent, ensure confidentiality and anonymity and adhere to General Data Protection Regulation (GDPR) (Gov.UK, 2018) requirements, to protect the participants. Consider how you will store and record your data; what policies and procedures do you need to adhere to, and who is responsible for sponsoring your research/QI projects? Who would have access to the data? This should be limited to only those identified on the research/QI protocol (UK Research Integrity Office, 2023).

- Collaborative writing of the findings/results, with dedicated, regular time to write up results/findings. Resources are finite, and sourcing funding, time and expenses, for example, may be a requirement of your project. You will need to factor in the time and potential for these.

- Ensuring that you as an advanced practitioner remain on-board with the research project from the planning phases through to the publication of any results/findings and outputs. Consider how you will disseminate your findings/results. Where and how will you do this? (UK Research Integrity Office, 2023).

PIT STOP!

Review the UK Research Integrity Office Checklist for researchers at the following link:
https://ukrio.org/wp-content/uploads/UKRIO-Recommended-Checklist-for-Researchers.pdf

Maintaining a commitment and focus to research is a challenge when clinical pressures impact on the time available, but it is so rewarding to see your research change practice (Valentino & Juanico, 2020). Understanding the challenges associated with integrating the research pillar is important. Brysiewicz and Oyegbile (2021) propose the START model to help you address challenges in research and keep on track. To give you a flavour, they identify the following steps:

- **S**tart simple
- **A**rrange your team
- consider the **R**elevance
- **T**imelines

PIT STOP!

You may wish to consider reading the article identified earlier:
Brysiewicz, P., & Oyegbile, Y. (2021). Addressing "research-phobia" among nurses in the clinical area. *Professional Nursing Today, 25*(1), 21–23.
The areas they consider are applicable across all professions.

As your role progresses, it is important that you recognise the contribution that research and QI make to improving care and changing healthcare in response to evidence. It is therefore imperative that future managers ensure that policies and guidance include protected time for advanced practitioners to develop, nurture and promote education and training around research and QI.

We, as a team, have overcome some of the barriers by working in partnership and inviting some AP students to collaborate in participatory research. In participatory research, control over the process and agenda shifts from the researcher to the participants (for us, this was AP trainees). The work we have been involved in allowed the trainees to actively analyse and reflect on the information generated during the research (in this case, we looked at what trainees needed before starting their AP courses). We found that this approach empowered both participants and us as researchers to work together to identify the realities facing trainees. This then led to us cocreating the 'Aspiring Advanced Practice' programme talked about in Chapter 7. Consider participatory research processes as a way of being more collaborative in your approach to research. We have found it a way of engaging all involved in AP.

The Research Journey

The research journey and pillar can be challenging, but it is fulfilling and worthwhile. It requires as much attention as all of the other three pillars of AP, as an understanding of research supports your practice across all pillars.

Research: The Basics

Research methods and methodology refer to the systematic and scientific approaches used to explore and investigate problems and gather data for a specific purpose. It involves different methods and procedures to identify, collect, analyse and interpret data, to answer research questions or solve research problems.

There are underlying assumptions as research methodology is guided by philosophical and theoretical frameworks. These frameworks shape the entire research process, influencing choices related to research design, data collection and analysis. The assumptions are referred to as ontological and epistemological perspectives. Ontology refers to our philosophical assumptions about reality, whereas epistemological assumptions are those around what we know, and how we know it (University of Sheffield, 2024).

Research methods are the specific techniques and procedures used to collect and analyse data. They vary based on the research project's requirements. Quantitative research methodology involves collecting and analysing numerical data using statistical methods. It aims to study cause-and-effect relationships and make predictions. Qualitative research methodology is at the other end of what can be viewed as a continuum and focuses on nonnumerical data (such as words, images and observations). It aims to explore complex phenomena and gain in-depth understanding (Dahlberg & McCaig, 2013). Remember that understanding these concepts is crucial for designing effective research studies!

There are different data collection tools that you could choose to use, depending on the methodology and methods that you have chosen. The methods listed in the next section have benefits and challenges and it is advisable that you read widely to ensure that the tool that you choose is the most appropriate, and can be managed within the remits and limits of your project.

Qualitative Data Collection Methods

Braun and Clarke (2013), Dingwall and Staniland (2020) and Pope and Mays (2020) are useful texts for understanding qualitative methods. We give here brief examples of data collection methods for information:

   Interviews: These involve one-on-one or group conversations where, as a researcher, you would ask open-ended questions to explore your participants' experiences, opinions and motivations.

Focus groups: These are small group discussions led by a facilitator or researcher to delve into specific topics or issues. Participants share their perspectives and interact with each other.

Observations: This is where, as a researcher, you would directly observe behaviour, events or phenomena in natural settings. This method provides rich contextual information.

Ethnographies: These are in-depth studies involving immersion in a specific cultural context. Ethnographers participate in daily life to understand cultural practices and norms.

Quantitative Data Collection Methods

Teater et al. (2017) and Creswell and Creswell (2018) are useful texts for understanding quantitative methods. We give here brief examples of a few data collection methods for information:

Surveys: These are structured questionnaires with close-ended questions (multiple choice, rating scales) distributed to a sample of participants. Surveys can be conducted online, in person or over the phone.

Experiments: These involve controlled situations where variables are manipulated to establish cause-and-effect relationships. They are commonly used in scientific research. Examples are randomised controlled trials.

Observations (quantitative): This is a systematic recording of observable behaviours or events. Researchers use predefined categories or scales to quantify data.

Archival research: This involves analysing existing records, documents or databases (for example, historical records, organisational data) to extract quantitative information.

Mixed-Methods Approach: Sometimes, researchers combine both qualitative and quantitative methods to gain a comprehensive understanding. This approach allows triangulation, where findings from different methods validate each other and add richness to the data collected (Dahlberg & McCaig, 2013).

Remember that the choice of data collection method depends on your research or QI goals, available resources and the specific questions you aim to answer. Whether you are exploring human experiences or testing hypotheses, these methods play a crucial role in advancing your research knowledge, adding to evidencing your research pillar and ultimately in improving patient care.

Ethics

When embarking on a research project in healthcare, ethical considerations play a pivotal role in ensuring the integrity of your study and safeguarding the rights and well-being of participants.

PIT STOP!

Review the six principles of ethics in research using the following link:

https://www.ukri.org/councils/esrc/guidance-for-applicants/research-ethics-guidance/
framework-for-research-ethics/our-core-principles/#:~:text=Our%20six%20key%20
principles%20for%20ethical%20research%20are%3A,and%20accountability%20
should%20be%20clearly%20defined%20More%20items

The use of the word 'participants' is important, as when conducting a research study, patients become participants. Let's delve into some key ethical aspects.

INFORMED CONSENT

Informed consent involves obtaining voluntary and well-informed agreement from research participants before their involvement in the study. You will need to provide information so that participants understand the purpose, risks, benefits and procedures of the research. They should have the autonomy to choose whether to participate or withdraw without coercion. This is possible through providing a participant information sheet. Examples are available on the HRA and National Institute for Human and Health Research (NIHR) websites.

ANONYMITY AND CONFIDENTIALITY

You will need to protect participants' identities by avoiding any association between data and specific individuals. This could require you to provide pseudonyms or unique identifiers/codes to protect anonymity. You will also need to consider how to safeguard participants' information by ensuring that only authorised personnel have access to data. All data collected will need to be stored safely and align to data retention policies from the institution that you work within, or that you are studying at. You will need to have informed your participants that the information (data) that they share will be used (anonymously) in different formats.

You will need to seek approval from a research ethics committee or review boards and submit research proposals in the required format to ensure ethical compliance. You will need to ensure that you obtain ethical approval prior to commencement of your research and potentially service improvement project. Please seek advice from your local ethics committees or university.

Remember, ethical research does not only uphold scientific integrity but also respects the dignity and rights of those who contribute to advancing healthcare knowledge.

PIT STOP!

Consider reviewing the HRA and NIHR website for guidance and advice on ethical considerations:

https://www.hra.nhs.uk/
https://www.nihr.ac.uk/

Dissemination

Once you have completed a research, QI or service improvement project, it is important that you share the results and findings, to improve practice. Dissemination of the data can take numerous forms such as conference attendance and presentation, publishing your findings and results in journals and sharing via local networks. Attendance at conference can support networking and the development of your contacts, which may result in further research.

Research Opportunities

Depending on where you live and work, there may be a variety of opportunities to undertake research education additional to your research modules and/or dissertation. There may also be opportunities to take part in some research projects. If you are a trainee undertaking an AP programme, you will normally be offered some education, usually modular, with research as the focus. However, you may feel you would like more support before independently undertaking research. A variety of routes to support your continuous professional development exist. This includes free online courses through accredited online courses and modules as part of educational postgraduate programmes. Your local university AP programme lead may also be aware of ongoing research projects and opportunities. In many cases, universities, health and social care organisations and other stakeholders work in partnership to undertake research. This is an area that you may wish to explore, to expand your knowledge and network, to support the development of your research pillar.

Depending on career aspirations, there are specific research degrees that you may wish to consider undertaking, such as a master's in research (MRES) or master's in philosophy (MPhil) in health or health sciences, and there are also a variety of doctoral and PhD opportunities, some of which may be funded. The National Institute for Health and Care Research (NIHR) identifies a range of learning and support which can help develop the research workforce to transform the care and treatment that patients receive. There is support and funding for researchers who work on and deliver patient-focused research studies in a wide range of clinical settings. Currently, there are over 10,000 research delivery staff who are partly or fully funded by the NIHR (NIHR, 2023). NIHR offers a variety of different research routes with online accredited learning programmes, with innovative programmes involving Massive Open Online Courses (MOOCs) which take you through the research journey, including how research improves treatment and cures, the impact of clinical research and the how and why's of doing research (NIHR, 2024).

There are also additional e-learning modules for individuals with minimal experience covering new skills and knowledge to encourage confidence building and interest to engage with research and research opportunities. There are continuing professional development modules for those interested in shorter training courses which offer formal, structured activities and may offer qualifications, formal coaching and supervision learning opportunities, and other academic training programmes which can support your developing career as a researcher.

> **PIT STOP!**
>
> **Further Reading**
>
> Take some time to explore the NIHR website and opportunities available. It might also be beneficial to have conversations with colleagues in your practice area to identify interest in undertaking research and colleagues at your local higher education institute to consider what support might be available for you.
>
> https://www.nihr.ac.uk/

International Advanced Practice Research

Internationally, like in the UK, research is a key aspect of AP roles. However, the UK is the world leader in the development of the multiprofessional approach to AP. Most countries around the world have focused on developing nurses as APs; therefore, discussion around the international arena in this chapter focuses on nurses as an example. At the time of writing, around 81 countries have developed or are developing APN roles, for example, nurse practitioners and clinical nurse specialists (Miller et al., 2024). This section provides a brief discussion on APNs and research in addition to an example of a research development journey. It is hoped that as other countries see the success of the multiprofessional approach to AP, international collaborative research opportunities will develop.

Providing healthcare systems that meet patient needs, developing appropriate policies and workforce strategies and ensuring high-quality patient care need to be embedded in the evidence base. The ICN (2020) identifies that APNs should be involved in research and research activities as part of their roles. Nurses, like many other healthcare professions, have extensive experience and knowledge about the needs of their patients and the services that provide healthcare. This knowledge is a clarion call to engage in research activities and ensure all healthcare provision they provide is quality assured and evidence based with the goal of enhancing patient care. Bryant-Lukosius and Martin-Misener (2016) encourage APNs to recognise that their roles are incredibly powerful mechanisms that can change service delivery and patient care. Participating in research activities is key to doing this.

The World Health Organization (2020), in their 'State of the World's Nursing' report, recognised the role of APNs in ensuring that patient quality is provided at the highest level internationally. Without APN participation in research activities, the evidence base and research findings will not include their voice and expertise (ICN, 2020). Indeed, Clarke et al. (2021) stated that APNs have an additional responsibility to participate in research activities by virtue of their responsibilities as leaders. This also applies to allied health advanced practitioners.

In 2020, the first international Academy of Advanced Practice Nurse Research and Enterprise was established by the ICN Nurse Practitioner/Advanced Practice

Nurse Network (ICN NP/APN Network). The ICN NP/APN Network is an international resource for all APNs and interested parties, for example, policy makers, researchers and educators (https://icnnpapnnetwork.wildapricot.org/). The Network is passionate about supporting knowledge development and transfer in all aspects of the APN role, including education, policy, research, leadership and clinical practice. Currently, the Network has membership in over 141 countries (Gray et al., 2024). The Academy's main roles include fostering research in all aspects of AP nursing. They are working with colleagues across the world to support projects which add to the body of knowledge which continues to support the development and growth of AP (Gray et al., 2024).

The following example is Melanie Rogers' journey through research culminating in her becoming the director of the first global Academy of Advanced Practice research. Partly written in the first person, it includes some tips she has learnt.

I work as an AP in primary care as well as being a professor of advanced practice. I have always been committed to providing holistic care to the highest standard possible and that has driven my interest and dedication to research activities as I have seen the difference it makes.

My research journey began many years ago when I worked in accident and emergency (A&E). I was appalled to see how patients who self-harmed were sometimes treated by colleagues. They were made to feel guilty about self-harming and told they were wasting the resources of A&E. I wanted to do something about the way patients were treated and asked a couple of colleagues to join me in developing a quality improvement plan. Despite being a junior nurse at that time, I utilised our Trust librarian and undertook a literature search on supporting patients in A&E who self-harmed to see what the literature said about the needs of these patients. With my colleagues, we undertook a literature review and presented our findings to other colleagues at a team meeting. We then ran a focus group with colleagues exploring their perceptions of patients who self-harmed.

This identified similarities from the literature review and helped us recognise some of the ways we could challenge these perceptions, leading to providing a number of teaching sessions to all staff about self-harm and the needs of patient when they come to A&E.

Finally, we partnered with mental health services to write a new standard of care which was piloted and implemented into the Trust. This was evaluated after a year through an audit and further focus groups. The outcome of this was that care had improved in our department.

This initial foray into research helped me recognise that even without very much research knowledge, it was possible to make a difference to care by working with colleagues who knew more about research processes. This experience helped me to feel more confident about quality improvement projects and led to further projects with colleagues in the department. I also implemented a monthly journal club to help myself and colleagues keep up to date with evidence-based practice, as I found it easier talking through articles than reading them on my own.

Top Tips:

- Look at areas of practice where you are currently working which could benefit from improving.
- Find a few colleagues who will work with you to look at the literature and evidence base.
- Talk to your local librarian who can support you with the literature search process.
- Gain management and colleague support for changes to practice whether through service evaluation processes, team meetings or teaching sessions, for example.
- Use mentoring and journal clubs to help you develop your research skills and knowledge. This will help you grow in confidence.
- Find a way to make learning about research enjoyable. Think about your learning style and tailor your learning to this. For example, you may learn more when you have practical examples and can talk to colleagues who are interested in research about the skills needed to improve care.
- Consider how you will develop the research pillar as a student and as a qualified advanced practitioner.
- Take opportunities you are given to undertake empirical research or QI projects; small studies and projects are just as important as large ones.
- Consider developing international collaborations which can enhance your understanding of healthcare globally.
- Look for opportunities to develop the four pillars of AP in ways that fit with your professional vision.
- Consider roles where the four pillars are integrated and where you can hone each of the pillars.
- If you are struggling in your clinical role to integrate research, consider how you can use the evidence base to continually improve your practice.

In relation to AP education, having an educator who makes research interesting is key. Such educators encourage students to consider the evidence base and help you consider the impact of providing care that was not evidence based. These educators teach the skills necessary in a way which is interesting and enjoyable. Additionally, they can support you to undertake small empirical studies or QI projects. Finally, AP educators can introduce you to international APN colleagues who can talk to you about their roles.

Conclusion

In order to support the integration of the research pillar into AP, we need to demystify research activities for advanced practitioners. This includes increasing the opportunities for trainees and qualified advanced practitioners to undertake research activities as part of their roles. Universities can support this, through offering opportunities via assessment and collaboration with wider service improvement and research projects.

A greater and wider understanding of and around the importance of research needs to be developed. Incentives and support are needed by employers to enable advanced practitioners and trainee advanced practitioners to focus some of their practice on the research pillar with the aim of improving services and patient care. Advanced practitioners need to develop the skills and confidence to do this, and be able to implement evidence-based practice and research findings. Additionally, disseminating research findings will go a long way to boosting advanced practitioners' morale and confidence in research activities and will ensure more role models who can support peers to develop their research acumen. Understanding that today's research is tomorrow's standard of care should encourage every advanced practitioner to recognise that research is fundamental to the development and longevity of AP.

References

Backhouse, A., & Ogunlayi, F. (2020). Quality improvement into practice. *BMJ (Clinical research ed.), 368*, m865. https://doi.org/10.1136/bmj.m865.

Braun, V., & Clarke, V. (2013). *Successful qualitative research*. Sage.

Bryant-Lukosius, D., & Martin-Misener, R. (2016). *Advanced practice nursing: An essential component of country level human resources for health*. Policy Paper for the International Council of Nurses. International Council of Nurses.

Brysiewicz, P., & Oyegbile, Y. (2021). Addressing "research-phobia" among nurses in the clinical area. *Professional Nursing Today, 25*(1), 21–23.

Carrier, J., & Jones, A. (2023). Evidence-based healthcare. In J. Carrier (Ed.), *Managing long-term conditions and chronic illness in primary care. A guide to good practice* (3rd ed.). London: Routledge.

Clarke, V., Lehane, E., Mulcahy, H., & Cotter, P. (2021). Nurse practitioners' implementation of evidence-based practice into routine care: A scoping review. *Worldviews Evidence Based Nursing, 18*(3), 180–189. https://doi.org/10.1111/wvn.12510

Creswell, J. W., & Creswell, J. D. (2018). *Research design: Qualitative, quantitative & mixed methods approaches* (5th, international student ed.). Sage.

Dahlberg, L., & McCaig, C. (2013). Introduction to research and evaluation basics. In L. Dahlberg & C McCaig (Eds.), *Practical research and evaluation. A start-to-finish guide for practitioners* (pp. 13–28). London: Sage.

Dean, S. (2023). Advanced clinical practitioners and the research pillar. *International Journal for Advancing Practice, 1*(1). https://doi.org/10.12968/ijap.2023.1.1.42 (Accessed April 26, 2023)

Department of Health, Social Service and Public Safety Northern Ireland (DHSS). (2023). *Advanced nursing practice framework*. https://www.health-ni.gov.uk/publications/advanced-nursing-practice-framework (Accessed April 20, 2024)

Dingwall, R., & Staniland, K. (2020). *Qualitative research methods for nurses*. Sage.

Dugani, S. B., Geyer, H. L., Maniaci, M. J., Schenzel, H. A., & Burton, M. C. (2020). Perspectives on and barriers to research among clinical practice provider and physician hospitalists. *The Nurse Practitioner, 45*(9), 41–47. doi:10.1097/01.NPR.0000694720.63033.a5

Evidence-Based Medicine Working Group. (1992). Evidence-based medicine. A new approach to teaching the practice of medicine. *JAMA, 268*, 2420–2425.

Faubion, D. (2024). *What is evidence-based practice in nursing? (With examples, benefits, & challenges)*. https://www.nursingprocess.org/evidence-based-practice-in-nursing-examples.html (Accessed March 17, 2024)

Fielding, C., Riley, J., Sutherland, C., Swift, K., & Gordon, A. (2022). Research as part of the advanced clinical practitioner role. *British Journal of Nursing, 31*(7), 372–374. doi:10.12968/bjon.2022.31.7.372.

Gabbay, J., & le May, A. (2016). Editorials. Mindlines: Making sense of evidence in practice. *British Journal of General Practice, 66*, 402-403.

Gabbay, J., & Le May, A. (2011). *Practice-based evidence for healthcare: Clinical mindlines*. Abingdon: Routledge.

Gov.Uk. (2018). *General Data Protection Regulation (GDPR). The data protection act.* Available online at: Data protection: The Data Protection Act. https://www.gov.uk/data-protection (Accessed April 24, 2024)

Gray, D., Rogers, M., & Ladd, E. (2024). Collaborating for excellence in advanced practice nurse research: The International Council of Nurses Nurse Practitioner/Advanced Practice Nurse Network Academy. In M. Rogers, J. Roussel, D. Lehwaldt, & M. Acorn (Eds.), *Advanced practice nurse networking to enhance global health* (pp. 229–239). Springer.

Hallas, D., & Melnyk, B. (2003). Evidence-based practice – A paradigm shift. *Journal of Pediatric Health Care, 17*(1), 46–49.

Health and Care Professions Council (HCPC). 2021. *Advanced practice final independent research report.* https://www.hcpc-uk.org/resources/policy/advanced-practice-full-research-report/ (Accessed March 17, 2024)

Health Education and Improvement Wales. (2023). *Framework for advanced nursing, midwifery and allied health professional practice in Wales.* https://heiw.nhs.wales/workforce/workforce-development/professional-framework-for-enhanced-advanced-and-consultant-clinical-practice/

Health Research Authority. (2023). *UK policy framework for health and social care research.* https://www.hra.nhs.uk/planning-and-improving-research/policies-standards-legislation/uk-policy-framework-health-social-care-research/ (Accessed April 14, 2024)

Healthcare Improvement Scotland. (2023). *Scottish Patient Safety Programme (SPSP): Working with health and social care services to improve the safety and reliability of care and reduce harm.* https://ihub.scot/improvement-programmes/scottish-patient-safety-programme-spsp/ (Accessed April 20, 2024)

Healthcare Quality Improvement Partnership. (2015). *A guide to quality improvement methods.* https://hqip.org.uk/wp-content/uploads/2018/02/guide-to-quality-improvement-methods.pdf (Accessed March 17, 2024)

Healthcare Quality Improvement Partnership. (2024a). *Quality improvement expertise and support.* https://www.hqip.org.uk/services/quality-improvement/ (Accessed March 17, 2024)

Healthcare Quality Improvement Partnership. (2024b). *Data, insights and service evaluation.* https://www.hqip.org.uk/services/data-insights/ (Accessed March 17, 2024)

Hooks, C., & Walker, S. (2020). An exploration of the role of advanced clinical practitioners in the East of England. *BJN, 29*(15). https://www.britishjournalofnursing.com/content/professional/an-exploration-of-the-role-of-advanced-clinical-practitioners-in-the-east-of-england (Accessed March 17, 2024)

HS England (2025) *Multi-professional framework for advanced Practice in England.* Birmingham: Centre for Advancing Practice.

Improvement Cymru. (2024). *What is improvement?* https://phw.nhs.wales/services-and-teams/improvement-cymru/improvement/ (Accessed April 14, 2024)

Improvement Cymru Academy. (2024). *Improvement Cymru Academy toolkit guide.* https://phw.nhs.wales/services-and-teams/improvement-cymru/improvement-cymru-academy/resource-library/academy-toolkit-guides/process-mapping/ (Accessed March 17, 2024)

Institute for Healthcare Improvement. (2024). *Driving health care forward through insights and innovations.* https://www.ihi.org/ (Accessed March 17, 2024)

International Council of Nurses, Schober, M., Lehwaldt, D., Rogers, M., Steinke, M., Turale, S., et al. (2020). *Guidelines on advanced practice nursing 2020.* https://www.icn.ch/system/files/documents/2020-04/ICN_APN%20Report_EN_WEB.pdf (Accessed October 20, 2023)

Institute of Medicine. (1990). *Medicare: A strategy for quality assurance* (Vol. 1). Washington, DC: National Academies Press.

Kelley, D. P., Wilder, D. A., Carr, J. E., Rey, C., Green, N., & Lipschultz, J. (2015). Research productivity among practitioners in behavior analysis: Recommendations from the prolific. *Behavior Analysis in Practice, 8*, 201–206.

Kilpatrick, K., Savard, I., Audet, L. A., Kra-Friedman, A., Atallah, R., Jabbour, M., et al. (2023). A global perspective of advanced practice nursing research: A review of systematic reviews protocol. *PLoS One, 18*(1), e0280726. https://journals.plos.org/plosone/article?id=10.1371/journal.pone.0280726

Kristensen, N., Nymann, C., & Konradsen, H. (2016). Implementing research results in clinical practice – The experiences of healthcare professionals. *BMC Health Services Research, 16*, 48. https://pubmed.ncbi.nlm.nih.gov/26860594/

Langley, G. L., Moen, R., Nolan, K. M., Nolan, T. W., Norman, C. L., &, Provost, L. P. (2009). *The improvement guide: A practical approach to enhancing organizational performance* (2nd ed.). San Francisco, CA: Jossey-Bass Publishers.

Mackavey, C., Henderson, C., de Zwart van Leeuven, E., Maas, L., & Ladd, A. (2024a). The advanced practice nurse role's development and identity: An international review. *International Journal for Advancing Practice, 2*(1). https://doi.org/10.12968/ijap.2024.2.1.36

Mackavey, C., Henderson, C., & Stout, T. (2024b). Stepping outside national borders: International active learning educational collaboration events. *International Nursing Review, 71*(1). https://doi.org/10.1111/inr.12927

Mackey, P. A., Perez, S. T., Frederixon, M. A., Northern, J. B., Garcia, H. J., Boyd, K. L., et al. (2016). Academic rank barriers for physician assistants and nurse practitioners. *Journal for Nurse Practitioners, 12*(5), e211–e218.

Mann, C., Timmins, S., Evans, C., Pearce, R., Overton, C., Hinsliff-Smith, K., & Conway, J. (2023). Exploring the role of advanced clinical practitioners (ACPs) and their contribution to health services in England: A qualitative exploratory study. *Nurse Education in Practice, 67*, 103546. https://europepmc.org/article/MED/36739736 (Accessed March 17, 2024)

Miller, M., Roussel, J., Rogers, M., & Lehwaldt, D. (2024). The global phenomenon of advanced practice nurses. In M. Rogers, J., Roussel, D. Lehwaldt, & M. Acorn (Eds.), *Advanced practice nurse networking to enhance global health* (pp. 19–42). Springer.

Morris, Z. S., Wooding, S., & Grant, J. (2011). The answer is 17 years, what is the question: Understanding time lags in translational research. *Journal of the Royal Society of Medicine, 12*. https://journals.sagepub.com/doi/full/10.1258/jrsm.2011.110180

National Institute for Health and Care Excellence (NICE). (2018). *Principles for putting evidence-based guidance into practice.* https://www.nice.org.uk/Media/Default/About/what-we-do/Into-practice/Principles-for-putting-evidence-based-guidance-into-practice.pdf (Accessed January 22 2025)

National Institute for Health and Care Research (NIHR). (2023). *Health and care professionals.* NIHR. https://sphr.nihr.ac.uk/

National Institute for Health and Care Research. (2024). *NIHR MOOCs. What are Massive Open Online Courses?* https://enrich.nihr.ac.uk/nihr-launches-free-online-course-what-is-health-research/ (Accessed April 14, 2024)

Ndirangu-Mugo, E., Kimani, R., Onyancha, C., Mutwiri, B., Kamob, I., Tallam, E., et al. (2024). Scopes of practice for advanced practice nursing and advanced practice midwifery in Kenya: A gap analysis. *International Nursing Review, 71*, 276–284. https://doi.org/10.1111/inr.12947

NHS Education Scotland. (2024). *Advanced practice toolkit.* https://learn.nes.nhs.scot/63343/advanced-practice-toolkit (Accessed March 17, 2024)

NHS England. (2022). *Plan, Do*, Study, Act (PDSA) cycles and the model for improvement. NHS England.

NHS England. (2024a). *Improving patient safety culture – A practical guide.* https://www.england.nhs.uk/long-read/improving-patient-safety-culture-a-practical-guide/ (Accessed March 18, 2024)

NHS England. (2024b). *Clinical audit.* https://www.england.nhs.uk/clinaudit/ (Accessed April 16, 2024)

NHS England. (n.d.). *Lean Six Sigma: Some basic concepts.* https://www.england.nhs.uk/improvement-hub/wp-content/uploads/sites/44/2017/11/Lean-Six-Sigma-Some-Basic-Concepts.pdf (Accessed March 17, 2024)

NHSE. (2025). *Multi-professional framework for advanced practice in England.* London, England. In press.

Nursing and Midwifery Council (NMC). (2024a). *Review of advanced practice. options appraisal.* https://www.nmc.org.uk/globalassets/advanced-practice-review/advanced-practice-review-options-appraisal-paper-for-publication-18032024.pdf?_t_id=rYSMkpZPgM-vDKRimNjqiQ%3d%3d&_t_uuid=U4OBqb1VQ_-bWHwiXIheOw&_t_q=advanced+practice&_t_tags=language%3aen%2csiteid%3ad6891695-0234-463b-bf74-1bfb02644b38%2candquerymatch&_t_hit.id=NMC_Web_Models_Media_DocumentFile/_b4d22e31-acf0-4492-8a63-be5a5fd05e8c&_t_hit.pos=8 (Accessed April 14, 2024)

Nursing and Midwifery Council (NMC). (2024b). *Advanced practice: Our recommendations for additional regulation.* https://www.nmc.org.uk/news/news-and-updates/advanced-practice-our-recommendations-for-additional-regulation/ (Accessed April 14, 2024)

Pope, C., & Mays, N. (2020). *Qualitative research in healthcare.* Wiley.

Robinson, T., Bailey, C., Morris, H., Burns, P., Melder, A., Croft, C., et al. (2020). Bridging the research–practice gap in healthcare: A rapid review of research translation centres in England and Australia. *Health Research Policy and Systems, 18*, 117. https://doi.org/10.1186/s12961-020-00621-w (Accessed April 21, 2024)

Stallter, C., & Gustin T. S. (2021). Evaluating advanced practice nurses' burnout and potential helping modalities. *Journal for Nurse Practitioners, 17*(10), 1297–1299. doi:10.1016/j.nurpra.2021.07.003 (Accessed April 20, 2024)

Teater, B., Devaney, J., Forrester, D., Scourfield, J., & Carpenter, J. (2017). *Quantitative research methods for social work: Making social work count.* Palgrave Macmillan.

The Deming Institute. (2022). *PDSA cycle.* https://deming.org/explore/pdsa/ (Accessed March 17, 2024)

The Health Foundation. (2021). *Quality Improvement made simple.* https://www.health.org.uk/publications/quality-improvement-made-simple (Accessed April 20, 2024)

The Health Foundation. (2023). *A guide to making the case for improvement.* https://www.health.org.uk/publications/a-guide-to-making-the-case-for-improvement (Accessed April 21, 2024)

UK Research and Innovation. (2021). *Framework for research ethics.* https://www.ukri.org/councils/esrc/guidance-for-applicants/research-ethics-guidance/framework-for-research-ethics/our-core-principles/#:~:text=Our%20six%20key%20principles%20for%20ethical%20research%20are%3A,and%20accountability%20should%20be%20clearly%20defined%20More%20items (Accessed April 21, 2024)

UK Research Integrity Office. (2023). *Recommended checklist for researchers.* https://ukrio.org/wp-content/uploads/UKRIO-Recommended-Checklist-for-Researchers.pdf (Accessed April 20, 2024)

University of Sheffield. (2024). *Epistemology.* https://www.sheffield.ac.uk/philosophy/research/themes/epistemology (Accessed April 16, 2024)

University of Tennessee (UTC). (2018). *Quality improvement vs research.* https://www.utc.edu/sites/default/files/2020-05/irb-qi-qivsresearchguidance.pdf (Accessed April 14, 2024)

Valentino, A., & Juanico, J. F. (2020). Overcoming barriers to applied research: A guide for practitioners. *Behaviour Analysis in Practice, 13*, 894–904. https://doi.org/10.1007/s40617-020-00479-y (Accessed March 17, 2024)

World Health Organization. (2020). *State of the world's nursing report 2020 – Investing in education, jobs and leadership.* World Health Organization.

CHAPTER 7

Aspiring to Advanced Practice—How to Get Started

Jonathan Thomas ■ Angie Banks ■ Melanie Rogers ■ Charlotte Barker

CHAPTER OUTLINE

In this chapter, we will discuss how you can develop and prepare for advanced practice (AP). We will provide some examples of how to prepare to embark upon AP studies as well as drawing on the work that has been undertaken across the UK to help prepare registrants aspiring to advanced level practice. The latter part of the chapter will examine equality and diversity in application to AP.

Introduction

Within Chapter 1, the birth and development of advanced practice (AP) within the UK were discussed. The evolvement of AP has happened at pace; however, there remains no consistent UK pathway to this advanced level of practice (Palmer et al., 2023).

The enhanced, advanced and consultant level framework (Health Education and Improvement Wales (HEIW), 2023) has provided a roadmap for a suggested progression from registrant through to consultant level practice in Wales, which does encapsulate advanced level practice, but it is recognised that this journey is not linear (HEIW, 2023). Although variation exists across the four UK countries, as has been discussed in Chapter 1, the policy frameworks provide the direction for the development of this role in each UK country (NHS England (NHSE), 2025; HEIW, 2023; Northern Ireland Practice & Education Council for Nursing and Midwifery, 2023; Scottish Government, 2017).

The aim of this chapter is to provide a discussion about how registrants can develop and prepare for AP study. This chapter will provide some examples of how to prepare to embark upon AP studies as well as drawing on the work that has been undertaken across the UK to help prepare registrants who are aspiring to advanced level practice. The latter part of the chapter will examine equality and diversity in application to AP.

Journey to AP—Organisation Factors

Progressing to an advanced level of practice could be viewed as a journey with both challenges and opportunities that need to be navigated along the way. The journey begins with an employer and a service level need aligned to strategic plans for implementation and development of AP within organisations. Many employers will have specific workforce policies regarding the implementation of AP roles into practice (NHS Lothian, 2021), while other employers might recognise AP within their workforce planning strategy but lack the formalised processes for implementation.

Bryant-Lukosius and Dicenso (2004) recognised the need for a robust approach to AP role development and produced the advanced practice nursing (APN) role development, implementation and evaluation (PEPPA framework). This framework focuses on the principles and values of AP nursing utilising a collaborative inclusive process that enables consideration of healthcare providers and the systems they work in. Although specific to nursing, this framework will be useful for other professions. In more recent developments, within England, the Centre for Advancing Practice has produced a maturity matrix. The governance matrix for AP (NHS England, n.d.) supports organisations which assess the governance of AP in the workforce, and this includes the recognition for a need for advanced practitioners in a service and the development of a business case. Furthermore, an employer readiness checklist for AP has been developed (HEE, 2022a).

PIT STOP!

The governance of AP produced by the Centre for Advancing Practice (NHS England) and the resources to support this can be found here:

https://advanced-practice.hee.nhs.uk/our-work/governance/

As highlighted within other chapters of this book, the Centre for Advancing Practice is only applicable to England, so the maturity matrix and check list are likely to only be utilised within English organisations. Each AP framework across the four nations of the UK can provide a degree of guidance to employers; however, the strategic direction to support the implementation of AP can be challenging for the aspiring advanced practitioner to navigate. Furthermore, this can lead to disparities within an organisation amongst different teams and specialities. The Nuffield Trust Report on AP (Palmer et al., 2023) recognises that AP development has been complex due to the balance between workplace demand and expectations for AP versus national policy. Furthermore, the number of UK organisations with responsibility for AP makes this rather complex and challenging (Palmer et al., 2023). This has been reflected within Fothergill et al.'s (2022) evaluation of advanced clinical practitioner roles across England. Fothergill et al. (2022) noted a plethora of inconsistencies from job titles to scope of practices and governance arrangements for advanced practitioners in England.

The independent sector, such as general practices, will also have their own approaches to supporting their workforce to transition into AP roles. Third sector (charity) AP roles are not yet visible in the literature. The different approaches amongst employers echo a lack of standardisation to developing and accessing AP education (Mannix & Jones, 2020).

TABLE 7.1 ■ UK Variations to AP Workforce Planning

Scotland	Papers 2 of the Transforming Roles Programme Advanced Nursing Practice (Scottish Government, 2017) is a policy framework that sets the direction for employers on developing advanced nursing practice roles.
England	The Centre for Advancing Practice (CfAP) in England has developed employer guidance to assess readiness for AP and the governance matrix. Across England, CfAP has developed seven regional faculties, all of which have local work streams which support employers with AP workforce development.
Wales	The enhanced, advanced and consultant level framework (HEIW, 2023) sets out guidance for workforce planning which links to HEIW's workforce planning capability self-assessment framework.
Northern Ireland	The Northern Ireland Practice & Education Council for Nursing and Midwifery (NIPEC) published an analysis and recommendations for expanding advanced nursing practice across Northern Ireland (NIPEC, 2023).

AP, Advanced practice; *HEIW*, Health Education and Improvement Wales.

Across the UK, there have been key drivers at a national level to support employers with AP workforce planning, as set out in Table 7.1.

As noted from Chapter 1, with the current plans for regulation of AP within the nursing and midwifery workforce (Nursing and Midwifery Council, 2024), the pathway to developing and implementing AP roles might have more clarity. However, this would only be applicable for nursing and midwifery, so there might be the potential for further confusion and disparity between nursing, midwifery and allied health professionals.

PIT STOP!

Review your country's and employer's policies and guidance around AP workforce planning. This might identify key elements you need to consider or that need to be in place prior to before embarking on the AP journey.

Causality Dilemma

The causality dilemma with what comes first can be applied to the starting point for AP in terms of being employed within a trainee AP role versus not currently employed in one of these roles. Across the UK, this remains fragmented, with different approaches being witnessed (Palmer et al., 2023). Within England, the AP apprenticeship scheme is only open to trainee advanced practitioners, who are employed and working in that role. The apprenticeship scheme ensures funding along with other criteria the employer must agree to. Although the apprenticeship scheme for AP is only available in England, other areas of the UK have adopted trainee AP roles; although they may not be termed 'apprenticeship', they might have similar approaches. Whilst it might be appealing to be employed within a trainee AP role, there are potential challenges that can be faced. Box 7.1 provides a case study of a trainee AP and the challenges encountered.

> **BOX 7.1 ■ Example of a Trainee Advanced Practitioner's Journey**
>
> Joe is a physiotherapist and has been fortunate to secure a trainee AP post within stroke care at their local hospital. Joe's working week as a trainee AP includes 1 day attending university to undertake the MSc award, 1 day practice supervision time and then 3 days working as a physiotherapist within the stroke unit, but not as a trainee AP for these 3 days. The details of these 3 days have been vague, and management has not provided any direction or clarity. Joe is trying to juggle being a trainee AP and a physiotherapist during these 3 days, which is challenging.
>
> Juggling the demands of their current role, university study and family life has resulted in Joe failing a core module on the MSc programme on two attempts. Based on this failed module, Joe has been formally withdrawn from the MSc programme, which means he is no longer able to continue to achieve the MSc award.
>
> Being in a trainee AP role, Joe is required to successfully complete an MSc AP programme.

The case study highlighted in Box 7.1 captures a situation that can happen; however, there are many factors that have attributed to this outcome. The employer is required to plan service developments such as role advancement and should have discussed and clarified role expectations, which should include a discussion with human resources (HR) and amendments to job descriptions if/as necessary. Governance arrangements need to be clear from the onset as highlighted by Fothergill et al. (2022). Appointing staff into trainee advanced practitioner roles requires consideration of academic ability and the support needed to ensure progression. This approach may be enhanced if higher education institutions are involved with recruitment processes.

Workplace support is vital to ensure a smooth transition to AP roles (HEE, 2021). However, intrinsic factors such as Joe's motivation and consideration of a 'last minute' approach to studying may have contributed to a failing grade and need to be considered in this case as well. Despite all these considerations, Joe is employed as a trainee advanced practitioner but is no longer enrolled in an MSc AP programme; this would have various possible outcomes ranging from job loss or redeployment to a requirement to commence another MSc AP programme at a different university.

The second case study (Box 7.2) provides a narrative of a registrant who is not employed as a trainee advanced practitioner working as a paramedic whilst juggling undertaking an MSc AP programme.

The case study in Box 7.2 is often a true reflection of many students' journey through to advanced practitioner. This case highlights the challenges of a lack of organisational workforce planning for AP. The lack of structured approach to workforce planning and implementation policies resulted in Mike, an experienced paramedic, leaving the organisation. Despite supporting Mike to undertake the MSc, the organisation lost a key member of staff due to poor workforce planning. The emotional and physical impact of studying and working full time needs consideration; as has been highlighted in this case, it may lead to a negative experience of role development. Such considerations can have a huge impact on any student undertaking any post graduate qualification.

BOX 7.2 ■ Case Study of a Nontrainee Advanced Practitioner

Mike has been employed as a paramedic for 14 years and has decided he wants to undertake the MSc AP programme at his local university. The Ambulance NHS Trust supports the funding of paramedics to undertake the MSc award. The service has no clear pathway for paramedics to transition to AP roles; the expectation is that they can undertake the MSc award and when an advanced paramedic practitioner role becomes available, applicants can apply for these roles.

Since Mike has no evidence of degree level study, the university advises him that he needs to undertake a degree level module to help develop his academic skills prior to starting the MSc. Successful completion of this degree level module allows Mike to enrol on the MSc AP programme. Study leave to attend the university appears haphazard as the employing organisation has only granted Mike 20 study days per year. All practice supervision needs to be undertaken in Mike's own time.

The 3-year MSc programme remains challenging for Mike to complete due to lack of employer support for adequate study and practice supervision time. However, Mike manages to successfully complete and achieve the MSc award. Unfortunately, there are no advanced paramedic practitioner roles for Mike within the ambulance service. Mike has no alternative but to leave the ambulance service to take up an advanced practitioner role at a local primary care centre.

Enhanced to Advanced Level Practice

Enhanced level practice has been an emerging trend across the UK over the past few years. HEE (2022b) regards the enhanced level practitioner as someone working beyond novice/competent but who is not working at an advanced level. Examples of enhanced level practice can include an extended scope practitioner in physiotherapy, an emergency nurse practitioner or a proton principal radiographer (HEE, 2022b). Within England, enhanced clinical practitioner apprenticeship programmes have been developed with education being delivered at degree level, this being level 6 or level 9 for Scotland (see Chapter 1 for education levels across the UK). Likewise, in Wales, the enhanced level practice role has been recognised and is regarded as a specific level of practice (HEIW, 2023). Both England and Wales recognise that the enhanced level role can support the journey towards AP; however, they also appreciate that enhanced clinical practitioners might not want to progress to advanced level practice. An example of a registrant's journey to AP could be a physiotherapist who then becomes a first contact practitioner (enhanced level practice) and then progresses through practice and education to become a musculoskeletal advanced practitioner.

Preparing Yourself to Undertake an MSc AP Programme

Before deciding to embark on an AP journey and apply for an MSc programme, there are many factors to consider, which have been captured in Table 7.2.

Trainee Advanced Practitioner Supportive Resource

In 2021, a small group of AP educators from different universities across the UK collectively identified the need for trainee AP student support resource. The faculty

TABLE 7.2 ■ **Factors to Consider Before Starting the AP Journey**

Factor	Discussion
Employment	The starting point with the AP journey is to review whether the employer supports AP. If the employer does not support AP or has plans to develop AP, then you need to explore what your future options might be. Do you stay in the clinical environment that has no AP vision or do you move clinical areas/employers? ! Speak to your employer about your career plans and see if they align with the employing organisation.
Clinical experience	Clinical experience is an important factor that needs to be considered. Individual universities will have specific entrance criteria which will dictate the number of years postregistration experience required for an AP programme and some might dictate the clinical experience needed. For a generic MSc AP programme, having diverse clinical exposure through different roles before settling on a specific role prior to MSc application might support the applicant to be in an ideal place since they can draw on this experience and knowledge. ! Review your local university MSc AP programme website as this will normally display the entrance requirements. You may also wish to speak to the MSc programme lead for clarification and further discussions.
Education requirements	Different universities will have different entrance criteria. If you have no evidence of degree level study, some universities might offer a place based on clinical experience. Alternatively, if you have completed a degree many years previously and have been out of academic study for some time, it might be worth considering undertaking a stand-alone module to help prepare you for MSc studies. ! Speak to the MSc programme lead and explore these options.
Apprenticeship requirements	With the apprenticeship schemes in England, they have many requirements including holding grade C or above in GCSE English and Mathematics. ! Speak to the relevant AP faculty regions, employer and MSc course lead about apprenticeship entrance requirements.
Know the MSc	You need to gain an understanding of the MSc AP programmes available to you. Your employer might have service level agreements with two or more universities while others might only be linked to one. Explore the modules offered within the MSc programme in terms of the learning outcomes, the syllabus and assessment frameworks. ! Speak to current students who are enrolled on to the MSc programme you are considering applying for. Gauge their thoughts and opinions of how best to prepare. Also speak to the MSc programme lead.
Is this the ideal time	An MSc AP programme is challenging, and this can impact upon both home and work life. If there is something at home or at work that might impact upon you while studying for the MSc, then consider if this is an ideal time for you. For example, you might have planned surgery in 3 months' time which has an anticipated 3-month recovery period, or the department you work within is being restructured in 6 months' time. That might never be an ideal time, but having minimal impact from home and work life will help. ! Reflect and discuss with family and colleagues to explore if this is the right time.
Know your AP framework	As highlighted throughout the book, the four nations of the UK all have their own AP frameworks. Become familiar with your home countries AP framework and local AP policies.

AP, Advanced practice.

involved concurred that this support should be offered prior to students commencing AP programmes to help them feel more prepared for their studies.

The faculty identified some of the main areas of concern which AP students consistently raise on starting MSc AP programmes. These concerns included limited anatomy and physiology knowledge, context-specific understanding of AP development within the UK and critical writing skills, a core component of MSc-level education.

This led to the development of a national precourse workbook which supports students commencing MSc AP programmes. Providing a UK-wide AP resource demonstrates a robust and consistent national approach to the development of AP student support. The national precourse workbook highlights key areas for development and aims to facilitate a proactive approach to student learning; this is achieved by providing additional resources to students to help them assimilate key knowledge prior to starting their AP programmes of education. Access to the web address for the precourse workbook is in the Pitstop.

PIT STOP!

The precourse workbook is freely available and is hosted via the Association of Advanced Practice Educators (APPE) website. Please access the website and review the precourse workbook.

https://aape.org.uk/huuiuydcqrgccgndfa3qudehz/

The workbook has been accessed by over 3600 students and has been evaluated as an excellent resource. This UK-wide multidisciplinary collaboration is consistently updated in response to AP student and faculty feedback. The aim of this supportive free resource is to enable students to feel more prepared for their MSc-level studies and provides an expectation for students.

Aspiring Advanced Practice Study Days

Building upon feedback from the precourse workbook, the University of Huddersfield and Sheffield Hallam University, with the support from HEE Northeast and Yorkshire region AP faculty, developed a 2-day face-to-face aspiring AP course. The course aimed to facilitate an introduction to AP training and was offered to students across the region irrespective of where they were going to study. Faculty across the region were also invited to attend and support the course.

In addition to opportunities for students to ask questions and discuss topical issues through panels, didactic sessions were also provided and covered the following topics:

- Studying at master's level and the required skills for academic writing
- Demystifying the role of an advanced practitioner, both in training and on qualification
- Understanding and developing knowledge of anatomy and physiology relevant to AP training

- Developing a personal toolkit of e-resources that are useful for students throughout their training
- Preparing for training and how organisations could and should prepare and support students
- The role of AP e-portfolios
- An introduction to the four pillars of AP

A total of 80 to 120 students from regional universities have attended the aspiring AP course.

The course has run for 2 consecutive years and plans are in place to offer the course at different universities across the region. Faculty from most universities are now involved in the delivery of the course each year and the aims are to ensure that each university representative is present at the course to address any institution-specific questions. In addition to ensuring rotation of delivery point for the course, it is anticipated that different universities or colleagues will take leadership of the course and delivery.

Feedback from the course has been positive, as seen in Box 7.3.

UK-Wide Benchmarks

Building upon the success of this 2-day aspiring AP course, work continues across the devolved countries of the UK. Scotland and Wales are currently collaborating with colleagues in the Northeast and Yorkshire region of England to produce an equivalent aspiring AP course to engender lifelong learning and demonstrate collaboration between and across professional associations and universities in the UK. This will enable the Scottish and Welsh university colleagues to increase networking across the two nations, creating a culture of mutual respect and reciprocation between students and educators. The long-term aim would be a four-nation

---

BOX 7.3 ■ Examples of Feedback From the Aspiring AP Course

What was good about the Aspiring Advanced Clinical Practice (ACP) course?

'It has been a good insight into the course and expectations.'
'It has inspired me to want to learn more and develop as an AP.'

How did you feel about the trainee AP role before attending the course?

'I was apprehensive and unsure if I could do this.'
'I felt really anxious and not very well informed.'

Did your thoughts and feelings change after attending the Aspiring AP programme?

'Yes, I realised it would be hard but feel ready to grab the opportunity by both hands.'
'It has confirmed that this is the right step for me.'
'It has made me feel able to be more assertive about prioritising my own learning needs!'

approach to initiatives like this one to ensure parity to all prospective students. Collaboration is key to ensuring aspiring AP is recognised as an important area for universities to focus upon. Similarly, steps have begun to explore some of these approaches with our international partners.

Attracting and Increasing Student Diversity

Within Bolton and Lewis' (2024) briefing paper, they identified that there are many underrepresented student groups within the higher education system; such groups include those from low socioeconomic backgrounds, certain ethnic groups, mature students and students with disabilities. Key to AP role development is the requirement to provide culturally competent care (Mackavey et al., 2024). To consider this further, we will consider specific challenges relevant to the UK starting with equality and diversity issues.

The National Health Service (NHS) has one of the most ethnically diverse workforces within the public sector, as evidenced by the findings from the Office for National Statistics (ONS) (2019). Concurrently, the proactive response to issues of racism and discrimination has become a prominent focal area within organisations across the UK. There has been a sustained and steadfast dedication to confronting workplace disparities and mitigating discriminatory practices, with the overarching objective of cultivating an equitable and all-encompassing professional environment. A notable nationwide initiative, 'The Race Equality Plan', as outlined by the Department of Health (2004), underscored the imperative of confronting racial discrimination within the recruitment and employment of healthcare staff. Subsequently, in 2015, the introduction of the Workforce Race Equality Standard (WRES) mandated the systematic collection of workforce data to identify disparities in the treatment and opportunities afforded to staff from Black and minority ethnic (BME) backgrounds. More recently, NHS England has instituted the Equality, Diversity and Inclusion Plan (NHS England, 2023). Likewise, the Welsh Government (2021) has produced a workforce equality, diversity and inclusion strategy and similar plans are seen across Scotland and Northern Ireland.

PIT STOP!

Review your own country's equality, diversity and inclusion plan.

Although the latest WRES (NHS England, 2022) report illustrates an increased representation of ethnically diverse staff across the NHS, with figures ascending from 19.1% in 2018 to 24.2% in 2022, a conspicuous disparity persists when contrasting their representation within the distinct Agenda for Change bands. This disparity is particularly salient at Band 7 and beyond and is notably exacerbated within clinical roles, wherein the ratio of underrepresentation continues to escalate. Moreover, the data show that individuals from a minority ethnic background perceive fewer opportunities for professional advancement in comparison to their White counterparts and are more likely to experience harassment, bullying or abuse.

Despite the plethora of initiatives, policies and regulatory directives implemented, the data substantiate the enduring disparities and an exasperatingly slow progression with respect to achieving workforce parity. The BME Leadership Network (2022) 'Shattered Hopes' report indicated that individuals of minority ethnic backgrounds encountered challenges when engaging in discussions about racism and this difficulty was exacerbated by the pronounced lack of diversity in leadership roles, resulting in staff members experiencing a sense of apprehension and fear when expressing their concerns.

What Do the Data Show for the Advanced Practice Workforce?

At present, a comprehensive dataset assessing the diversity and professional experiences of the AP workforce is conspicuously absent. Numerous England-based regional faculties have undertaken initiatives aimed at enhancing data collection on equality and diversity within the profession. This includes the Northeast and Yorkshire Faculty, which found that approximately 8% of advanced practitioners across the region were from a minority ethnic background. However, it is essential to exercise caution in accepting the accuracy of these data, as these were acquired through a query of the electronic staff record (ESR) system utilising search terms such as 'advanced practitioner', 'advanced clinical practitioner' and 'advanced nurse practitioner'. An investigation conducted by Fothergill et al. (2022) discerned a significant variability in role titles and the extensiveness of practice associated with advanced practitioners. Consequently, the search criteria employed are apt to be insufficient in capturing or representing the complete spectrum of the AP workforce within the region. Additionally, it should be noted that ESR exclusively encompasses NHS secondary care organisations, thereby excluding advanced practitioners working in primary care from the dataset.

Why Does Equality, Diversity and Inclusion Matter In Healthcare?

First and foremost, the pursuit of equality, diversity and inclusion within a healthcare workforce is grounded in moral and ethical values. The NHS, as a publicly funded healthcare system, serves the entirety of the British population and was established on the principles of social justice and equity (NHS England, 2022). Therefore, it has a moral responsibility to ensure that its workforce is representative of the communities it serves.

Diversity within the workforce is a pivotal domain in promoting health equity. Health disparity signifies variances in the quality of care that individuals receive and the extent to which they can engage in health-promoting lifestyles (The King's Fund Report, by Raleigh, 2023). During the COVID-19 pandemic, inequalities were thrust into the spotlight when data revealed that individuals belonging to minority ethnic groups experienced a disproportionate impact (Phiri et al., 2021).

However, these disparities are not a recent occurrence, and evidence substantiates that ethnic minority groups consistently encounter poorer outcomes and less favourable experiences in comparison to the broader population (Ajayi Sotubo, 2021).

Health inequalities extend beyond individuals from ethnic minority backgrounds. According to Public Health England (2021), they can be categorised into four distinct groupings encompassing socioeconomic status and deprivation, geographical factors, protected characteristics and socially marginalised segments of the population. It is not uncommon for individuals to encounter a blend of these factors, resulting in diverse health profiles and risk levels within any given population. This is described by Holman et al. (2021) as intersectionality and refers to the interconnected and overlapping systems of discrimination, privilege and disadvantage that individuals may experience based on multiple aspects of their identity and social positioning. This concept recognises that a person's health outcomes and experiences are influenced by a combination of various factors, such as race, gender, socioeconomic status, age, sexual orientation, disability and more. Understanding intersectionality theory within health disparities has the potential to provide direct and practical benefits in the realm of population-level interventions, particularly in the context of policy adjustments and workforce planning, to guarantee the implementation of the distinctive requirements of communities impacted by inequalities (Bauer, 2014).

Representation of communities is critical to addressing health inequalities by facilitating a better understanding of the cultural nuances of a wide array of patients (NHS England, 2023). This concept is frequently described as cultural competence in the realm of healthcare. Cultural competence denotes the provision of effective and high-quality healthcare to patients who exhibit a range of diverse belief systems, attitudes, values and behaviours (Kaihlanen et al., 2019). It requires the implementation of systems capable of customising healthcare delivery in accordance with cultural and linguistic disparities, alongside a comprehensive grasp of the potential ramifications stemming from cultural differences on the provision of healthcare services.

As AP students, your comprehension of your patients' culture, values and preferences constitutes a pivotal aspect of patient-centred care. Patient's health beliefs serve as a predictive determinant of health-related behaviours, including medication adherence, utilisation of healthcare services and lifestyle decisions (Kennedy et al., 2017). For example, diminished levels of COVID-19 vaccine adoption within ethnic minority communities have been ascribed to scepticism regarding its effectiveness and the mechanisms responsible for its distribution, primarily stemming from incidents of historical medical mistreatment and institutionalised racism (Razai et al., 2021).

PIT STOP!

The Care Quality Commission provides an excellent resource on cultural competence, which can be accessed here:

https://www.cqc.org.uk/guidance-providers/adult-social-care/culturally-appropriate-care#:~:text=Culturally%20appropriate%20care%20(also%20called,be%20determined%20by%20cultural%20heritage.

A workforce that reflects the demographic diversity of the patient population is well positioned to establish enhanced communication, a pivotal element in facilitating accurate diagnoses and formulation of effective treatment plans (Howick et al., 2018). Communication errors, occurring within the interprofessional context and during clinician–patient interactions, have the potential to lead to adverse patient outcomes and a provision of care that falls below the accepted standards (General Medical Council, 2018). Studies indicate that lapses in communication are not solely attributable to poor transmission or insufficient information exchange. Rather, they can be due to a prevailing organisational culture that does not value or appreciate diverse viewpoints (Sutcliffe et al., 2004). Differing perspectives can enhance communication efficacy and foster heightened capacities for innovative and creative problem-solving. Engaging with a diverse array of viewpoints improves outcomes in all aspects of health and social care.

There exists an extensive body of research that substantiates the notion of a race concordance hypothesis, wherein it is suggested that individuals from racial minority backgrounds exhibit a preference for healthcare providers who share the same race and ethnicity (Moore et al., 2023). A diverse AP work force means that irrespective of the individual, there will be an advanced practitioner who shares common identifiers, facilitating effective communication and an enhanced capacity to address their specific requirements.

Diversity not only enhances patient outcomes and experiences but also positively influences employees and teams. As observed by The King's Fund (West et al., 2015), discrimination is most prone to manifest at the team level. However, it is precisely at this organisational tier where opportunities for enacting transformative change can be maximised. The advantages inherent in a diverse team, underpinned by a foundation of inclusivity and a sense of belonging, are emphasised by the Equality, Diversity and Inclusion Plan (NHS England, 2023). Employees who experience a sense of value and respect tend to exhibit diminished rates of health-related issues, heightened levels of professional contentment and increased levels of engagement and motivation. Moreover, this improvement in morale significantly enhances the propensity for staff retention and facilitates the attraction of new talent, owing to the widened outreach and enlarged pool of skilled individuals achieved through embracing diversity.

A workforce marked by diversity, inclusivity and a steadfast dedication to these core principles not only offers healthcare services that are responsive to the intricate requirements of patients, encompassing dimensions of equity and intersectionality, but also concurrently fosters heightened staff engagement, reduced turnover rates and heightened levels of innovation within healthcare organisations and teams.

Why Is This Important to AP?

Considerable empirical evidence substantiates the presence of systemic and organisational discrimination within the healthcare sector (British Medical Association, 2021). The enduring effects of discrimination substantially and comprehensively compromise the health, well-being and overall work-related quality of life among a significant portion of NHS staff. Moreover, such discrimination also exerts an adverse influence on patients' experiences and, subsequently, their healthcare outcomes.

Effectively addressing this issue necessitates a paradigm shift that extends beyond individual change, encompassing a cultural transformation. The role of leaders within healthcare institutions is pivotal in shaping the ethos and culture, thereby bearing a significant responsibility for fostering inclusivity in the workplace.

Advanced practitioners bring to the healthcare milieu a distinctive array of expertise and a multifaceted skill set, significantly enriching the capacity of healthcare teams. Situated as senior members within a multidisciplinary team (MDT), advanced practitioners are well positioned to exert influence and provide comprehensive clinical and organisational leadership (Elliott et al., 2016). They can hold pivotal roles in establishing an environment that supports the sharing of perspectives and facilitation of effective communication within interprofessional teams. They are instrumental in enhancing the cognitive capacity of team members to embrace and integrate diverse viewpoints. The presence of a diverse AP team conveys several significant advantages, including enhanced patient care and outcomes, a more effective healthcare delivery system and the establishment of equitable opportunities for staff.

Conclusion

In conclusion, this chapter has highlighted that the journey into AP is neither linear nor consistent. This is further complicated by different approaches to organisational workforce planning, along with various AP drivers amongst the four countries of the UK. Despite attempts to provide policy and guidance, the aspiring advanced practitioner can face obstacles from enrolling in an MSc AP programme through to workplace and practice-based supervision, as captured within the two case studies. There are national initiatives to support the aspiring AP journey such as the student workbook and the dissemination of the aspiring AP course across other parts of the UK. However, despite these initiatives, it is still observed that those from underrepresented groups face challenges in both accessing education and career progression. A lack of diversity with senior leadership teams has recognised and this needs to be addressed. In addition to this, there is a clear need for the development of cultural competence not only within the AP workforce but also across the health and social care sector.

References

Ajayi Sotubo, O. (2021). A perspective on health inequalities in BAME communities and how to improve access to primary care. *Future Healthcare Journal, 8*(1), 36–39. doi:10.7861/fhj.2020-0217

Bauer, G., R. (2014). Incorporating intersectionality theory into population health research methodology: Challenges and the potential to advance health equity. *Social Science and Medicine, 110*, 10–17.

BME Leadership Network. (2022). *Shattered hopes Black and minority ethnic leaders' experiences of breaking the glass ceiling in the NHS*. NHS Confederation. https://www.nhsconfed.org/system/files/2022-06/Shattered-hopes-BME-leaders-glass-ceiling-NHS.pdf. Accessed December 10, 2023.

British Medical Association. (2021). *BMA condemns Sewell race report.* https://www.bma.org.uk/news-and-opinion/bma-condemns-sewell-race-report. Accessed December 10, 2023.

Bryant-Lukosius, D., & Dicenso, A. (2004). A framework for the introduction and evaluation of advanced practice nursing roles. *Journal of Advancing Nursing, 48*(5), 530–540.

Department of Health. (2004). *The race equality action plan*. Department of Health. https://webarchive.nationalarchives.gov.uk/ukgwa/+/www.dh.gov.uk/en/Publicationsandstatistics/Bulletins/DH_4072494. Accessed December 10, 2023.

Elliott, N., Begley, C., Sheaf, G., & Higgins, A. (2016). Barriers and enablers to advanced practitioners' ability to enact their leadership role: A scoping review. *International Journal of Nursing Studies, 60*, 24–45.

Fothergill, L. J., Al-Oraibi, A., Houdmont, J., Conway, J., Evans, C., Timmons, S., et al. (2022). Nationwide evaluation of the advanced clinical practitioner role in England: A cross-sectional survey. *BMJ Open, 12*(1). doi: 10.1136/bmjopen-2021-055475.

General Medical Council. (2018). *A scoping review of evidence relating to communication failures that lead to patient harm*. https://www.gmc-uk.org/-/media/documents/a-scoping-review-of-evidence-relating-to-communication-failures-that-lead-to-patient-harm_p-80569509.pdf. Accessed December 10, 2023.

Health Education and Improvement Wales. (2023). *Professional framework for enhanced, advanced and consultant clinical practice*. https://heiw.nhs.wales/workforce/workforce-development/professional-framework-for-enhanced-advanced-and-consultant-clinical-practice/. Accessed November 14, 2023.

Health Education England. (2021). *Workplace supervision for advanced clinical practice*. https://advanced-practice.hee.nhs.uk/workplace-supervision-for-advanced-clinical-practice-2/. Accessed April 6, 2024.

Health Education England. (2022a). *Employer readiness for advanced practice*. https://advanced-practice.hee.nhs.uk/wp-content/uploads/sites/28/2022/03/AP-Readiness-Checklist-London-2022-23-2.pdf. Accessed November 28, 2023.

Health Education England. (2022b). *Enhanced clinical practice apprenticeship (ECP)*. https://haso.skills-forhealth.org.uk/wp-content/uploads/2022/08/2022.08.03-ECP-Apprenticeship-Employer-Guidance.pdf. Accessed January 16, 2024.

Holman, D., Salway, S., Bell, A., Beach, B., Adebajo, A., Ali, N., et al. (2021). Can intersectionality help with understanding and tackling health inequalities? Perspectives of professional stakeholders. *Health Research Policy and Systems, 19*(1), 97. https://doi.org/10.1186/s12961-021-00742-w

Howick, J., Moscrop, A., Mebius, A., Fanshawe, T. R., Lewith, G., Bishop, F. L., et al. (2018). Effects of empathic and positive communication in healthcare consultations: A systematic review and meta-analysis. *Journal of the Royal Society of Medicine, 111*(7), 240–252.

Kaihlanen, A., M., Hietapakka, L., & Heponiemi, T. (2019). Increasing cultural awareness: Qualitative study of nurses' perceptions about cultural competence training. *BMC Nursing, 18*, 38. https://doi.org/10.1186/s12912-019-0363-x

Kennedy, B. M., Rehman, M., Johnson, W. D., Magee, M. B., Leonard, R., & Katzmarzyk, P. T. (2017). Healthcare providers versus patients' understanding of health beliefs and values. *Patient Experience Journal, 4*(3), 29–37.

Mackavey, C., Henderson, C., & Stout, T. (2024). Stepping outside national borders: International active learning educational collaboration events *International Nursing Review, 71*, 1.

Moore, C., Coates, E., Watson, A., de Heer, R., McLeod, A., & Prudhomme, A. (2023). "It's important to work with people that look like me": Black patients' preferences for patient-provider race concordance. *Journal of Racial and Ethnic Health Disparities, 10*(5), 2552–2564. https://doi.org/10.1007/s40615-022-01435-y

Mannix, K., & Jones, C. (2020). Nurses' experience of transitioning into advanced practice roles. *Nursing Times, 116*(3) 35–38.

NHS England. (n.d.). *Governance of advanced practice*. https://advanced-practice.hee.nhs.uk/our-work/governance/. Accessed April 6, 2024.

NHS England. (2022). *NHS Workforce Race Equality Standard (WRES) 2022 data analysis report for NHS trusts*. https://www.england.nhs.uk/wp-content/uploads/2023/02/workforce-race-equality-standard.pdf. Accessed December 10, 2023.

NHS England (2025) *Multi-professional framework for advanced Practice in England*. Birmingham: Centre for Advancing Practice.

NHS England. (2023). *NHS equality, diversity, and inclusion plan.* NHS England. https://www.england.nhs.uk/wp-content/uploads/2023/06/B2044_NHS_EDI_WorkforcePlan.pdf. Accessed January 10, 2024.

NHS Lothian. (2021). *Advancing practice policy.* https://policyonline.nhslothian.scot/wp-content/uploads/2023/03/Advancing_Practice_Policy.pdf. Accessed January 20, 2024.

Northern Ireland Practice & Education Council for Nursing and Midwifery. (2023). *Advanced nursing practice in Northern Ireland. Analysis and recommendations.* https://www.health-ni.gov.uk/sites/default/files/publications/health/doh-nipec-anp.pdf. Accessed April 6, 2024.

Nursing and Midwifery Council. (2024). *Advanced practice review.* https://www.nmc.org.uk/about-us/our-role/advanced-practice-review/. Accessed April 7, 2024.

Office for National Statistics. (2019). *Who works in the public sector?* Office for National Statistics. https://www.ons.gov.uk/economy/governmentpublicsectorandtaxes/publicspending/articles/whoworksinthepublicsector/2019-06-04#ethnic-diversity-in-public-sector-occupations-varies-considerably. Accessed December 10, 2023.

Bolton, P., & Lewis, J. (2024). Equality of access and outcomes in higher education in England. House of Commons Library. UK Parliament. https://commonslibrary.parliament.uk/research-briefings/cbp-9195/. Accessed January 19, 2025.

Palmer, W., Julian, S., & Vaughan, L. (2023). *Independent report on the regulation of advanced practice nursing and midwifery.* Nuffield Trust.https://www.nuffieldtrust.org.uk/research/independent-report-on-the-regulation-of-advanced-practice-in-nursing-and-midwifery. Accessed April 6, 2024.

Phiri, P., Delanerolle, G., Al-Sudani, A., & Rathod, S. (2021). COVID-19 and Black, Asian, and minority ethnic communities: A complex relationship without just cause. *JMIR Public Health Surveillance, 7*(2). https://doi.org/10.2196/22581

Public Health England. (2021). *Addressing health inequalities through collaborative action.* https://assets.publishing.service.gov.uk/media/615213efe90e077a2db2e804/health_inequalities_briefing.pdf. Accessed December 10, 2023.

Raleigh, V. (2023). *The health of people from ethnic minority groups in England.* The King's Fund. https://www.kingsfund.org.uk/insight-and-analysis/long-reads/health-people-ethnic-minority-groups-england. Accessed January 19, 2025.

Razai, M. S., Osama, T., McKechnie, D. G. J., & Majeed, A. (2021). COVID-19 vaccine hesitancy among ethnic minority groups. *British Medical Journal. 372,* n513. https://doi.org/10.1136/bmj.n513

Scottish Government. (2017). *Transforming nursing, midwifery and health professions roles: Advance nursing practice.* https://www.gov.scot/publications/transforming-nursing-midwifery-health-professions-roles-advance-nursing-practice/#:~:text=The%20second%20paper%20outlines%20guidance,nursing%20practice%20in%20NHSS%20cotland.&text=The%20Chief%20Nursing%20Officer%20is,traditional%20boundaries%20of%20professional%20roles. Accessed April 8, 2024.

Sutcliffe, K. M., Lewton, E., & Rosenthal, M. M. (2004). Communication failures: An insidious contributor to medical mishaps. *Academic Medicine: Journal of the Association of American Medical Colleges, 79*(2), 186–194. https://doi.org/10.1097/00001888-200402000-00019

Welsh Government. (2021). *Workforce equality, diversity and inclusion strategy: 2021 to 2026.*

West, M., Randhawa, M., & Dawson, J. (2015). *Making the difference: Diversity and inclusion in the NHS.* The King's Fund. https://www.kingsfund.org.uk/insight-and-analysis/reports/making-difference-diversity-inclusion-nhs

CHAPTER 8

Introduction to the Importance of Anatomy, Physiology and Pathophysiology

John Knight ■ Zubeyde Bayram-Weston ■ James Taylor

CHAPTER OUTLINE

Advanced practitioners require a comprehensive understanding of anatomy, physiology and pathophysiology to underpin effective clinical practice in relation to their assessment and diagnostic thinking. Within this chapter, inflammation is explored as this underpins many pathologies. The chapter begins with an exploration of homeostasis and how the immune system works to protect the human body from pathogens. This will explore the immune system, which includes the nonspecific and specific responses to these pathogens. A key component of the nonspecific immune responses is the inflammatory response, which can be observed within many pathologies. Some common pathologies will be presented within the cardiovascular, renal and neurological systems, with a discussion of how inflammation leads to disease development in these systems. Through an understanding of the inflammatory process, it is anticipated that this will provide the foundations for the advanced practitioner to explore other pathologies that are underpinned by inflammation.

Introduction

To be an effective advanced practitioner, a thorough understanding of anatomy, physiology and pathophysiology is essential. Knowledge of these subjects underpins and informs virtually all areas of clinical practice. Clearly, a single chapter in a textbook could never explore all relevant topics in these vast subject areas. However, there are many high-quality textbooks and research articles available for readers who wish to explore and build upon their current knowledge; some of these are highlighted as recommended texts throughout this chapter. The aim of this chapter is to revisit some key aspects of anatomy, physiology and pathophysiology in the context of the inflammatory response. We have chosen this approach because inflammation is present in virtually all pathologies routinely encountered in advanced clinical practice.

Organisation of the Human Body

At its simplest, the human body can be regarded as a highly integrated colony of around 50 trillion (50 million million) cells which are organised into the four major tissue types:

- Epithelial—absorption, secretion, protection
- Connective—support, binding, transport, protection
- Muscle—movement
- Nervous—coordination

These tissues all have their unique structural and functional characteristics which are revealed under the microscope (Lowe et al., 2019). Tissues form the building blocks of organs; for example, the stomach consists of a lining of epithelial tissue and a wall composed of connective tissue and muscle, which is innervated with nervous tissue to regulate its activity. Groups of several organs often work together in organ systems to perform specific functions essential to life; for example, the digestive system includes the oesophagus, stomach, small and large intestines together with accessory organs such as the liver and pancreas. These collectively allow digestion of complex food molecules (macromolecules) into simple components which can be absorbed and utilised by the body.

Tissue samples are frequently collected in clinical practice to help screen for disease. Broadly speaking, there are two major categories of tissue sample.

- Biopsies—These are tissue samples collected from living patients. The most common biopsy is a simple blood sample which can be used to examine multiple parameters, including glucose, electrolyte, waste product and hormone concentrations together with inflammatory markers and evidence of infection.
- Necropsies—These samples are collected from deceased patients. This frequently happens during autopsies to help establish cause of death.

Organ Systems and Homeostasis

To survive, and perform optimally, the cells which form the human body must be maintained under very strict environmental conditions. Variables such as temperature, pH, oxygen saturation, electrolyte and nutrient composition must be maintained within tight physiological ranges. It is easy to forget that the ultimate purpose of all our organ systems is to maintain this strict homeostatic control of our internal environment. When homeostasis is not maintained, pathological states arise; for example, in patients with type I diabetes, the hormone insulin is no longer produced, and the blood glucose concentration increases leading to hyperglycaemia which precipitates all of the symptoms and potential complications of diabetes (Knight & Nigam, 2017a).

THE PERPETUAL BATTLE

The human body is continually exposed to a multitude of diverse microorganisms in the environment; these include bacteria, viruses, fungi and other infectious agents such as prions (abnormal pathogenic agents). Additionally, larger parasitic organisms such as worms, flukes, fleas, mites and ticks attempt to infest the body (van Seventer & Hochberg, 2017).

Most of the microorganisms we are exposed to are nonpathogenic and unlikely to cause infection. However, large numbers of bacteria, viruses and fungi have been identified as being human pathogens and if they gain access to the body can quickly lead to infection and potentially life-threatening disease. It is important to remember that some infections may also precipitate a variety of cancers and autoimmune diseases; for example, the human papillomavirus (HPV) is known to lead to malignant transformations initiating cervical and pharyngeal (throat) cancers (Zhang et al., 2020), while bacterial infections such as certain streptococcal infections may trigger the autoimmune disease rheumatic fever, which may subsequently lead to serious valve damage to the heart valves (Auala et al., 2022).

To deal with the continual assault from pathogens in the environment, the body is equipped with an exquisite array of immune defences.

Immunity and the Inflammatory Response

The immune system can be broadly divided into two branches.

SPECIFIC IMMUNE RESPONSES

As implied by their name, these target a specific pathogen for destruction and typically rely on molecules called antibodies which bind to the pathogen and mark it out for destruction by a process called opsonisation.

> **PIT STOP!**
>
> For a focused overview of specific immunity, refer to the article by Nigam and Knight (2020) as per the reference list.

NONSPECIFIC IMMUNE RESPONSES

Our nonspecific defences form the first line of defence against infection; these can be divided into four distinct layers.

Mechanical Defences

The skin forms the major mechanical barrier to infection. The epidermis is the outermost layer and is composed of cells termed 'keratinocytes' which have accumulated the dense protein keratin. To appreciate the nature of this protein, look at your fingernails, which are almost pure keratin. The keratinised nature of the epidermis provides a tough external barrier which few potential pathogens can penetrate. The accumulation of keratin also disrupts the internal structure of the cells so that they can no longer metabolise and release energy; as a result the cells in the outermost layers die and begin to slough away. This also provides additional protection since any potentially pathogenic microorganisms on the skin surface are shed along with the dead outer skin cells. However, the mechanical barrier afforded by the skin is prone to damage, and breaches in skin integrity caused by cuts, grazes, burns, insect/animal bites and nonhealing wounds (e.g., pressure ulcers) all provide a potential route for pathogens into the body (Coates et al., 2018).

In areas where a body cavity opens out to the surface such as the mouth, nose and reproductive tracts, there is no keratinised skin present. Here, mechanical protection is provided by the mucous membranes. These produce a continual basal secretion of transparent watery mucus which is produced by resident goblet cells (Benedetto et al., 2019). Mucus is incredibly sticky and serves to trap pathogens and thereby functions as an effective mechanical barrier. If a mucus membrane is irritated, the goblet cells also show induced mucus secretion with much greater amounts produced. This is seen in many upper respiratory tract infections, such as the common cold, leading to the characteristic streaming nose. Induced secretion is also a characteristic of allergies (Banafea et al., 2022); indeed, nasal congestion and a runny nose are common features of allergies affecting the upper respiratory tract such as pollen allergies (hay fever) and perennial rhinitis. Although freshly produced mucus is transparent, when it has trapped particulates such as dust, bacterial and viral particles, and pollutants, it takes on a darker typically greenish colour. When infection is present, leukocytes (white blood cells) typically move in to manage the infection; this results in the formation of pus, which gives the mucus a characteristic yellow colour. Advanced practitioners often become experts on the nature of mucus since sputum samples are commonly collected to identify pathogens. The nature of the mucus can also give important clues to the current state of the patient's body; for example, dry mucous membranes or thickened mucus is often seen in patients who are dehydrated. Smoking is known to not only contaminate mucus with particulates but also cause mucus dehydration leading to much thicker mucus in the airway (Lin et al., 2020b).

The final mechanical barrier to infection is found lining the nasal cavity and the bronchial tree. This is a specialised area of ciliated epithelium which forms the mucociliary escalator. Air inhaled into the respiratory tract will be laden with particulates including dust and a variety of pathogens; these stick to mucus within the airway. The cilia function as mobile hairs which lift and move contaminated mucus towards the pharynx (throat), where it is swallowed before entering the sterilising acidic secretions of the stomach (O'Neil & Jefferson, 2019).

Chemical Defences

Any pathogens that have breached the mechanical defences are then confronted by a diverse array of chemical defences.

Hydrochloric acid in the stomach typically has a pH of between 2.5 and 3.5; as well as activating digestive enzymes, its primary function is to sterilise food entering the stomach. We tend to think that the food we put into our mouths is clean, but even if it has just been cooked and plated, it will have accumulated a multitude of microorganisms from the atmosphere. Stomach acid is very effective at killing the vast majority of pathogens, although some, such as *Helicobacter pylori* (a bacterium associated with gastric ulceration), have evolved and can withstand the low pH of the gastric juices (Ansari & Yamaoka, 2017)

Body fluids contain an enzyme called lysozyme. This is a general antibacterial compound and attacks the peptidoglycan components of bacterial cell walls resulting in bacterial lysis (bursting) and death. Lysozyme is found in the majority of bodily fluids including plasma, lymph, cerebrospinal fluid, saliva and mucus. It is found in particularly high concentrations in the tear film that covers the eyes; here, it is essential to initiate lysis of bacteria which come into contact with the eyes while they are open. Lysozyme is such an effective antibacterial molecule that it is often used in wound dressings and impregnated into a variety of medical devices including meshes used in treating vaginal prolapsed and dental implants (Ferraboschi et al., 2021).

Metal binding proteins (MBPs) are also found in the plasma and other bodily fluids such as mucus and milk; as implied by their name, these function to bind to (chelate) certain free metal ions such as iron and copper which are required as co-factors for many bacterial enzymes. In this way, MBPs deprive bacteria of these essential cofactors, slowing the rate at which they can metabolise and replicate (Permyakov, 2021). As with lysozyme, MBPs can be added to wound dressings to limit and reduce infection at wound sites (Wang et al., 2022).

Lactic acid is produced by a variety of lactobacillus species which live in the female reproductive tract. These 'friendly bacteria' are essential to female reproductive health since the secretion of lactic acid ensures a low pH in the vagina of around 3.9; this makes it very difficult for potential pathogens such as the yeast *Candida albicans* and pathogenic bacteria to colonise and grow rapidly (Amabebe & Anumba, 2018). Unfortunately, the populations of lactobacilli can be depleted when antibiotics are prescribed, and this can lead to the vaginal pH tending towards neutral and thereby allow pathogens to thrive. This is observed most frequently with *C. albicans*, which can begin to replicate rapidly leading to vaginal thrush (Lin et al., 2021).

Interferons are small proteins which are produced by virally infected cells. They act as warning signals to alert healthy cells in the immediate environment so that they can adopt strategies to prevent their own infection (Negishi et al., 2018).

Cellular Defences

The leukocyte (white blood cell) populations that circulate throughout the body all originate from the red bone marrow, which functions as the organ of haematopoiesis (Knight et al., 2020). Leukocyte populations can be broadly split into granular leukocytes (three major types) and agranular leukocytes (two major types).

PIT STOP!

Review where granular and agranular leukocytes originate from.

Granular Leukocytes. *Neutrophils:* These are the most common leukocytes, accounting for 50% to 70% of the total leukocyte population. These cells are also known as polymorphonuclear leukocytes (PMNLs) because they have a distinctive multilobed nucleus which is easily recognisable under a microscope. Neutrophils function as contact phagocytes and will trap and engulf potential pathogens before killing and digesting them intracellularly (Burn et al., 2021). During the process of inflammation (see later), neutrophils can leave small blood vessels to enter areas of injury and infection; when this happens the combination of actively phagocytosing neutrophils, pathogen and tissue fluid forms the yellowish thick fluid commonly referred to as pus (Lämmermann, 2016).

Basophils: Found in relatively small numbers (1%) and the rarest leukocyte. Basophils are readily recognisable under a microscope since the entire cell is full of darkly staining granules of histamine and heparin (Shah et al., 2021). Histamine is a powerful inflammatory mediator (see the following section on inflammation) while heparin functions as one of the natural anticoagulants and helps ensure that blood does not randomly clot (Knight et al., 2020).

Eosinophils: Characterised by having a bilobed nucleus and usually easily recognisable under the microscope because they take up the orange-coloured stain eosin. Approximately 5% to 7% of leukocytes are eosinophils; these cells play an essential role in attacking and destroying parasites such as worms. Eosinophils are also regarded as being antiinflammatory cells because they generate the enzyme histaminase which breaks down histamine (Rahimi et al., 2018; Saraswathi et al., 2003).

Agranular Leukocytes. *Lymphocytes:* These are found in relatively high numbers in the blood, typically accounting for 20% to 30% of the total leukocyte population. They are also found in large numbers in lymphoid organs such as the spleen, thymus and lymph nodes. Lymphocytes are easily recognisable because almost the entire cell is filled up with a large nucleus. These cells are a cornerstone of the specific immune responses and are responsible for the generation of specific antibodies which bind to pathogens to opsonise them; this process effectively labels pathogens for destruction by phagocytic leukocytes (Nigam & Knight, 2020).

Monocytes: These are the largest leukocyte and are recognisable by their crescent/kidney-shaped nucleus. Monocytes tend to only remain circulating in the blood for short periods of time (1–3 days), after which they leave the blood vessels and enter many of the solid organs and tissues. These emigrated cells wander around the interstitial spaces (gaps between cells) and gradually enlarge to form much larger cells termed 'wandering macrophages'. Both monocytes and macrophages are highly phagocytic and because of their size have the ability of trapping and killing large numbers of pathogens. Some wandering macrophages eventually anchor themselves within their tissues, becoming fixed macrophages. When macrophages trap and kill pathogens, they release a cocktail of chemical signals called cytokines which help to up-regulate, modulate and fine-tune the immune responses (Austermann et al., 2022). A key cytokine released by macrophages is interleukin 1 (IL-1); this is also referred to as endogenous pyrogen because it initiates a fever response (pyrexia). Macrophages normally release IL-1 when encountering pathogens such as bacteria and viruses; IL-1 circulates in the blood before initiating the release of prostaglandins from the hypothalamus (Goyal et al., 2020). This initiates a resetting of the set point within the hypothalamic thermoregulatory centre, leading to an increase in body temperature. During a typical fever response, the core temperature may rise from 37°C to between 38°C and 40°C and occasionally higher. Pyrexia is a useful response since most bacteria that infect humans replicate optimally at around 37°C; the increase in temperature reduces the rate at which bacterial enzymes function, slowing the rate of bacterial replication. Phagocytic leukocytes involved in pathogen destruction function more efficiently during a fever response (Evans et al., 2015); this slowing of pathogen replication and enhanced pathogen killing can give the immune system the edge when battling an infection. Unfortunately, most of the enzymes that catalyse our internal biochemistry begin to slow during a fever response and some cells may even die; this usually leaves the patient feeling very unwell and lacking in energy, resulting in the characteristic malaise that is experienced with an infection-induced pyrexia (Geddes, 2020; Ogoina, 2011).

The Inflammatory Response

The inflammatory response has evolved primarily to limit the spread of infection. Inflammation can be defined as 'a normal response to, irritation, infection or injury' and most areas of inflammation are easily recognised by the presence of the five cardinal signs of inflammation (Stankov, 2011):

- redness
- swelling
- heat
- pain
- loss of function

The inflammatory response has four distinct stages.

The insult: Inflammation is usually triggered by some form of insult to the body, this could take the form of a cut, graze, burn (chemical or thermal), irritant or infectious agent.

In the example in Fig. 8.1, we look at a foreign object such as a splinter or rusty nail puncturing the skin and introducing bacteria.

Vascular stage: All objects in the environment are covered by surface microorganisms, and the rusty nail puncturing the skin in Fig. 8.1 will breach the mechanical barrier of the keratinised epidermis, introducing these together with any skin-borne microorganisms in the locality of the wound. Bacteria introduced into the lower (dermal) layer of the skin are now in a very favourable environment which is warm, rich in nutrients and oxygen; this usually results in rapid bacterial replication. In such conditions, bacteria could double in numbers every 30 minutes or so, with exponential growth of bacterial numbers eventually allowing more widespread infection; indeed, if bacteria enter

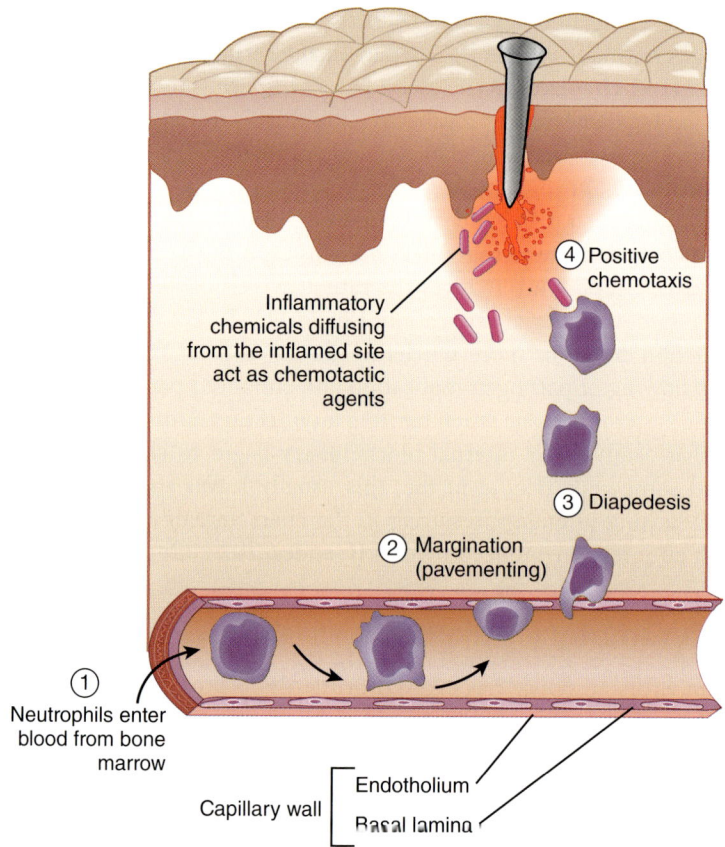

Fig. 8.1   Acute inflammatory response following a foreign object puncturing the skin.

the blood vessels, systemic infection leading to septicaemia and potentially sepsis and septic shock is possible. However, an effective inflammatory response can quickly deal with the infection at an early stage before more widespread infection can occur.

Within the dermis of the skin, and indeed within most of our solid organs and tissues, are large numbers of mast cells which act to trigger the inflammatory response (González & Alvarez-Twose, 2018). Mast cells are very similar in nature to the basophils circulating in our blood; their primary role is to generate the inflammatory mediator histamine and to store this as dark staining granules (Fig. 8.2A).

When the skin is damaged by the penetration of the rusty nail, cells are damaged, and their cell membranes disrupted. Damaged human tissue releases a variety of internal cellular components into the local environment, including histone proteins (from the nucleus), and organelles such as mitochondria and a variety of cytoplasmic molecules. Since these are all indicative of cellular damage, they are referred to as damage-associated

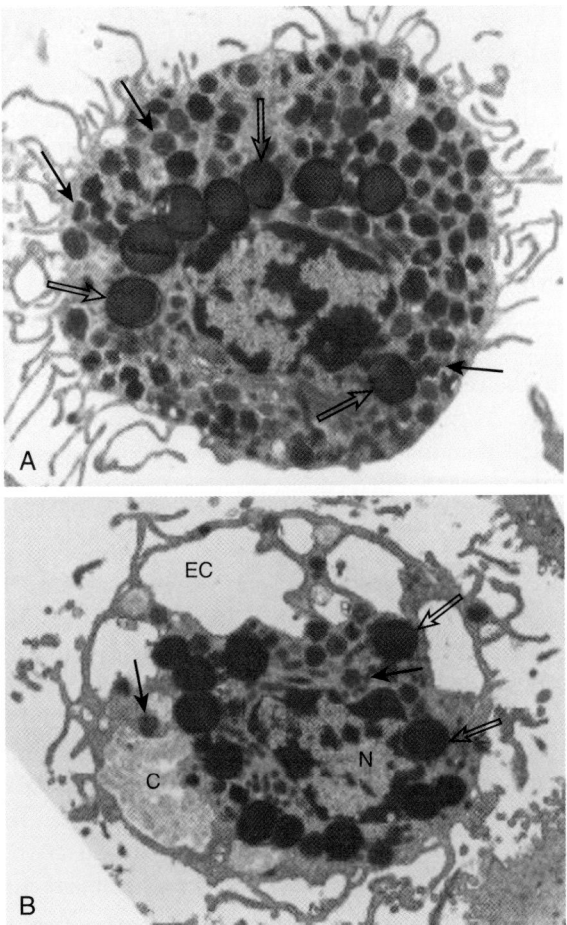

Fig. 8.2 Mast cells and Mast cell degranulation. (A) Intact mast cell (B) Mast cell following degranulation; histamine granules released into local environment. *(From Galli, S. J., Dvorak, A. M., & Dvorak, H. F. (1984). Basophils and mast cells: Morphologic insights into their biology, secretory patterns, and function. Progress in Allergy, 34, 1–141. Reproduced with permission from S. Karger AG, Basel.)*

molecular patterns (DAMPs). Additionally, the bacteria introduced by the rusty nail have their own distinctive molecules such as bacterial DNA, bacterial lipopolysaccharide (LPS) and a variety of toxins; these are referred to as pathogen-associated molecular patterns (PAMPs). Unsurprisingly, immune cells, including resident mast cells, have evolved to become highly adept at recognising the PAMPs and DAMPs present within wound sites (Agier et al., 2018) and respond by degranulating and releasing their histamine into the local environment (see Fig. 8.2B). Histamine is a powerful vasodilator and binds to receptors in the smooth muscle layer of blood vessels to induce relaxation and vessel dilation (Thangam et al., 2018). Histamine is primarily responsible for the redness and the heat seen at sites of inflammation. The effects of histamine can easily be demonstrated on yourself by gently slapping the inside of your forearm. Within a couple of minutes, the resident mast cells will release their histamine and the slapped area will appear red and warm to the touch as the local blood vessels dilate. Histamine also increases vascular permeability (Ashina et al., 2015); this effect may be enhanced in the presence of other inflammatory mediators and pathogens (Morsing et al., 2020; Wautier & Wautier, 2022). With increased vessel permeability, fluid can leak into the inflamed area, resulting in swelling at the injured site. The formation of inflammatory exudate means that the blood flowing through the small blood vessels at the injured site becomes more viscous and the rate of blood flow slows, allowing phagocytic leukocytes, particularly neutrophils, to make contact with and adhere to the vessel lining (see Fig. 8.1).

The cellular stage: As neutrophils attach, they begin to flatten and elongate by a process termed 'margination' (also known as pavementing). Eventually, these cells begin the process of diapedesis, whereby they gradually squeeze through the tiny pores of local capillary walls and enter the general location of the injury (Norris, 2018). Other mediators of inflammation produced act as chemotactic agents; the group of lipid mediators termed 'leukotrienes' are particularly important in this role. Leukotrienes and other chemotactic agents are produced by the physically damaged tissues and diffuse through the local tissues setting up a concentration gradient (Ellett et al., 2022). In Fig. 8.1, these chemotactic molecules are represented by the tiny pink dots close to the point where the nail is puncturing the skin. The neutrophils then begin to migrate up this concentration gradient and eventually make contact with the bacteria that have been introduced at the wound site. These are quickly phagocytosed and killed intracellularly, limiting the infection to the local area (Burn et al., 2021). This injury site will often accumulate a small amount of pus, highlighting that these events have taken place; this is often seen when we accidently get a wooden splinter in our skin (perhaps when gardening) and subsequently remove it with tweezers.

The pain experienced at sites of inflammation is produced as a result of direct stimulation of pain receptors (nociceptors) in the wound site and via the action of inflammatory mediators. Prostaglandins in particular are known to interact with sensory nerve endings, making them even more sensitive to painful stimuli (Baral et al., 2019), for example, the nail puncturing the skin in Fig. 8.1.

Resolution: This is the final stage of the inflammatory response and usually involves the complete removal of pathogens and damaged human cells from the site of injury and the subsequent initiation of wound healing. Gradually, the concentration of inflammatory mediators at the wound site decreases and the sign of inflammation subsides. Cells called fibroblasts are activated and begin to generate the collagen and elastin fibres forming scar tissue (Alfaro et al., 2022). In a healthy person, following resolution and wound healing, the wound site may be undetectable, or it may be marked by the presence of a white scar formed from the deposition of collagen; in most cases, any scar will itself fade over time.

Inflammatory conditions are usually denoted by the suffix 'itis'; there is a multitude of these routinely encountered in clinical practice, including appendicitis, tonsillitis, bronchitis, conjunctivitis, sinusitis and laryngitis as some examples.

Acute and Chronic Inflammation

The example of a nail puncturing the skin that we have examined is a classic example of acute inflammation, and these types of injuries and associated infection usually resolve quickly within days or weeks. Sometimes, inflammatory reactions may become chronic and persist for months, years or even for the rest of a person's life. Common chronic inflammatory conditions include chronic obstructive pulmonary disease (COPD), osteoarthritis, inflammatory bowel disorders such as Crohn's disease and autoimmune diseases such as rheumatoid arthritis and systemic lupus erythematosus (Pahwa et al., 2022). It is true to say that the vast majority of conditions encountered in clinical practice have inflammation associated with them, to varying degrees; for the remainder of this chapter, we will revisit some routinely encountered pathologies and examine the role of inflammation in their aetiologies.

The Cardiovascular System

The cardiovascular system consists of the heart and blood vessels and functions primarily as the major transport system. Every day the heart is responsible for circulating around 7200 L of blood around the body (Knight et al., 2020). From this fluid medium, cells obtain the oxygen, water and essential nutrients that allow them to carry out their designated metabolic functions. Simultaneously, waste products such as carbon dioxide, urea and uric acid are released from cells into the blood to be transported to the lungs and kidneys for elimination. We are born with arteries that are elastic and compliant, but as we age, there is a tendency for these vessels to become less compliant (Knight & Nigam, 2017b); this occurs as a result of increased collagen deposition in the vessel wall and progressive occlusion by the deposition of fatty plaque.

Atherosclerosis: The process of vessel occlusion by fatty plaque is recognised as being inflammatory in nature and is termed 'atherosclerosis'. Atherosclerotic occlusion is usually initiated by damage to the delicate inner lining of arteries. This inner lining is called the endothelium and is composed of a single layer of thin flat (squamous) cells with a thickness of around 10 microns. Many things are known to damage this fragile endothelial layer, including:

- **Smoking**: A multitude of chemicals in tobacco smoke are highly toxic (Hahad et al., 2021).
- **Hypertension:** Physical damage (Gallo et al., 2022).

■ **Hyperglycaemia**: Elevated blood glucose in undiagnosed or poorly managed patients with diabetes mellitus can osmotically damage the endothelium or lead to accumulation of advanced glycation end-products (AGEs), which are toxic (Gero, 2018).

The largest circulating leukocyte is the monocyte (see section on agranular leukocytes earlier), and these can detect DAMPs associated with endothelial damage. Monocytes attach themselves to regions of damaged endothelium and gradually begin a process of rolling (Fig. 8.3). Eventually, these monocytes migrate beneath the damaged endothelial layer and gradually enlarge and mature into macrophages. This population of macrophages actively phagocytose lipids (particularly low-density lipoprotein cholesterol) circulating in the blood; this gradually causes them to enlarge and puff up (a bit like popcorn) to form foam cells which are the major component of the fatty plaque (Jebari-Benslaiman et al., 2022). Despite being referred to as fatty plaque, this material is hard and has a consistency similar to candle wax. Atherosclerosis is therefore associated with hardening of the vessel wall and loss of elasticity and compliance (Fan & Watanabe, 2022).

Clearly, following a healthy lifestyle that avoids smoking and effectively manages any existing hypertension and diabetes can significantly slow the process of atherosclerotic occlusion. Additionally, limiting the intake of unhealthy saturated fats and monitoring cholesterol and blood lipid profiles are also of great benefit. Unfortunately, many people in developed counties have unhealthy lifestyles with low levels of exercise and diets rich in high-fat, high-glycaemic index food; this contributes to high levels of obesity. Frequently, obesity, poor glycaemic control and hypertension are found together; this collection of clinical features is often referred to as metabolic syndrome. Such patients are at particular risk of developing significant blood vessel disease (Dobrowolski et al., 2022). Atherosclerotic occlusion can affect arteries throughout the body but is often particularly apparent in the coronary arteries (coronary artery disease (CAD)), the arteries of the arms and legs (peripheral arterial disease (PAD)), the renal arteries (prerenal disease) and the carotid arteries that run up through the neck, increasing the risk of stroke; these pathologies are discussed further in the next sections.

CORONARY ARTERY DISEASE

Atherosclerotic occlusion of the coronary arteries leads to CAD. Mild to moderate occlusion may cause no observable symptoms initially, but as occlusion progresses, the active cardiac muscle cells of the myocardium are deprived of adequate oxygen, forcing them to undergo anaerobic respiration. This leads to the accumulation of lactic acid and is commonly associated with the characteristic central chest pain referred to as angina pectoris; this is usually accompanied by evidence of ischaemic changes on EGC recordings (Ford & Berry, 2020). This is usually first experienced on exertion (stable angina), but as occlusion becomes more significant, pain may be experienced when resting (unstable angina). Angina should always be investigated, and if occlusion is significant, stents may be fitted or bypass surgery recommended.

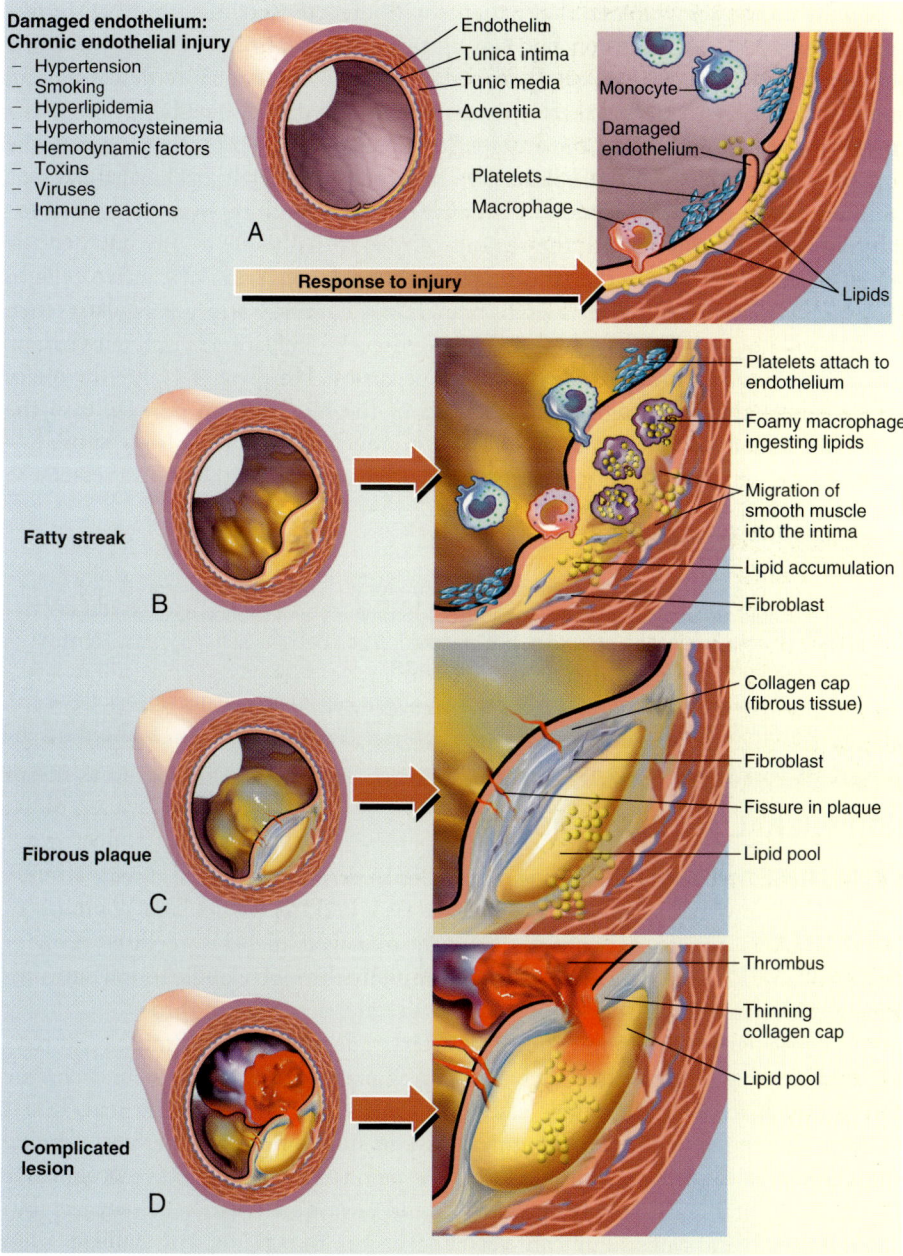

Fig. 8.3 Progression of atherosclerosis. (A) Damaged epithelium. (B) Sub endothelial monocytes/macrophages and beginnings of plaque formation) (C+D) Mature plaque and risk of plaque rupture and thrombosis *(From McCance, K. L., & Huether, S. E. (2014). Pathophysiology: The biologic basis for disease in adults and children (7th ed.). Elsevier.)*

It should also be remembered that patients with diabetes mellitus can have significant coronary artery occlusion but may not experience angina pain because their sensory nerve endings have been damaged and are no longer able to detect painful stimuli; this is often referred to as silent angina (Vigili de Kreutzenberg, 2021). The major risk with CAD is that the atherosclerotic plaque may rupture, triggering the formation of a blood clot (thrombosis). This may completely occlude the vessel, stopping blood flow to a portion of the myocardium, resulting in a myocardial infarction (MI). During an MI, the regions of myocardial tissue in proximity to the occluded vessels begin to die (the infarction) and larger areas of cardiac cells in the vicinity may be injured. If a small branch of a coronary artery is blocked, then the MI will not usually prove fatal since the coronary circulation is rich in collateral blood vessels, which can expand and restore perfusion. However, if a larger coronary artery is occluded, then significant portions of the myocardium may die and the heart can no longer function as an effective pump; this commonly leads to cardiogenic shock, which has a very high mortality (Samsky et al., 2021).

PIT STOP!

Acute coronary syndrome (ACS) is the umbrella term for an ST elevation MI, non-ST elevation MI and unstable angina. The underlying pathological process is atherosclerosis and chest pain might be the presenting symptom, but as noted, those patients suffering with diabetes mellitus might not experience chest pain with an ACS.

Review the clinical guidelines around the assessment and immediate management of a patient presenting with an ACS.

PERIPHERAL ARTERIAL DISEASE

Occlusion of arteries in the limbs is referred to as peripheral arterial disease (PAD), previously known as peripheral vascular disease. PAD is particularly common in heavy smokers and in patients with poorly managed diabetes mellitus (Gul & Janzer, 2023). PAD usually manifests itself initially through claudication (Latin for limping). Atherosclerotic occlusion of the major arteries that run through the lower limbs, particularly the femoral and tibial arteries, deprives the calf muscles of oxygenated blood and nutrients. As a result, during periods of exercise, the muscles are forced into anaerobic respiration, leading to the accumulation of lactic acid. This is associated with pain and the patient may have to stop periodically, perhaps rubbing the affected calf muscle or muscles, until the pain subsides, and they can continue (Spannbauer et al., 2019). Claudication should always be taken very seriously because it usually indicates significant vessel occlusion. In patients with diabetes mellitus, PAD may result in particularly poor blood flow to the feet, leading to a combination of clinical features commonly referred to as 'the diabetic foot'. Initially, the foot may show minor symptoms such as feeling cold due to poor blood flow; as PAD progresses, blood flow to the metabolically active nerves of the legs is restricted, leading to endoneural hypoxia, which may cause both sensory and autonomic peripheral neuropathies (Zozulińska-Ziółkiewicz & Araszkiewicz, 2019).

PIT STOP!

PAD can often be thought of as angina in the leg, and when an occlusion occurs, this is the same process as with an MI but within the arteries of the leg.

Review the guidelines for the assessment and the investigation for a patient who might have suspected PAD.

Peripheral neuropathies usually manifest in the 'diabetic foot' as a progressive loss of sensation; this may also be occurring simultaneously in the hands due to PAD affecting the upper limbs. Indeed, peripheral neuropathies are often described as having a 'glove and stocking' distribution (Lehmann et al., 2020). Lack of sensation in the feet may increase the chances of physical injury since patients may no longer become aware of pain (Volmer-Thole & Lobmann, 2016), for example, standing on a sharp object or abrasions inflicted from poorly fitting footwear.

Autonomic neuropathy is frequently associated with damage to sympathetic nerves which innervate the eccrine sweat glands of the feet. The feet have the thickest skin found anywhere in the human body, particularly the areas around the heels and the balls of the feet. For this reason, sweat production in the feet is usually very profuse to prevent skin desiccation. In patients with peripheral neuropathies affecting the autonomic nerves, the sweat glands never receive activating action potentials and so sweat production declines; this results in the skin drying and cracking (Hillson, 2017). Simultaneously, the reduced blood flow to the skin of the foot deprives the actively dividing cells of the epidermis of oxygen and nutrients; this is associated with a slowing of cell division and a gradual thinning of the skin. For these reasons, the skin of the 'diabetic foot' is usually characterised as being thin, dry and cracked.

As we have seen earlier in this chapter, the skin is the major mechanical barrier to infection, and the thin, dry, cracked skin of the diabetic foot provides a perfect site for opportunistic infection, whilst raised blood glucose concentrations allow for rapid replication of pathogens. Skin-borne bacteria such a staphylococcus and streptococcus species are common early colonisers of the 'diabetic foot' and these tend to infect the dermal layers. The presence of PAMPs and DAMPs within the infected foot triggers an inflammatory response. Infection and inflammation of the dermal layers of the skin are referred to as cellulitis; this is commonly observed in the 'diabetic foot' as diffuse, spreading areas of redness. Excess glucose also encourages fungal infections of the foot and toenails. Fungal nail infections usually lead to discoloured and brittle nails which progressively lose their integrity and may begin to 'scroll up' to become in-growing toenails; these may grow into the skin of the toes, causing further damage and inflammation, and contribute to the formation of diabetic foot ulcers (Grennan, 2019). In patients with advanced PAD, oxygen levels in the foot may fall significantly, encouraging the proliferation of anaerobic bacteria such as clostridium species. Chronic infection and ulceration can inflict significant tissue damage and may lead to areas of gangrene and tissue necrosis that can be serious enough to necessitate amputation (Lin et al., 2020a).

The Urinary System: Dysfunction

Following numerous changes and refinement of the terminology associated with this area in recent years, dysfunction of the renal system is currently classified as follows:

- Acute kidney diseases and disorders (AKD)
- Acute kidney injury (AKI)
- Chronic kidney disease (CKD)

Despite being categorisations in their own right, there is much overlap between these disorders. While diagnosed with one categorisation, for example, it is possible for a patient to develop superimposed characteristic signs and symptoms of another, a situation with important implications for the approach to treatment (Taylor, 2023a). To support effective treatment through more accurate diagnosis, the Kidney Disease: Improving Global Outcomes (KDIGO) organisation provides the current, most widely accepted defining criteria for each categorisation (Table 8.1).

Attributed to a variety of causes, kidney dysfunction, in particular AKI, is categorised according to the nature of the primary underlying cause, described as being either prerenal, intrarenal or postrenal. Some of the more common causes of kidney dysfunction are related to changes in blood flow or pressure and the toxicity or particular use of certain medications. Where the kidneys are no longer able to effectively remove waste products and excess fluid volume from the blood, toxins accumulate within the body with various complications for the wider body systems.

A characteristic feature of intrarenal AKI is the presence of cellular damage to the kidneys. Although pre- and postrenal AKIs are not inherently associated with damage on this level, if treatment is not effective, both conditions can result in the development of cellular damage to the kidneys and therefore the development of intrarenal AKI, with additional complications (Makris and Spanou, 2016; Taylor, 2023b).

TABLE 8.1 ■ **KDIGO Criteria for Kidney Dysfunction**

Category	Defining Criteria
AKD	**For ≤3 months:** GFR: <60 mL/min per 1.73 m^2 **or** ≥35% reduction **or** SCr: >50% increase **or** indicators for kidney damage
AKI	**For ≤3 months:** SCr: >0.3 mg/dL increase in 2 days **or** >50% increase in 1 week **or** oliguria for >6 hours (<0.5 mL/kg per hour for >6 hours)
CKD	**For >3 months:** GFR: <60 mL/min per 1.73 m^2 **or** indicators for kidney damage

AKD, Acute kidney diseases and disorders; *AKI*, acute kidney injury; *CKD*, chronic kidney disease; *GFR*, glomerular filtration rate; *KDIGO*, Kidney Disease: Improving Global Outcomes; *SCr*, serum creatinine.
From Levey, A. S., Eckardt, K. U., Dorman, N. M., Christiansen, S. L., Hoorn, E. J., Ingelfinger, J. R. et al. (2020). Nomenclature for kidney function and disease: Report of a Kidney Disease: Improving Global Outcomes (KDIGO) Consensus Conference. Kidney International, 97, 1117–1129. https://doi.org/10.1016/j.kint.2020.02.010.)

THE URINARY SYSTEM, IMMUNITY AND INFLAMMATION

The urinary tract is often considered as two regions, with the upper urinary tract concerned with the kidneys and the lower urinary tract concerned with the ureters, bladder and urethra. Across these regions, a multitude of cell types are responsible for mediating the immune response of the urinary system. Within the renal interstitium and locality of the tubular epithelium and blood vessels, macrophages and dendritic cells are found (Abraham & Miao, 2015). Comprising several epithelial layers, the bladder, through its mast cells and macrophages, offers a vital early means of defence to infection of the urinary tract, with detection facilitating the recruitment of macrophages and neutrophils to the area (Abraham & Miao, 2015).

The renal tubular epithelial cells of the tubulointerstitium play an important role in acute and chronic kidney dysfunction through interaction with immune cells and the production of proinflammatory molecules (Hong et al., 2020). Protection of the renal tubular cells from damage during AKI is facilitated through the actions of the innate and adaptive immune responses, which are also involved in recovery from the condition. Monocytes, macrophages, T and B lymphocytes and neutrophils are all involved in AKI, with the T lymphocytes playing a key role in the suppression of inflammation and the remodelling and repair of tissue after AKI (Bonavia & Singbartl, 2018).

AKI has also been shown to compromise the functioning of the innate immune system, leading to increased susceptibility to infection, with dysfunction of the immune system exacerbating the condition (Singbartl & Joannidis, 2015). Additionally, increased production of cytokines from the kidneys and their reduced clearance cause a state of systemic inflammation (Singbartl & Joannidis, 2015).

A thorough understanding of the pathophysiology and, in particular, the aetiology and any characteristic signs and symptoms of the forms of kidney dysfunction leads to more timely diagnosis and treatment, and is therefore paramount in ensuring more successful patient outcomes (Taylor, 2023b).

Prerenal AKI

The causes of prerenal AKI are most commonly associated with ischaemia of the kidneys, leading to a reduced glomerular filtration rate (GFR) (the rate at which filtration is occurring within the kidneys). This resultant reduction in overall kidney function allows waste products to accumulate within the blood.

The kidneys receive approximately 25% of the cardiac output, and so are particularly susceptible to changes in blood volume or pressure, particularly where there are any sudden changes. A reduction in blood volume here can have a significant impact on overall GFR and so lead to the development of prerenal AKI (Makris & Spanou, 2016; Taylor, 2023b). However, the nephrons are only affected where a decrease in blood volume is prolonged (Kellum et al., 2021). Timely detection and initiation of treatment are essential in preventing the development of complications including acute tubular necrosis (ATN) and intrarenal AKI (Cook et al., 2022; Taylor, 2023b).

Some of the more common causes of ischaemia of the kidneys include surgery, severe trauma and sepsis (Harwood et al., 2022), as well as renal artery stenosis (RAS). RAS describes the partial or complete occlusion of one or both of the renal arteries (or their branches) supplying the kidneys. In causing decreased renal blood flow, RAS is associated with hypertension and an overall reduction in GFR and kidney function. As hypertension is known to increase the risk of stroke and MI, careful management of blood pressure should form part of the wider approach to treatment to prevent further complication.

Additionally, as a result of increased blood pressure, those with RAS are also at increased risk of developing CKD, which, unlike AKI, is irreversible. Studies have indicated that the development of CKD in those with RAS is primarily linked to the actions of lymphocytes and recruitment of phagocytic macrophages as part of the inflammatory response. Macrophages generate a range of damaging chemicals, including reactive oxygen species and a range of chemokines which serve to drive renal fibrosis (Al-Suraih & Grande, 2014).

In >90% of cases, atherosclerosis is the primary cause of RAS (see section on atherosclerosis earlier), with less common causes including fibromuscular dysplasia, compression of the renal artery and vasculitis (Gunawardena, 2021). In certain cases, the insertion of a stent into the renal artery can help reverse the hypertension associated with RAS and so serve to restore kidney function and prevent progression of the condition to CKD (Wang et al., 2016).

For those with atherosclerotic RAS (ARAS), there is also an increased tendency for atherosclerosis of other regions, with these individuals typically at increased risk of developing coronary and cerebrovascular events (Gunawardena, 2021).

Intrarenal AKI

Characterised by cellular damage of the kidneys, intrarenal AKI is mainly associated with damage of the glomerular capillaries or tubules of the nephrons. This is most often seen as a result of conditions such as nephritis, prolonged hypertension and ATN.

The most common cause of intrarenal AKI is ATN, a condition whereby ischaemia (and the resultant restricted oxygen supply) causes necrosis of the endothelial cells. The loss of nephrons which results, combined with the actions of the inflammatory response, reduces GFR and overall kidney function (Ronco et al., 2019; Taylor, 2023b). As mentioned previously, some of the common causes of ischaemia include trauma and sepsis. For ATN, the primary cause of ischaemia is the result of surgery, accounting for approximately 40% to 50% of all ATN cases (Cook et al., 2022).

Another major cause of intrarenal AKI and which presents risk of further complication is tubulointerstitial nephritis (TIN), a condition estimated to be the cause of 15% to 20% of all AKI diagnoses worldwide (Casals et al., 2023). TIN is a condition characterised by inflammatory cell infiltration of the interstitium of the kidney. Commonly drug induced (principally antimicrobials and nonsteroidal antiinflammatory drugs) or the result of infection or certain inflammatory disorders such as inflammatory bowel disease, TIN presents with nonspecific symptoms during the early stages leading to delayed diagnosis and treatment, often associated with worse outcomes (Joyce et al., 2017). Pathologically, TIN is primarily associated with infiltration of lymphocytes and eosinophils and oedema of the interstitium. Over time, these acute inflammatory responses can cause substantial impairment of GFR and overall kidney function through tubular atrophy and interstitial fibrosis, a situation that is the result of the build-up of extracellular matrix (Joyce et al., 2017).

Of additional concern in TIN, complicated by the distinct lack of clear, specific signs and symptoms, is that failure to promptly detect and treat the condition during the early stages can result in the development of CKD. During TIN, macrophages help facilitate repair of the resultant cellular damage. Over time, however, their action can also contribute to systemic inflammation and the release of fibrogenic cytokines, with tubular damage and loss of nephrons eventually bringing about significant reduction in kidney function and the development of CKD (Joyce et al., 2017).

Postrenal AKI

The causes of postrenal AKI arise from partial or complete obstruction of the urinary tract between the tubules of the kidney and the urethra. Any blockage within the urinary tract can cause increased pressure within the tubules, leading to reduced kidney function. Depending on the particular obstruction, locality and severity, a condition called hydronephrosis may result (Taylor, 2023b). Caused by the accumulation of urine within the kidney, hydronephrosis results in the kidney becoming swollen, causing an increase in pressure, which, over time, can lead to damage of the nephrons, a reduction in GFR and the development of intrarenal AKI.

Restriction of the urinary tract with reduced capacity to effectively remove urine from the body, causing an increase in intrarenal pressure, also inherently affects normal renal blood flow. This can cause a reduction in the volume of blood being filtered through the glomeruli and so further compromise GFR and overall kidney function, with the increased risk of developing intrarenal AKI (Makris & Spanou, 2016). Fundamentally associated with obstruction of the urinary tract, some of the main causes of postrenal AKI are seen as a result of urinary tract infection (UTI) and renal calculi.

UTI describes infection within any part of the urinary system. Most often the result of bacterial infection (particularly the gut bacterium, *Escherichia coli*), UTI can more rarely also be caused by fungi. They are most often seen in females due to the shorter length of the urethra, which allows relatively easier access to the bladder, particularly for motile bacteria such as *E. coli*. Where the infection reaches the bladder, cystitis is the result. Once in the bladder, the bacteria typically undergo rapid replication, with potentially greater consequence for the wider urinary system, including infection of the kidneys and pyelonephritis (Flores-Mireles et al., 2015).

Mediated by cells of the immune system found in the bladder, one of the primary ways by which the body seeks to combat cystitis is through shedding of the epithelial cells which line the wall of the bladder (Wu et al., 2020). Driving this important process capable of greatly reducing bacterial load are mast cells of the lamina propria, the thin connective layer of the bladder which separates the urothelium on the inside from the muscularis propria on the outside (Choi et al., 2016). Here, inflammasome signalling mechanisms resulting in the secretion of IL-1β by the epithelial cells cause the mast cells to secrete their granules, which, once taken up by the epithelial cells, triggers the process of cytolysis (Choi et al., 2016).

It has also been suggested that part of the reason for the shedding of epithelial cells is that it serves as a means of regulating the inflammatory response, given the negative effects that a high level of proinflammatory mediators can have (Abraham & Miao, 2015). Additionally, although a vital means by which bacterial load can be reduced, the shedding of epithelial cells increases the risk of further complication, through exposure of the lower tissue to the array of waste compounds within urine. To limit this exposure, once the cells of the upper layer have been shed, the urothelium is signalled to undergo high-level proliferation to restore the upper layer and the vital barrier role it provides (Abraham & Miao, 2015).

Besides the spread of bacterial infection, cystitis can also be caused by dysfunction of the immune system. The adaptive immune response within the bladder displays some fundamental differences from that seen of kidney infection and pyelonephritis, with cystitis inducing minimal antibody production. In contrast, kidney infections and pyelonephritis induce the production of far greater levels (Wu et al., 2020).

In pyelonephritis the epithelial cells of the urinary tract again play a crucial role, where they provide an important means of initial defence against an infection. Here, the epithelial cells secrete a range of antibacterial compounds and proinflammatory cytokines, with IL-1, IL-6 and IL-8 being some of the earliest cytokines detectable within urine. These cytokines help to facilitate the recruitment of phagocytes to the site of infection (Abraham & Miao, 2015). Another key means of defence to kidney infection is provided primarily by the epithelial cells which line the ascending limbs of the loops of Henle of the nephrons. The epithelial cells here produce a glycoprotein called uromodulin (Tamm–Horsfall protein) which binds to uropathogenic *E. coli*. This binding causes the bacteria to clump together and prevents their interaction with the surface epithelial cells. Aggregation of the bacteria in this way allows for their earlier and more effective removal in the urine (Abraham & Miao, 2015). Uromodulin has also been shown to play important roles in the overall inflammatory response through the recruitment of leukocytes and is known to inhibit the formation of calcium crystals, therefore playing a key role in preventing kidney stone formation (Immler et al., 2020).

More commonly referred to as kidney stones, renal calculi arise from the aggregation of crystals within the urinary tract. Worldwide, the majority of calculi are composed of calcium oxalate mixed with calcium phosphate (80%), while less common are those composed of struvite (10%), uric acid (9%) and cystine (1%) (Khan et al., 2016). Some of the key risk factors for the development of renal calculi are diabetes and obesity, conditions associated with increased risk of hypertension, with the potential for this to develop kidney dysfunction and wider complication (Khan et al., 2016). Renal calculi are themselves a key risk factor associated with the development of diabetes, along with cardiovascular disease, bone fractures and CKD (Stamatelou & Goldfarb, 2023).

Studies have indicated links between renal calculi and an increase in the expression of genes associated with immunity and the inflammatory response (Khan et al., 2021). Macrophages, for example, have been found to be heavily involved in renal calculi, with genes found to be associated with both formation and suppression of calculi (Thongboonkerd et al., 2021). Renal calculi inflict mechanical damage to the urinary tract, triggering inflammation. If not treated promptly, calculi can result in increased frequency of UTI, blood in the urine and partial or complete obstruction of the urinary tract, which over time can lead to intrarenal AKI and further complication (Wang et al., 2021).

PIT STOP!

As an advanced practitioner working within clinical practice, you will need to appreciate and understand the renal system even if you do not work within the renal speciality. Many drugs are renally excreted, so if a patient has renal failure, you will need to consider this factor. Likewise, there are medications that are renal toxic. You might not be a prescriber or working within renal medicine, but you might encounter the patient with abnormal renal function within your area of clinical practice.

Cerebrovascular Accident

A cerebrovascular accident (CVA) (also known as a stroke) is a clinical syndrome characterised by a sudden onset of a focal neurologic deficit that persists for at least 24 hours and results from an abnormality of the cerebral circulation (Haines & Mihailoff, 2017). Stroke is the second leading cause of death after cardiovascular disease (Vijayan & Reddy, 2016). The incidence of stroke increases with age and is higher in older men than in women (Horodinschi et al., 2019). The significant risk factors include hypertension, hypercholesterolemia, diabetes, smoking, heavy alcohol consumption and oral contraceptive use (Kuriakose & Xiao, 2020).

The main signs and symptoms observed during a stroke correlate with the brain area supplied by the affected blood vessels. There are two major categories of stroke, based on pathogenesis.

- **Ischaemic:** Caused by blockage of cerebral blood vessels by a clot or embolus
- **Haemorrhagic:** Caused by a bleed within the brain

In ischaemic stroke, vascular occlusion disrupts blood flow to a specific brain region. This produces a relatively characteristic pattern of neurological damage resulting in various degrees of loss of function in the affected region (Campbell & Khatri, 2020). Not all signs are present in every patient due to the extent of the injury and the presence or absence of collateral blood vessels. Individual variations in the vascular anatomy, blood pressure and the exact location of the occlusion can significantly affect outcomes between patients (Musuka et al., 2015). The pattern of damage and neurological deficits with cerebral haemorrhage are often less predictable and dependent upon the size of the affected blood vessel, location and extent of the bleed and also on factors such as intracranial pressure, brain oedema, compression of brain tissue and the potential of blood being released into ventricles or subarachnoid space (Kuriakose & Xiao, 2020; Mtui et al., 2015).

Several vascular, cardiac and haematologic disorders can lead to focal cerebral ischaemia. The most common is atherosclerosis of the large carotid arteries within the neck and at the base of the brain (Mtui et al., 2015). As we have previously examined, atherosclerosis is triggered by endothelial damage and results in the deposition of fatty plaque and vessel hardening. Damaged endothelial cells also provide a focal point for platelet aggregation and activation and the formation of blood clots leading to cerebral thrombosis (Neubauer & Zieger, 2022). Fatty plaque, particularly in the carotid arteries, may break away from the vessel lining resulting in fatty emboli which may block cerebral vessels (Mtui et al., 2015).

In haemorrhagic stroke, epidural and subdural haematomas can occur as a result of head injury (Hansen, 2014). Epidural haematomas arise from damage to an artery (usually the middle meningeal artery), which can be ruptured by a blow to the temporal bone (Hansen, 2014). Blood separates the dura from the skull, compressing the brain tissue below (Hansen, 2014).

Subdural haematomas generally arise from venous blood that leaks from torn cortical veins before collecting in the subdural space (Hansen, 2014). Subarachnoid haemorrhage may also occur from head trauma or from leakage of blood from another compartment into the subarachnoid space or, most commonly, from the rupturing of an arterial aneurysm (Hansen, 2014). Berry aneurysms (resembling a holly berry) most frequently occur as a result of a hereditary or genetic weakness in the walls of large vessels at the base of the brain and occur most frequently at the point where blood vessels bifurcate (D'Souza, 2015). These types of aneurysms most frequently become symptomatic in adulthood, generally after the third decade (D'Souza, 2015). The rupture suddenly increases intracranial pressure, which can interrupt cerebral blood flow. This results in loss of consciousness in half of the patients (D'Souza, 2015). With very large haemorrhages, overall cerebral ischaemia can cause severe brain damage and often result in death (D'Souza, 2015; Pohl et al., 2021). Intraparenchymal haemorrhage may occur as a result of a significant increase in blood pressure or a variety of disorders that weaken vessels (Mtui et al., 2015). This disturbs the function of surrounding brain tissue and nearby vessels causing local ischaemia. Chronic hypertension is the most common influencing factor (D'Souza, 2015).

PIT STOP!

TIAs and CVAs are common clinical pathologies that the advanced practitioner will encounter in practice. Review the current clinical guidelines for the assessment of the patient presenting with a suspected TIA or stroke including recognition of signs and symptoms and assessment tools.

Transient ischaemic attack (TIA) is associated with brain dysfunction by a regional reduction in blood flow causing either transient or minor visible clinical symptoms. Twenty percent of stroke patients display a TIA in hours to days prior to the stroke. Eighty percent of strokes after TIA are preventable; therefore, early diagnosis and treatment are crucial. TIA is mainly a clinical diagnosis and is characterised by a sudden onset of a focal neurologic deficit assumed to be on a vascular origin. The most clinical determination is that the neurologic symptoms are either focal (localised) or nonfocal (nonlocalised) (Coutts, 2017). Specific clinical features such as diabetes mellitus (Johnston et al., 2000), hypertension (Hill et al., 2004) and weakness or speech disturbances (Rothwell et al., 2005) have been associated with recurrent stroke after TIA.

Multiple Sclerosis

Myelin is a lipid-rich material that surrounds the axon of the neuron to insulate them and increase the rate of saltatory conduction (Bayram-Weston et al., 2022). Multiple sclerosis (MS) attacks the myelin sheaths of the bundle of the axons in the brain, spinal cord and optic nerves. The name is derived from the Greek word for 'hardening', which describes the lesions that develop around bundles of axons, and sclerosis is multiple because the disease attacks many sites in the nervous system at the same time (Bear et al., 2020; Reich, 2018). The importance of myelin in the normal conduction of nerve impulses is revealed in MS. Patients with MS usually complain of weakness, lack of coordination and impaired vision and speech (Halabchi et al., 2017). The disease is unpredictable, usually marked by remissions and relapses that occur over the years. The precise cause of MS is still not understood; however, the cause of sensory and motor disturbances is now quite clear. There are a few theories around different influencing factors for MS, for example, vitamin D deficiency and infection with Epstein–Barr virus (EBV), the virus that causes glandular fever (Brütting et al., 2021). Vitamin D is synthesised in the skin by conversation of 7-dehydrocholesterol to vitamin D by ultraviolet (UV) light from the sun. Research has shown that people with higher vitamin D levels are less likely to develop MS https://www.ninds.nih.gov/health-information/disorders/multiple-sclerosis. Indeed, low levels of vitamin D increase the risk of developing MS in neonates (Nielsen et al., 2017). It has been suggested that vitamin D induces T cells with immunosuppressive properties, which may have a role in preventing the auto-immune response (Murdaca et al., 2019).

EBV has long been associated with MS. It has been suggested that it activates self-reactive T and B cells, leading to autoantibody production as well as reducing the self-tolerance breakdown threshold while enabling autoreactive B cells to survive (Liu et al., 2022) Patients with MS have EBV antibody levels higher than the general population (Belbasis et al., 2015).

MS is a neuroinflammatory disease that affects myelin but also can damage the nerve cell bodies. Pathologically, the plaques are the result of an autoimmune attack on the focal areas of central nervous system (CNS) myelin. As the disease progresses, the brain's cortex tends to atrophy (shrink). Plaques can be as small as a pinhead or as large as a golf ball. The demyelination can occur at any site of CNS (Bear et al., 2020).

A genetic tendency with unknown environmental exposures is thought to trigger the immune response. MS is relatively common, especially in young adults, and can be a seriously devastating chronic disorder. The symptoms of MS generally begin over one to several days (Lassmann, 2018). Symptoms come and go in most people with MS. The presence of symptoms is called an attack or exacerbation. Recovery from symptoms is referred to as remission (Doshi & Chataway, 2016). MS is now classified into benign, relapsing-remitting (the most common form), progressive-relapsing, primary progressive and secondary progressive (Momsen et al., 2022). The first symptoms of MS often include vision problems, weakness, stiff muscles, often painful muscle spasms and tingling or numbness in the arms, legs, trunk of the body or face. Over time, difficulty staying balanced when walking, dizziness, mental fatigue, mood changes and bladder control problems can occur. The diagnosis of MS is based on the integration of clinical, imaging and laboratory findings. These diagnostic criteria, known as McDonald Criteria 2017 version, are the most widely used guidelines for MS diagnosis (Thompson et al., 2018).

A variety of immunosuppression strategies are currently used as treatment approaches, including interferon beta 1, glatiramer acetate, natalizumab, fingolimod and mitoxantrone. Glucocorticoids can be used for a sudden attack but should not be used long-term (Yamout, 2018). Although MS can cause severe disability, it is rarely fatal and most people with MS have a normal life expectancy (Thompson et al., 2018).

Our understanding of the pathophysiology of MS is derived from both findings in animal models and observations in human cases. MRI scans with patients with MS suggest that disruption of the blood–brain barrier (BBB) may be an early event in acute lesions (Liu et al., 2022). Lymphocytes are activated and adhere to the endothelial cells of the BBB and, along with inflammatory mediators and cytokines, cause the tight junctions of the BBB to relax (Liu et al., 2022). Then, activated T and B lymphocytes can enter the CNS and have distinctive actions. Activated T lymphocytes release proinflammatory cytokines such as IL-2, interferon-gamma and tumour necrosis factor. These stimulate and activate inflammatory macrophages and microglia which then attack myelin proteins, as highlighted in Fig. 8.4 (Liu et al., 2022). B lymphocytes progressively release myelin-specific antibodies which target myelin by binding to it and marking it out for destruction by the immune system (Liu et al., 2022). It has also been suggested that they also target oligodendrocytes (the major myelin-containing cells of the CNS), causing reduced numbers. As a result, infiltration of these cells across the BBB leads to inflammation, demyelination, gliosis and axonal degeneration, creating the lesions seen in MS (Liu et al., 2022).

Alzheimer Disease

Alzheimer disease (AD) is the most common cause of dementia, accounting for more than 50% of cases (two-thirds of dementia cases) (Alzheimer's Association Report, 2021; Kumar et al., 2022). It is a neurodegenerative disease that progressively

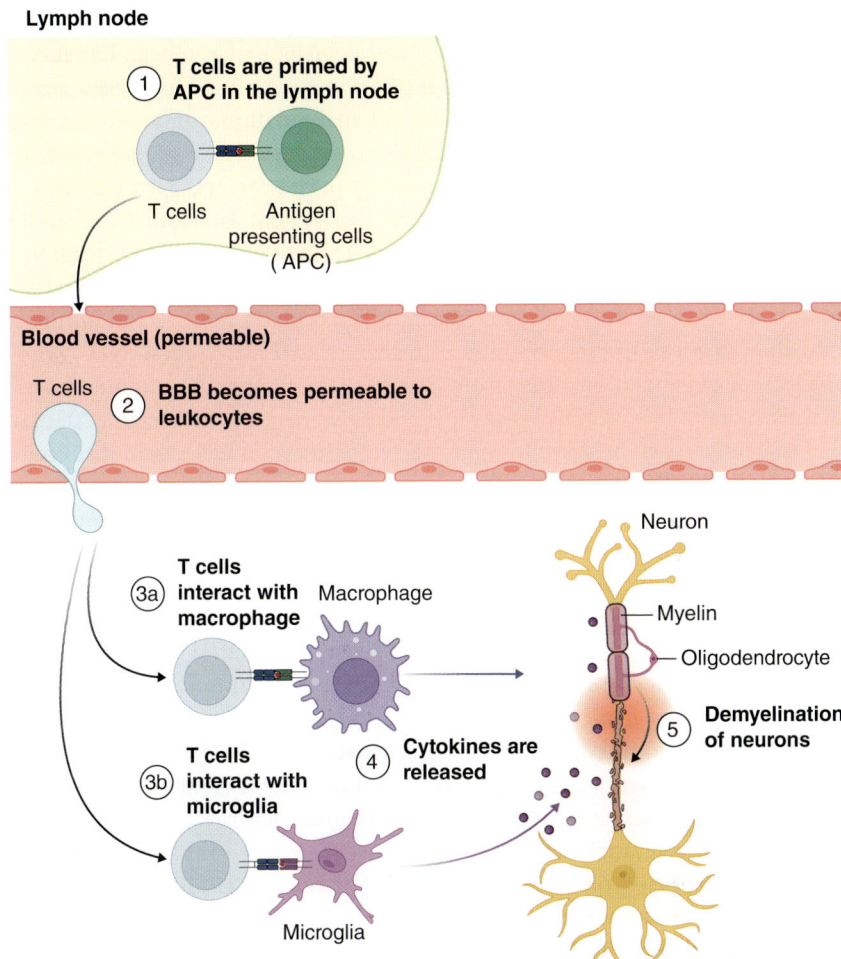

Fig. 8.4 Activated T cells in the pathogenesis of multiple sclerosis. *BBB,* Blood–brain barrier. *APC,* Antigen Presenting Cells. *(From Liu, R., Du, S., Zhao, L., Jain, S., Sahay, K., Rizvanov, A., Lezhnyova, V., Khaibullin, T., Martynova, E., Khaiboullina, S., & Baranwal, M. (2022). Autoreactive lymphocytes in multiple sclerosis: Pathogenesis and treatment target. Frontiers in Immunology, 13, 996469. https://doi.org/10.3389/fimmu.2022.996469.)*

worsens in a course of 5 to 10 years. It usually begins with impairment of learning and recent memory. Early clinical features include (Kumar et al., 2022):

- **Anomia**: The inability to remember the right words such as names of objects.
- **Aphasia**: The affected person is unable to speak, write or understand speech or writing.
- **Acalculia** (loss of the ability to accomplish simple calculation) ultimately develops, causing loss of employability and managing finances.

Spatial disorientation causes patients to become lost easily, and many patients progressively find they have problems performing simple daily tasks such as cooking, cleaning and self-care such as tying shoelaces and buttoning a shirt (Alzheimer's

Association Report, 2021). In its later stages, social skills are lost and psychiatric symptoms such as paranoia, hallucinations and delusions may appear. Patients with end-stage AD will require 24-hour care. Severe dementia often causes complications such as immobility, swallowing disorders and malnutrition, ultimately leading to death (Alzheimer's Association Report, 2021).

MRI brain scans usually reveal severe atrophy of the cerebral cortex with widening of the sulci and enlargement of the ventricular system. In addition, other structures including the amygdala, olfactory bulb tract, cingulate gyrus and thalamus are affected in AD (Chandra et al., 2019). MRI images have shown that the medial temporal lobe areas are most severely affected. The primary sensory and motor areas and the upper regions of the prefrontal cortex are relatively well preserved. Although the pattern of degeneration varies from case to case, it generally commences in the medial temporal lobe and travels upwards and forwards (Chandra et al., 2019).

AD is characterised by disruption of the cytoskeleton (a collection of supporting filaments within cells) structure within the neurons of the cerebral cortex which are vital for cognitive function (Adav & Sze, 2016). AD's underlying brain pathology was first described in 1907 by the German physician Alois Alzheimer in his paper titled 'A Characteristic Disease of the Cerebral Cortex'. Alzheimer examined the patient's brain under the microscope, and he made particular note of changes in the 'neurofibrils' elements of the cytoskeleton (Selkoe, 2004). The severity of the dementia in AD is well correlated with the number and distribution of what are now commonly known as neurofibrillary tangles. It is now understood that these filaments consist of the microtubule-associated protein *tau*. In AD, the tau detaches from the microtubes and accumulates in the soma. This disruption of cytoskeleton causes the axons to weaken, thus threatening the normal flow of nerve impulse in the affected neurons (Adav & Sze, 2016; Bear et al., 2020; Kumar et al., 2022).

Attention is focused on another protein that accumulates in the brain of AD patients called *amyloid* (Greek *amylon*, starch; *eidos*, resemblance). We know today that the abnormal deposition of amyloid is the first step in the process that leads to neurofibrillary tangle formation and dementia (Bear et al., 2020). In general, all pathological changes observed in AD are most prominent in the hippocampus, cortex and forebrain. Hippocampus is a part of the limbic system and crucial for learning and memory (Rao et al., 2022). The subregion of the hippocampus is responsible for memory formation, especially episodic memory, a type of long-term memory that involves conscious collection of previous experiences (Knierim, 2015). An early study has shown that the neuropathological abnormality in AD includes neuronal loss and gliosis at the hippocampus (Ball et al., 1985). Therefore, amyloid beta peptide (Aβ) deposition in these brain regions has been associated with cognitive decline and memory function (Hampel et al., 2021). The current therapeutic intervention is focused on strategies to reduce the deposition of amyloid in the brain. It has been suggested that the deposition of amyloid weakens the walls of small cortical vessels and causes lobar haemorrhages, often affecting several sites (Raman et al., 2016). In addition, some studies have shown that activated microglia (immune cells in the brain, brain-resident macrophages) are accumulated and surround Aβ plaques. This migration and activated microglia response to Aβ plaques leads to phagocytosis of Aβ, however, as microglia clean up Aβ fibres, and this event is followed by microglial cell death. When microglial cells are dying, they release their content including Aβ fibres into the extracellular space and contribute to Aβ plaque growth (Baik et al., 2016). Apart from microglia, astrocytes (glial cells of the CNS responsible for maintaining CNS integrity, forming the BBB, house-keeping functions that promote neuronal well-being) are major contributors in the neuroinflammation (Medeiros & LaFerla, 2013; Preman et al., 2021). In AD, these immune cells become progressively dysfunctional in regulating metabolic and immunoregulatory pathways, thus promoting chronic inflammation.

Conclusion

In this chapter, we have highlighted the importance of a detailed grasp of key aspects of anatomy and physiology for advanced practice. Knowledge of these areas of bioscience is usually initially gained when studying for professional qualifications at the undergraduate level. It is then continually built upon as the healthcare worker's career develops and a greater diversity of patients and their needs are encountered. Inflammation is a common theme present in most pathological conditions, and in this chapter, we have explored the role of inflammation in a variety of diverse diseases and medical conditions.

References

Abraham, S. N., & Miao, Y. (2015). The nature of immune responses to urinary tract infections. *Nature Reviews Immunology*, *15*, 663. https://doi.org/10.1038/NRI3887

Adav, S. S., & Sze, S. K. (2016). Insight of brain degenerative protein modifications in the pathology of neurodegeneration and dementia by proteomic profiling. *Molecular Brain*, *9*(1), 92. https://doi.org/10.1186/s13041-016-0272-9

Agier, J., Pastwińska, J., & Brzezińska-Błaszczyk, E. (2018). An overview of mast cell pattern recognition receptors. *Inflammation Research*, *67*(9), 737–746.

Alfaro, S., Acuña, V., Ceriani, R., Cavieres, M. F., Weinstein-Oppenheimer, C. R., & Campos-Estrada, C. (2022). Involvement of inflammation and its resolution in disease and therapeutics. *International Journal of Molecular Sciences*, *23*(18), 10719. doi:10.3390/ijms231810719

Al-Suraih, M., Grande, J. P. (2014). Management of renal artery stenosis: What does the experimental evidence tell us? *World Journal of Cardiology*, *6*, 860. https://doi.org/10.4330/WJC.V6.I8.855

Alzheimer's Association Report. (2021). Alzheimer's disease facts and figures. *Alzheimer's & Dementia: The Journal of the Alzheimer's Association*, *17*(3), 327–406. https://doi.org/10.1002/alz.12328

Amabebe, E., & Anumba, D. O. C. (2018). The vaginal microenvironment: The physiologic role of lactobacilli. *Frontiers in Medicine*, *13*(5), 181. doi:10.3389/fmed.2018.00181

Ansari, S., & Yamaoka, Y. (2017). Survival of *Helicobacter pylori* in gastric acidic territory. *Helicobacter*, *22*(4), 10.1111/hel.12386. doi:10.1111/hel.12386

Ashina, K., Tsubosaka, Y., Nakamura, T., Omori, K., Kobayashi, K., Hori, M., Ozaki, H., & Murata, T. (2015). Histamine induces vascular hyperpermeability by increasing blood flow and endothelial barrier disruption in vivo. *PLoS One*, *10*(7), e0132367. doi:10.1371/journal.pone.0132367

Auala, T., Zavale, B. G., Mbakwem, A. Ç., Mocumbi, A. O. (2022). Acute rheumatic fever and rheumatic heart disease: Highlighting the role of group A Streptococcus in the global burden of cardiovascular disease. *Pathogens*, *11*(5), 496. http://dx.doi.org/10.3390/pathogens11050496

Austermann, J., Roth, J., & Barczyk-Kahlert, K. (2022). The good and the bad: Monocytes' and macrophages' diverse functions in inflammation. *Cells*, *11*(12), 1979. doi:10.3390/cells11121979

Baik, S. H., Kang, S., Son, S. M., & Mook-Jung, I. (2016). Microglia contributes to plaque growth by cell death due to uptake of amyloid β in the brain of Alzheimer's disease mouse model. *Glia, 64*(12), 2274–2290. https://doi.org/10.1002/glia.23074

Ball, M. J., Fisman, M., Hachinski, V., Blume, W., Fox, A., Kral, V. A., Kirshen, A. J., Fox, H., & Merskey, H. (1985). A new definition of Alzheimer's disease: A hippocampal dementia. *Lancet* (London, England), *1*(8419), 14–16. https://doi.org/10.1016/s0140-6736(85)90965-1

Banafea, G. H., Bakhashab, S., Alshaibi, H. F., Pushparaj, P. M., & Rasool, M. (2022). The role of human mast cells in allergy and asthma. *Bioengineered, 13*(3), 7049–7064.

Baral, P., Udit, S., & Chiu, I. M. (2019). Pain and immunity: Implications for host defence. *Nature Reviews Immunology, 19*, 433–447.

Bayram-Weston, Z., Andrade-Sienz, M., & Knight, J. (2022). Nervous system 1: Introduction to the nervous system. *Nursing Times, 118*, 3.

Bear, M. E., Connor, B., & Paradiso, M. (2020). *Neuroscience: Exploring the brain.* Jones and Bartlett Publishers.

Belbasis, L., Bellou, V., Evangelou, E., Ioannidis, J. P., & Tzoulaki, I. (2015). Environmental risk factors and multiple sclerosis: An umbrella review of systematic reviews and meta-analyses. *The Lancet Neurology, 14*(3), 263–273. https://doi.org/10.1016/S1474-4422(14)70267-4

Benedetto, R., Cabrita, I., Schreiber, R., & Kunzelmann, K. (2019). TMEM16A is indispensable for basal mucus secretion in airways and intestine. *FASEB Journal, 33*(3), 4502–4512. doi:10.1096/fj.201801333RRR

Bonavia, A., & Singbartl, K. (2018). A review of the role of immune cells in acute kidney injury. *Pediatric Nephrology, 33*, 1629–1639. https://doi.org/10.1007/S00467-017-3774-5

Brütting, C., Stangl, G. I., & Staege, M. S. (2021). Vitamin D, Epstein-Barr virus, and endogenous retroviruses in multiple sclerosis – Facts and hypotheses. *Journal of Integrative Neuroscience, 20*(1), 233–238. https://doi.org/10.31083/j.jin.2021.01.392

Burn, G. L., Foti, A., Marsman, G., Patel, D. F., & Zychlinsky, A. (2021). The neutrophil. *Immunity, 54*(7), 1377–1391.

Campbell, B. C. V., & Khatri, P. (2020). Stroke. *Lancet (London, England), 396*(10244), 129–142. https://doi.org/10.1016/S0140-6736(20)31179-X

Casals, J., Acosta, Y., Caballero, G., Morantes, L., Zamora, C., Xipell, M., et al. (2023). Differentiating acute interstitial nephritis from immune checkpoint inhibitors from other causes. *Kidney International Reports, 8*, 672–675. https://doi.org/10.1016/j.ekir.2022.12.017

Chandra, A., Dervenoulas, G., & Politis, M. (2019, June). Alzheimer's Disease Neuroimaging Initiative. Magnetic resonance imaging in Alzheimer's disease and mild cognitive impairment. *Journal of Neurology, 266*(6), 1293–1302. doi:10.1007/s00415-018-9016-3

Choi, H. W., Bowen, S. E., Miao, Y., Chan, C. Y., Miao, E. A., Abrink, M., et al. (2016). Loss of bladder epithelium induced by cytolytic mast cell granules. *Immunity 45*, 1269. https://doi.org/10.1016/J.IMMUNI.2016.11.003

Coates, M., Blanchard, S., & MacLeod, A. S. (2018). Innate antimicrobial immunity in the skin: A protective barrier against bacteria, viruses, and fungi. *PLoS Pathogens, 14*(12), e1007353. doi:10.1371/journal.ppat.1007353

Cook, N., Shepherd, A., Dunleavy, S., & McCauley, C. (2022). *Essentials of pathophysiology for nursing practice* (2nd ed.). SAGE Publications Ltd.

Coutts, S. B. (2017). Diagnosis and management of transient ischemic attack. *Continuum (Minneapolis, Minn.), 23*(1, Cerebrovascular Disease), 82–92. doi:10.1212/CON.0000000000000424

Dobrowolski, P., Prejbisz, A., Kuryłowicz, A., Baska, A., Burchardt, P., Chlebus, K., et al. (2022). Metabolic syndrome – A new definition and management guidelines. *Archives of Medical Science, 18*(5), 1133–1156.

Doshi, A., & Chataway, J. (2016). Multiple sclerosis, a treatable disease. *Clinical Medicine (London, England), 16*(Suppl. 6), s53–s59. https://doi.org/10.7861/clinmedicine.16-6-s53

D'Souza, S. (2015). Aneurysmal subarachnoid hemorrhage. *Journal of Neurosurgical Anesthesiology, 27*(3), 222–240. doi:10.1097/ANA.0000000000000130

Ellett, F., Marand, A. L., & Irimia, D. (2022). Multifactorial assessment of neutrophil chemotaxis efficiency from a drop of blood. *Journal of Leukocyte Biology, 111*(6), 1175–1184.

Evans, S. S., Repasky, E. A., & Fisher, D. T. (2015). Fever and the thermal regulation of immunity: The immune system feels the heat. *Nature Reviews Immunology, 15*(6), 335–349.

Fan, J., & Watanabe, T. (2022). Atherosclerosis: Known and unknown. *Pathology International, 72*, 151–160.

Ferraboschi, P., Ciceri, S., & Grisenti, P. (2021). Applications of lysozyme, an innate immune defense factor, as an alternative antibiotic. *Antibiotics, 10,* 1534. http://dx.doi.org/10.3390/antibiotics10121534

Flores-Mireles, A. L., Walker, J. N., Caparon, M., & Hultgren, S. J. (2015). Urinary tract infections: Epidemiology, mechanisms of infection and treatment options. *Nature Reviews Microbiology, 13,* 284. https://doi.org/10.1038/NRMICRO3432

Ford, T. J., & Berry, C. (2020). Angina: Contemporary diagnosis and management. *Heart, 106,* 387–398.

Gallo, G., Volpe, M., & Savoia, C. (2022). Endothelial dysfunction in hypertension: Current concepts and clinical implications. *Frontiers in Medicine, 20*(8), 798958. doi:10.3389/fmed.2021.798958

Geddes, L. (2020). The fever paradox. *New Scientist (1971), 246*(3277), 39–41.

Gero, D. (2018). *Hyperglycemia-induced endothelial dysfunction. Endothelial dysfunction – Old concepts and new challenges.* InTech. doi:10.5772/intechopen.71433

González, D., & Alvarez-Twose, I. (2018). Mast cells as key players in allergy and inflammation. *Journal of Investigational Allergology and Clinical Immunology, 28,* 365–378.

Goyal, K., Garg, N., & Bithal, P. K. (2020). Central fever: A challenging clinical entity in neurocritical care. *Journal of Neurocritical Care, 13*(1), 19–31.

Grennan, D. (2019). Diabetic foot ulcers. *JAMA, 321*(1), 114. https://doi.org/10.1001/jama.2018.18323

Gul, F., & Janzer, S. F. (2023). Peripheral vascular disease. In *StatPearls* [Internet]. Treasure Island, FL: StatPearls Publishing. https://www.ncbi.nlm.nih.gov/books/NBK557482/

Gunawardena, T. (2021). Atherosclerotic renal artery stenosis: A review. *AORTA Journal, 9,* 99. https://doi.org/10.1055/S-0041-1730004

Hahad, O., Arnold, N., Prochaska, J. H., Panova-Noeva, M., Schulz, A., Lackner, K. J., et al. (2021). Cigarette smoking is related to endothelial dysfunction of resistance, but not conduit arteries in the general population—Results from the Gutenberg Health Study. *Frontiers in Cardiovascular Medicine, 8,* 674622. doi:10.3389/fcvm.2021.674622

Haines, D. E., & Mihailoff, G. A. (2017). *Fundamental neuroscience for basic and clinical applications* (5th ed.). Elsevier.

Halabchi, F., Alizadeh, Z., Sahraian, M. A., & Abolhasani, M. (2017). Exercise prescription for patients with multiple sclerosis; potential benefits and practical recommendations. *BMC Neurology, 17*(1), 185. https://doi.org/10.1186/s12883-017-0960-9

Hampel, H., Hardy, J., Blennow, K., Chen, C., Perry, G., Kim, S. H., et al. (2021). The amyloid-β pathway in Alzheimer's disease. *Mol Psychiatry, 26,* 5481–5503. https://doi.org/10.1038/s41380-021-01249-0.

Hansen, J. T. (2014). *Netter's clinical anatomy.* Elsevier.

Harwood, R., Bridge, J., Ressel, L., Scarfe, L., Sharkey, J., Czanner, G., et al. (2022). Murine models of renal ischemia reperfusion injury: An opportunity for refinement using noninvasive monitoring methods. *Physiological Reports, 10,* 1–11. https://doi.org/10.14814/PHY2.15211

Hill, M. D., Yiannakoulias, N., Jeerakathil, T., Tu, J. V., Svenson, L. W., & Schopflocher, D. P. (2004). The high risk of stroke immediately after transient ischemic attack: A population-based study. *Neurology, 62*(11), 2015–2020. https://doi.org/10.1212/01.wnl.0000129482.70315.2f

Hillson, R. (2017). Sweating in diabetes. *Practical Diabetes, 34,* 114–115.

Hong, S., Healy, H., & Kassianos, A. J. (2020). The emerging role of renal tubular epithelial cells in the immunological pathophysiology of lupus nephritis. *Frontiers in Immunology, 11,* 1–8. https://doi.org/10.3389/fimmu.2020.578952

Horodinschi, R. N., Stanescu, A. M. A., Bratu, O. G., Pantea Stoian, A., Radavoi, D. G., & Diaconu, C. C. (2019). Treatment with statins in elderly patients. *Medicina (Kaunas, Lithuania), 55*(11), 721. https://pubmed.ncbi.nlm.nih.gov/31671689/

Immler, R., Lange-Sperandio, B., Steffen, T., Beck, H., Rohwedder, I., Roth, J., et al. (2020). Extratubular polymerized uromodulin induces leukocyte recruitment and inflammation in vivo. *Frontiers in Immunology 11,* 1–16. https://doi.org/10.3389/fimmu.2020.588245

Jebari-Benslaiman, S., Galicia-García, U., Larrea-Sebal, A., Olaetxea, J. R., Alloza, I., Vandenbroeck, K., Benito-Vicente, A., & Martín, C. (2022). Pathophysiology of atherosclerosis. *International Journal of Molecular Sciences, 23*(6), 3346. https://doi.org/10.3390/ijms23063346

Johnston, S. C., Gress, D. R., Browner, W. S., & Sidney, S. (2000). Short-term prognosis after emergency department diagnosis of TIA. *JAMA, 284*(22), 2901–2906. https://doi.org/10.1001/jama.284.22.2901

Joyce, E., Glasner, P., Ranganathan, S., & Swiatecka-Urban, A. (2017). Tubulointerstitial nephritis: Diagnosis, treatment and monitoring. *Pediatric Nephrology, 32,* 587. https://doi.org/10.1007/S00467-016-3394-5

Kellum, J. A., Romagnani, P., Ashuntantang, G., Ronco, C., Zarbock, A., & Anders, H. J. (2021). Acute kidney injury. *Nature Reviews Disease* Primers, 7, 1–17. https://doi.org/10.1038/s41572-021-00284-z

Khan, S. R., Canales, B. K., & Dominguez-Gutierrez, P. R. (2021). Randall's plaque and calcium oxalate stone formation: Role for immunity and inflammation. *Nature Reviews Nephrology*, 17(6), 417–433. https://doi.org/10.1038/s41581-020-00392-1

Khan, S. R., Pearle, M. S., Robertson, W. G., Gambaro, G., Canales, B. K., Doizi, S., Traxer, O., & Tiselius, H.G. (2016). Kidney stones. *Nature Reviews Disease Primers*, 2, 1–50. https://doi.org/10.1038/NRDP.2016.8

Knierim J. J. (2015). The hippocampus. *Current Biology*, 25(23), R1116–R1121. https://doi.org/10.1016/j.cub.2015.10.049

Knight, J., & Nigam, Y. (2017a). Diabetes management 1: Disease types, symptoms and diagnosis. *Nursing Times*, 113(4), 40–44.

Knight, J., & Nigam, Y. (2017b). Anatomy and physiology of ageing 1: The cardiovascular system. *Nursing Times,* 113(2), 22–24.

Knight, J., Nigam, Y., & Cutter, J. (2020). *Understanding anatomy and physiology in nursing (transforming nursing practice series)*. Learning Matters SAGE.

Kumar, A., Sidhu, J., Goyal, A., & Tsao, J. W. (2022). Alzheimer disease. In *StatPearls*. StatPearls Publishing.

Kuriakose, D., & Xiao, Z. (2020). Pathophysiology and treatment of stroke: Present status and future perspectives. *International Journal of Molecular Sciences*, 21(20), 7609. https://doi.org/10.3390/ijms21207609

Lämmermann, T. (2016). In the eye of the neutrophil swarm – Navigation signals that bring neutrophils together in inflamed and infected tissues. *Journal of Leukocyte Biology*, 100(1), 55–63. doi:10.1189/jlb.1MR0915-403.

Lassmann, H. (2018). Multiple sclerosis pathology. *Cold Spring Harbor Perspectives in Medicine*, 8(3), a028936. https://doi.org/10.1101/cshperspect.a028936

Lehmann, H. C., Wunderlich, G., Fink, G. R., & Sommer, C. (2020). Diagnosis of peripheral neuropathy. *Neurological Research and Practice*, 2, 20. https://doi.org/10.1186/s42466-020-00064-2

Levey, A. S., Eckardt, K. U., Dorman, N. M., Christiansen, S. L., Hoorn, E. J., Ingelfinger, J. R., et al. (2020). Nomenclature for kidney function and disease: Report of a Kidney Disease: Improving Global Outcomes (KDIGO) Consensus Conference. *Kidney International*, 97, 1117–1129. https://doi.org/10.1016/j.kint.2020.02.010

Lin, C., Liu, J., & Sun, H. (2020a). Risk factors for lower extremity amputation in patients with diabetic foot ulcers: A meta-analysis. *PLoS One*, 15(9), e0239236. https://doi.org/10.1371/journal.pone.0239236

Lin, V. Y., Kaza, N., Birket, S. E., Kim, H., Edwards, L. J., LaFontaine, J., et al. (2020b). Excess mucus viscosity and airway dehydration impact COPD airway clearance. *European Respiratory Journal*. 55(1), 1900419. doi:10.1183/13993003.00419-2019

Lin, Y. P., Chen, W. C., Cheng, C. M., & Shen, C. J. (2021). Vaginal pH value for clinical diagnosis and treatment of common vaginitis. *Diagnostics (Basel)*, 11(11), 1996. doi:10.3390/diagnostics11111996

Liu, R., Du, S., Zhao, L., Jain, S., Sahay, K., Rizvanov, A., et al. (2022). Autoreactive lymphocytes in multiple sclerosis: Pathogenesis and treatment target. *Frontiers in Immunology*, 13, 996469. https://doi.org/10.3389/fimmu.2022.996469

Lowe, J. S., Anderson, P. G., & Anderson, S. I. (2019). *Stevens & Lowe's human histology* (5th ed.). Elsevier.

Makris, K., & Spanou, L. (2016). Acute kidney injury: Definition, pathophysiology and clinical phenotypes. *Clinical Biochemist Reviews*, 37, 98.

Medeiros, R., & LaFerla, F. M. (2013). Astrocytes: Conductors of the Alzheimer disease neuroinflammatory symphony. *Experimental Neurology*, 239, 133–138. https://doi.org/10.1016/j.expneurol.2012.10.007

Momsen, A. H., Ørtenblad, L., & Maribo, T. (2022). Effective rehabilitation interventions and participation among people with multiple sclerosis: An overview of reviews. *Annals of Physical and Rehabilitation Medicine*, 65(1), 101529. https://doi.org/10.1016/j.rehab.2021.101529

Morsing, S. K. H., Al-Mardini, C., van Stalborch, A. D., Schillemans, M., Bierings, R., Vlaar, A. P., van Buul, J. D. (2020). Double-hit-induced leukocyte extravasation driven by endothelial adherens junction destabilization. *Journal of Immunology (Baltimore, Md.: 1950)*, 205(2), 511–520.

Mtui, E., Gruener, G., & Dockery, P. (2015). *Fitzgerald's clinical neuroanatomy and neuroscience*. Elsevier.

Murdaca, G., Tonacci, A., Negrini, S., Greco, M., Borro, M., Puppo, F., & Gangemi, S. (2019). Emerging role of vitamin D in autoimmune diseases: An update on evidence and therapeutic implications. *Autoimmunity Reviews*, 18(9), 102350. https://doi.org/10.1016/j.autrev.2019.102350

Musuka, T. D., Wilton, S. B., Traboulsi, M., & Hill, M. D. (2015). Diagnosis and management of acute ischemic stroke: Speed is critical. *CMAJ: Canadian Medical Association Journal = Journal de l'Association Medicale Canadienne, 187*(12), 887–893. https://doi.org/10.1503/cmaj.140355

Negishi, H., Taniguchi, T., & Yanai, H. (2018). The interferon (IFN) class of cytokines and the IFN regulatory factor (IRF) transcription factor family. *Cold Spring Harbor Perspectives in Biology, 10*(11), a028423. doi:10.1101/cshperspect.a028423

Neubauer, K., & Zieger, B. (2022). Endothelial cells and coagulation. *Cell and Tissue Research, 387*(3), 391–398. https://doi.org/10.1007/s00441-021-03471-2

Nielsen, N. M., Munger, K. L., Koch-Henriksen, N., Hougaard, D. M., Magyari, M., Jørgensen, K. T., et. al. (2017). Neonatal vitamin D status and risk of multiple sclerosis: A population-based case-control study. *Neurology, 88*(1), 44–51. https://doi.org/10.1212/WNL.0000000000003454

Nigam, Y., & Knight, J. (2020). The lymphatic system 3: Its role in the immune system. *Nursing Times, 116*(12), 45–49.

Norris, T. L. (2018). *Porth's essentials of pathophysiology: Concepts of altered health states.* Philadelphia: Lippincott Williams & Wilkins.

O'Neil, L. M., & Jefferson, N. D. (2019). Direct visualization of laryngeal mucociliary clearance in adults. *Annals of Otology, Rhinology & Laryngology, 128*(11), 1048–1053. doi:10.1177/0003489419859376

Ogoina, D. (2011). Fever, fever patterns and diseases called 'fever' – A review. *Journal of Infection and Public Health, 4*(3), 108–124.

Pahwa, R., Goyal, A., & Jialal, I. (2022). Chronic inflammation. In *StatPearls* [Internet]. Treasure Island, FL: StatPearls Publishing. https://www.ncbi.nlm.nih.gov/books/NBK493173/

Permyakov, E. A. (2021). Metal binding proteins. *Encyclopedia, 1*(1), 261–292.

Pohl, M., Hesszenberger, D., Kapus, K., Meszaros, J., Feher, A., Varadi, I., et al. (2021). Ischemic stroke mimics: A comprehensive review. *Journal of Clinical Neuroscience: Official Journal of the Neurosurgical Society of Australasia, 93*, 174–182. https://doi.org/10.1016/j.jocn.2021.09.025

Preman, P., Alfonso-Triguero, M., Alberdi, E., Verkhratsky, A., & Arranz, A. M. (2021). Astrocytes in Alzheimer's disease: Pathological significance and molecular pathways. *Cells, 10*(3), 540. https://doi.org/10.3390/cells10030540

Rahimi, M., Mohammadzade, T., & Khanaliha, K. (2018). Eosinophils and parasitic infections. International *Journal of Enteric Pathogens, 6*, 108–112. doi:10.15171/ijep.2018.27

Raman, M. R., Kantarci, K., Murray, M. E., Jack, C. R., Jr, & Vemuri, P. (2016). Imaging markers of cerebrovascular pathologies: Pathophysiology, clinical presentation, and risk factors. *Alzheimer's & Dementia (Amsterdam, Netherlands), 5*, 5–14. https://doi.org/10.1016/j.dadm.2016.12.006

Rao, Y. L., Ganaraja, B., Murlimanju, B. V., Joy, T., Krishnamurthy, A., & Agrawal, A. (2022). Hippocampus and its involvement in Alzheimer's disease: A review. *3 Biotech, 12*(2), 55. doi:10.1007/s13205-022-03123-4

Reich, D. S., Lucchinetti, C. F., & Calabresi, P. A. (2018). Multiple sclerosis. *The New England Journal of Medicine, 378*(2), 169–180. https://doi.org/10.1056/NEJMra1401483

Ronco, C., Bellomo, R., Kellum, J. A. (2019). Acute kidney injury. *The Lancet, 394*, 1949–1964. https://doi.org/10.1016/S0140-6736(19)32563-2

Rothwell, P. M., Giles, M. F., Flossmann, E., Lovelock, C. E., Redgrave, J. N., Warlow, C. P., & Mehta, Z. (2005). A simple score (ABCD) to identify individuals at high early risk of stroke after transient ischaemic attack. *Lancet (London, England), 366*(9479), 29–36. https://doi.org/10.1016/S0140-6736(05)66702-5

Samsky, M. D., Morrow, D. A., Proudfoot, A. G., Hochman, J. S., Thiele, H., & Rao, S. V. (2021). Cardiogenic shock after acute myocardial infarction: A review. *JAMA, 326*(18), 1840–1850.

Saraswathi, T. R., Nalinkumar, S., Ranganathan, K., & Umadevi, R. (2003). Eosinophils in health and disease: An overview. *Journal of Oral and Maxillofacial Pathology, 7*(2), 31–33.

Selkoe, D. J. (2004). Cell biology of protein misfolding: The examples of Alzheimer's and Parkinson's diseases. *Nature Cell Biology, 6*(11), 1054–1061. https://doi.org/10.1038/ncb1104-1054

Shah, H., Eisenbarth, S., Tormey, C. A., Siddon, A. J. (2021). Behind the scenes with basophils: An emerging therapeutic target. *Immunotherapy Advances, 1*(1), ltab008. https://doi.org/10.1093/immadv/ltab008

Singbartl, K., & Joannidis, M., (2015). Short-term effects of acute kidney injury. *Critical Care Clinics, 31*, 751–762. https://doi.org/10.1016/J.CCC.2015.06.010

Spannbauer, A., Chwała, M., Ridan, T., Berwecki, A., Mika, P., Kulik, A., Berwecka, M., & Szewczyk, M. T. (2019). Intermittent claudication in physiotherapists' practice. *BioMed Research International, 2019*, 2470801. https://doi.org/10.1155/2019/2470801

Stamatelou, K., & Goldfarb, D. S. (2023). Epidemiology of kidney stones. *Healthcare, 11*, 1–25. https://doi.org/10.3390/healthcare11030424

Stankov, S. V. (2011). Definition of inflammation, causes of inflammation and possible anti-inflammatory strategies. *The Open Inflammation Journal, 5*, 1–9.

Taylor, J. (2023a). Renal system 2: Acute kidney injury and other types of kidney dysfunction. *Nursing Times, 119*(3), 1–6.

Taylor, J. (2023b). Renal system 3: Categorising, assessing and managing acute kidney injury. *Nursing Times, 119*(3), 1–4.

Thangam, E. B., Jemima, E. A., Singh, H., Baig, M. S., Khan, M., Mathias, C. B., Church, M. K., & Saluja R. (2018). The role of histamine and histamine receptors in mast cell-mediated allergy and inflammation: The hunt for new therapeutic targets. *Frontiers in Immunology, 9*, 1873. doi:10.3389/fimmu.2018.01873

Thompson, A. J., Baranzini, S. E., Geurts, J., Hemmer, B., & Ciccarelli, O. (2018). Multiple sclerosis. *Lancet (London, England), 391*(10130), 1622–1636. https://doi.org/10.1016/S0140-6736(18)30481-1

Thongboonkerd, V., Yasui, T., & Khan, S. R. (2021). Editorial: Immunity and inflammatory response in kidney stone disease. *Frontiers in Immunology, 12*, 1–3. https://doi.org/10.3389/FIMMU.2021.795559

van Seventer, J. M., & Hochberg, N. S. (2017). Principles of infectious diseases: Transmission, diagnosis, prevention, and control. *International Encyclopedia of Public Health*, 22–39. doi:10.1016/B978-0-12-803678-5.00516-6

Vigili de Kreutzenberg, S. (2021). Silent coronary artery disease in type 2 diabetes: A narrative review on epidemiology, risk factors, and clinical studies. *Exploration of Medicine, 2*, 1–19.

Vijayan, M., & Reddy, P. H. (2016). Stroke, vascular dementia, and Alzheimer's disease: Molecular links. *Journal of Alzheimer's Disease: JAD, 54*(2), 427–443. https://doi.org/10.3233/JAD-160527

Volmer-Thole, M., & Lobmann, R. (2016). Neuropathy and diabetic foot syndrome. *International Journal of Molecular Sciences, 17*(6), 917. https://doi.org/10.3390/ijms17060917

Wang, B., Zhao, J., Lu, W., Ma, Y., Wang, X., An, X., & Fan, Z. (2022). The preparation of lactoferrin/magnesium silicate lithium injectable hydrogel and application in promoting wound healing. *International Journal of Biological Macromolecules, 220*, 1501–1511.

Wang, W., Saad, A., Herrmann, S. M., Massat, A. E., McKusick, M. A., Misra, S., Lerman, L. O., & Textor, S. C. (2016). Changes in inflammatory biomarkers after renal revascularization in atherosclerotic renal artery stenosis. *Nephrology Dialysis Transplantation, 31*, 1437–1443. https://doi.org/10.1093/NDT/GFV448

Wang, Z., Zhang, Y., Zhang, J., Deng, Q., & Liang, H. (2021). Recent advances on the mechanisms of kidney stone formation (review). *International Journal of Molecular Medicine, 48*, 1–10. https://doi.org/10.3892/ijmm.2021.4982

Wautier, J. L., & Wautier, M. P. (2022). Vascular permeability in diseases. *International Journal of Molecular Sciences, 23*(7), 3645. https://doi.org/10.3390/ijms23073645

Wu, J., Hayes, B. W., Phoenix, C., Macias, G. S., Miao, Y., Choi, H. W., et al. (2020). A highly polarized Th2 bladder response to infection promotes epithelial repair at the expense of preventing new infections. *Nature Immunology, 21*, 683. https://doi.org/10.1038/S41590-020-0688-3

Yamout, B. I., & Alroughani, R. (2018). Multiple sclerosis. *Seminars in Neurology, 38*(2), 212–225. https://doi.org/10.1055/s-0038-1649502

Zhang, S., Xu, H., Zhang, L., & Qiao, Y., (2020). Cervical cancer: Epidemiology, risk factors and screening. *Chinese Journal of Cancer Research, 32*(6), 720–728. doi:10.21147/j.issn.1000-9604.2020.06.05

Zozulińska-Ziółkiewicz, D., & Araszkiewicz, A. (2019). Peripheral diabetic neuropathy: Better prevent than cure. *Polish Archives of Internal Medicine, 129*, 152–153.

CHAPTER 9

Introduction to Critical Writing

Helen Francis-Wenger ■ Clare Butler

CHAPTER OUTLINE

The aim of this chapter is to introduce the key concepts and skills required to develop criticality and synthesis required at master's level. With the use of pitstops, the chapter allows for the development and application of these key concepts such as literature searching, analysis and synthesis and academic writing. The chapter provides a clear step-by-step guide for those new to master's level study as well as providing a refresher for those who might have previously undertaken master's level study. An academic writing roadmap has been developed to support and guide the reading, thinking and writing stage at master's level.

Introduction

Master's level education provides you with the advanced skills, theoretical knowledge and research capabilities that are required for all elements of the four pillars of advanced practice (AP)—clinical, education, research and leadership and management. To develop this mastery, and find your own academic voice, you need to be able to read critically, think critically, analyse critically and compile critical evaluations.

This chapter is concerned with establishing the need for critical reading, thinking and writing and how this is applicable to your day-to-day work as an advanced practitioner, making it practical, influential and supportive. If you have received feedback on previous work that states 'you need to be more critical or synthesise more', it can often be unclear what is meant by this and how to achieve this. This chapter will help you understand criticality and synthesis, and developing these skills will stand you in good stead for managing complex evidence-based decisions and dealing with uncertainty in the clinical setting. Within this chapter, you will be guided through your journey towards writing critically, through a series of pitstops, using your own clinical problem in AP or academic assignment brief to illustrate where this link between critical reading, thinking and writing becomes demonstrable. At the end of the chapter, this will be unified through a 'writing roadmap' that aims to provide a structure and direction for your writing.

Criticality in AP

Stepping up to master's level study and writing can, and often does, present new challenges and expectations of ourselves and of others. Some of these expectations might be unsaid and not quantified or explicit. This is a direct demonstration of the interface between academia and critical writing and the role of the advanced practitioner. The journey takes time, and it is important that you allow yourself the time and space to improve and not to set your expectations so high initially, that it becomes unwieldy and difficult. Your critique will improve over time, and within the education setting, your tutors and lecturers will guide you and provide feedback to help you on this journey.

The role of criticality in AP must not be seen as just an academic exercise. Although the basis of master's level education, the lessons and skills learnt through this process are utterly transferable to our clinical practice, and the link between service delivery, in whatever field, is tangible to ensure that your practice as autonomous, complex decision makers is steeped in research, literature and, ultimately, facts.

As we demystify this element of AP, we will explore some fundamental elements involved in critical analysis, appraisal and writing; however, there is a significant volume of texts in existence that will bolt onto and extend your knowledge and skills further in this field.

As you enhance your skills of analysis and appraisal, you will inherently form your own unique formula to utilise these skills within your practice as an advanced practitioner. This formula will start in the world of academia but will transpose and embed itself in your practice so that the skills of critical reading, thinking and writing will lead to your own unique set of skills in critical evidence-based practice, steeped in rationale.

Critical analysis is a broad term that encompasses critical reading, critical thinking and critical writing. In our day-to-day life, the term 'critical' has a negative connotation. But in academia, it is a practice of analysing and evaluating ideas, arguments, evidence and our practice, adopting a sceptical and objective mindset.

PIT STOP!

Think about a concept of AP; this might be a clinical problem or academic assignment brief that you are facing. Use this as the basis for the pitstops you will see in the rest of this chapter as we take you through the journey towards writing critically.

Critical Reading

The first stage is critical reading, the most fundamentally important part of the process. The critical reading process starts with searching for relevant literature, and this must be approached in a systematic and structured way. Becoming familiar with accurate searching is essential to ensure a full exploration of the topic in hand.

With the advent and evolution of the internet, searching for literature often begins with an online search. Generic search engines such as Google and Google Scholar can provide an initial scope of a range of available literature, but often, this is unwieldy and provides an enormous amount of 'hits' that may or may not be relevant to your topic. It is therefore essential to use more subject-specific health and social care databases. These will often be available through your university or workplace and allow you to sift through the available relevant information. Most higher education institutes (HEIs) will have the facility and librarian support to provide detailed literature searches using the most contemporaneous and subject-specific databases.

Once you have established the subject-specific database you wish to use, you will then be prompted to use key search terms to find the plethora of research available about this topic. This is the stage at which you will need to start keeping records of the search terms you use, the Boolean operators ('OR', 'AND', 'NOT'), truncated words, variations in international spelling and the combinations of words you use. This is essential to ensure that if, in the future, you revisit this work, it is replicable.

Using an adjunct such as the PICOT acronym can also help you as you plan and to conduct effective literature searches (Aveyard et al., 2011; Stillwell et al., 2010), with the following as an example:

- **Population or problem**—The patient group/problem that you are investigating, the target of your line of enquiry.
- **Intervention or issue**—The intervention/issue you want to examine; in health, this often relates to treatments, diagnostics, therapies, experiences or perceptions.
- **Comparison, context or control**—This is the concept of comparison against another alternative/intervention/placebo (if applicable).
- **Outcome**—The desired or measurable outcome; in health, this may relate to changes in symptoms, patient experiences or quality of life.
- **Time**—The timeframe or duration over which the intervention and outcomes are being observed or measured (if applicable).

PIT STOP!

Apply PICOT to your search that you have undertaken surrounding your concept identified in the first pitstop.

Describe the Boolean operators that you have used and truncation of search terms to accurately reflect how you have undertaken your search. Remember to keep notes of all this information now and for future work, as it will be important so that you can revisit this stage of an assignment or piece of work in the future, thus making sure it is fully replicable.

Once you have completed your searches, and published work has been selected, you now need to start reading. You are 'reading' for a master's; therefore, you will be required to read widely. Much of what you read may not be used in the end product; however, no reading and learning is lost reading and learning, as it will all help formulate a structure of your arguments and will identify different uses of language and prose that may result in a shift in your mindset. This reading may inspire you; it may generate new streams of practice or research and it may ultimately cause a shift in direction of your initial thoughts and plans for your writing, and even practice.

When you begin to read, it can often be a challenge to establish what you are reading and whether it is evidence based. Evidence-based literature refers to scholarly works, often research studies that are based on rigorous empirical evidence and adhere to the principles of evidence-based practice. It is worth noting, however, that evidence-based literature can also include practice guidelines, expert consensus statements and other forms of evidence synthesis that provide recommendations for practice, based on a critical review of existing evidence. The following table should help to demystify the different types of healthcare literature you may read.

Basic research	Aims to expand knowledge and understanding in a specific field or discipline, for example, biological processes, diseases or health-related phenomena; it often takes place in laboratory settings and utilises experimental models. It does not develop an immediate solution or application but can provide a foundation for applied research and informs the development of new interventions, diagnostics or treatments.
Applied research	Aims to translate existing knowledge into practical applications to address specific clinical or healthcare challenges. It aims to improve patient care, enhance healthcare delivery or solve specific problems encountered in clinical practice. It often involves testing the effectiveness, safety or feasibility of interventions, treatments or diagnostic tools, for example, by conducting clinical trials or studying the impact of an intervention on patient outcomes. The findings from applied research are typically used to inform clinical decision-making or healthcare policy.
Practice guideline	A document that provides recommendations or guidance for healthcare professionals in making decisions about the appropriate management of patients. Practice guidelines are evidence based and are typically created by expert panels or professional organisations based on a rigorous review of the available scientific literature.
Service evaluation/ quality improvement study	A type of project that focuses on assessing and improving the quality, effectiveness and efficiency of a healthcare service. Unlike traditional research studies that aim to generate new knowledge or test hypotheses, service evaluations primarily aim to monitor, evaluate and improve existing services.
Audit	A systematic review and evaluation of clinical practices, procedures or processes within a healthcare setting. The primary purpose of an audit is to assess compliance with established standards, guidelines or protocols and identify areas for improvement in patient care, safety or service delivery.
Literature review	A critical and comprehensive summary and evaluation of existing research literature on a specific topic or research question. It involves identifying, selecting, analysing and synthesising published studies, books, articles and other relevant sources to provide an overview of the current knowledge on the subject. There are various types used in healthcare, for example, meta-analysis, narrative, systematic, scoping and integrative.

What you learn from critical techniques in reading in the academic context can be directly applied to making your own academic writing as robust as possible for other critical readers like you. The aim is to be intelligent, well informed, fair minded and ready to be convinced but expecting high standards of scholarship and clarity in what you read. Becoming a critical reader must entail becoming a discerning selector of those texts that promise, most centrally, to suit your study purposes. The internet makes it possible to access far more potentially relevant literature than you could ever read, so it is important to make effective choices about what and how much to read, and this is the first step in critical reading.

To help you decide what to read, first interrogate abstracts. Abstracts are invaluable because one of the most challenging aspects of working with the research literature is just how much of it there is. It is impossible to read every word fully just to see if it is relevant to your needs. This is where abstracts are very important when you are reading a research article; you can easily feel overwhelmed wondering if certain nuggets of information are in the text and you just missed it. Abstracts, however, give you the synopsis of the paper and therefore answer your scanning question of 'is this relevant?' You then need to decide if you go on to read more.

Wallace and Wray (2021) suggest that there are three useful reading strategies you can apply at this stage. As you get more practised, you may choose to use more than one strategy:

- **Scanning**, whereby you look through a text rapidly to locate specific sections or key words or phrases, then read these sections;
- **Skimming,** where you read quickly through sections of the text, to get a general sense of the content; or
- **Intensive reading,** whereby you carefully read every word from beginning to end.

It is important to note that these reading strategies are not mutually exclusive, and they can be combined based on your reading goals and the specific requirements of your academic tasks. For instance, you might start with scanning or skimming to quickly identify relevant texts, and then use intensive reading to thoroughly analyse and understand the selected texts in detail.

Critical reading is a dynamic process. You cannot avoid being affected by your own expectations, prejudices and previous knowledge which will shape your understanding of the literature you read. Hence, it becomes a unique and individualised process to you—the evolution of your own unique formula. When reading, we also need to realise that the authors will have prejudices, assumptions and beliefs and these too will tend to influence your understanding of a text. Therefore, a key critical reading skill is identifying the authors' underlying aims and agendas so that you can consider them in your evaluation of their work. Sometimes, you must think carefully and read between the lines to establish authors' values and aims.

Critical Thinking

The next stage is critical thinking. Critical thinking involves questioning and challenging assumptions. Critical thinkers look for evidence and for good reasons before believing something to be true, asking the most useful questions in the most productive sequence to yield a coherent and credible 'story'. Therefore, thinking critically entails asking questions and moving away from merely accepting what we read or hear 'at face value', and becoming curious and seeking to understand. By questioning assumptions, you can uncover potential limitations, biases or gaps in knowledge.

Critical thinkers consider multiple perspectives in various contexts, considering several perspectives and alternative viewpoints. Regardless of how persuasive one author is, you might feel that a single voice with a narrow focus does not carry much weight, so by considering multiple perspectives, you can gain a more comprehensive understanding of a subject and develop a more nuanced analysis.

Edward Glaser stated in 1941 that critical thinking calls for a persistent effort to examine any belief or supposed form of knowledge in the light of the evidence that supports it and the further conclusions to which it tends. In other words, Glaser emphasises the importance of 'following'—using persistence, considering an issue carefully and more than once; 'evidence'—evaluating the evidence put forward in support of the belief or viewpoint; and 'implications'—considering where the belief or viewpoint leads (Cottrell, 2013).

Wallace and Wray (2021) posit five very useful and tangible critical synopsis questions (Table 9.1) to ask yourself when reading. This will provide the critical thought required in this starting phase of a piece of academic work. We often ask these questions unknowingly and inherently, but the answers to these questions often detail the need to perform a more detailed exploration/critical appraisal of that particular piece. It is important to read with a view to identify the authors' main aims, arguments and conclusions whilst having an appreciation of the evidence they have utilised to make and draw together these arguments. All the while though, have your main aims in your thoughts about how these arguments and theories you are reading are relevant to your cause, whether it be an academic assignment or a change proposal in your field of work. Remember a key fact here—take notes while you are reading! As is often the case, as you become immersed in the literature, you may lose track of where you read a specific fact or commentary, and then have to revisit all the reading undertaken to find it again—not a productive use of your precious time. These five critical synopsis questions have been mapped onto the more detailed approach to critical writing. As will become clear, the extent to which you apply the in-depth level of engagement will vary depending on how central a given text is to what you are trying to achieve. These synoptic questions are all you

TABLE 9.1 ■ **Critical Synopsis Questions by Wallace and Wray (2021)**

Question A	Why am I reading this?
Question B	What are the authors trying to achieve in writing this?
Question C	What are the authors claiming that is relevant to my work?
Question D	How convincing are these claims, and why?
Question E	In conclusion, what use can I make of this?

need, even when you undertake a more detailed analysis. You can apply a structure for ordering your thoughts in response to any text you read. It is important, especially to begin with, that you write down your answer to each critical question rather than just thinking about them. This will help you develop a critical synopsis of each piece of literature that you are evaluating, in preparation for the writing stage. This will form part of the 'writing roadmap' that we will visit at the end of this chapter.

PIT STOP!

Provide answers to the five critical synopsis questions posed earlier to your reading. Be as detailed as you can as this will help define your critical thinking, identify your questioning and start challenging assumptions.

This may form the basis to your argument or themes for your critical writing.

As you become more practised, the critical thinking stage often happens inherently in the critical reading process. As you are progressing into the realms of AP, this is something that will be intrinsically entwined in your day-to-day job, not only from the patient-facing clinical perspective but also aligned to all four pillars of AP.

Critical Appraisal

Part of the role of becoming a critical thinker is to evaluate the quality, validity and relevance of the research studies or evidence that you have read. This is when we undertake critical appraisal; this skill is challenging at first, but there are several frameworks that can support you through this systematic process. Critical appraisal is part of the critical analysis process that specifically refers to the evaluation of research studies or evidence within an academic or scientific context. The primary purpose of critical appraisal is to evaluate the internal validity and methodological rigour of a study, as well as its external validity or generalisability to other settings or populations. Critical appraisal helps you as an advanced practitioner make informed judgements about the trustworthiness and applicability of research findings, relevant to your practice.

Herein lie the skills and process of carefully and systematically assessing the literature you have sourced through the stages mentioned earlier. This stage can only commence once you have located such evidence through a search, read widely, analysed and deemed the evidence to be appropriate enough for inclusion.

In existence are a plethora of different tools that you can use to fully interrogate and appraise the literature in front of you. These may be broken down to help you explore and evaluate systematic reviews, randomised control trials (RCTs), qualitative or quantitative research or other forms of evidence that met your search strategy. One key seminal tool is the CASP (Critical Appraisal Skills Programme, 2023) framework and is available at www.casp-uk.net for you to apply to your reading. This facilitates that intimate knowledge that you need to achieve of the research and will help formulate your arguments in preparation for your writing stage.

When conducting a critical appraisal, several key aspects of a study are typically interrogated. The goal here is to systematically assess the outcome of the scientific research or evidence and to assess it for trustworthiness, relevance, value and appropriateness:

- **Study design**—The type of study design used is assessed to determine its appropriateness for answering the research question.
- **Sample size and sampling**—The adequacy of the sample size and the process of participant selection are assessed to ensure that the study has sufficient statistical power and representative participants.
- **Data collection**—The methods used to collect data, such as surveys, interviews or observations, are evaluated to assess their appropriateness, reliability and validity.
- **Data analysis**—The statistical analyses performed on the data are assessed to determine if they are appropriate and accurately applied.
- **Internal validity**—The internal validity of a study refers to the degree to which the study design and execution minimise bias and confounding factors.
- **Results and discussion**—The presentation and interpretation of the results are examined to determine if they are transparent, coherent and logically connected to the research question.
- **Strengths and limitations**—The strengths and limitations of the study are identified and evaluated, for example, potential sources of bias, confounding factors, limitations in the study design and potential implications for the validity and generalisability of the findings.

PIT STOP!

Using the link to the Critical Appraisal Skills Programme, www.casp-uk.net, apply the checklist that is most applicable for one of the sources of literature you have read. Work through the checklist, making notes as this will provide you with a record of your decision-making which is important in ensuring your work is replicable and easy to audit.

The checklists are designed to support you in a systematic manner to ensure that you take all important factors into account as well as making your approach consistent due to using a framework.

We have discussed the use of critical questioning applied to our reading and thinking broadly and taken this to a narrower focus of appraisal that specifically pertains to the evaluation of research studies, articles or evidence. Now, you are at the stage to conduct a full critical analysis, including appraisal. Wallace and Wray (2021) define 10 critical analysis questions that build on the five synopsis questions, but in greater detail, as captured in Table 9.2.

Using a structure such as this is imperative to help your analysis of the text in front of you. This comprehensive and structured exploration and evaluation of your chosen texts will allow you to become exceedingly familiar with your texts and will form and inform the basis of your writing.

TABLE 9.2 ■ 10 Critical Analysis Questions by Wallace and Wray (2021)

	Critical Synopsis Question	Associated Critical Analysis Questions
	Exploration	
Question A	Why am I reading this?	1. What review questions am I asking of this text?
Question B	What are the authors trying to achieve in writing this?	2. How and why are the authors making this contribution?
Question C	What are the authors claiming that is relevant to my work?	3. What is being claimed that is relevant to answering my review question?
		4. How certain and generalised are the authors' claims?
	Evaluation	
Question D	How convincing are these claims, and why?	5. How adequate is the backing for these claims?
		6. How effectively does any theoretical orientation link with these claims?
		7. To what extent does any value stance adopted affect these claims?
Question E	In conclusion, what use can I make of this?	8. To what extent are claims supported or challenged by other's' work?
		9. To what extent are claims consistent with my experience?
		10. What is my summary evaluation of the text in relation to my review question?

Creating this takes a lot of time and effort, but as you become more practised, this will come naturally, and you will analyse and appraise the literature you are reading without necessarily writing each step down.

> **PIT STOP!**
>
> Moving on from the synoptic questions and critical appraisal, try answering the 10 questions given previously to provide you with a robust critical appraisal of the work you have been reading. You can then use this as a basis for your critical summary.

Synthesis

Synthesis is often what differentiates master's level from undergraduate level, going beyond a mere compilation of information. Pivotal in AP, synthesis ultimately allows the formulation of recommendations for practice based on the literature and allows the writer to answer the question 'what does the research evidence tell me about the issue, for my own practice?' It is essential to think about synthesis from the beginning of your planning stage and construct your arguments early, grouping together themes and lines of enquiry so that you begin to form a 'roadmap' provisionally of the direction of your writing. We will visit this in the 'writing roadmap' later in this chapter.

Synthesising demonstrates the breadth of your reading on that topic, again emphasising the point that you are 'reading for your master's'. It demonstrates your understanding of how certain topics and arguments are linked, but it also includes differences and distinctions, to support you own interpretations, as this shows how you have read widely in a nuanced way. Finding your own academic voice is essential in this stage. Do not be afraid to draw upon your personal and unique viewpoints to give you a greater level of engagement with what you are reading. When your own views align with or contrast to what you are reading, it relates to your field and makes it 'real' with regard to how your own practice and experiences might provide a unique and distinct perspective linking your thoughts to the scholarship in that field. Having an academic voice demonstrates your deeper questioning and criticality in your approach to what you read and how you have analysed it.

Synthesis is broadly undertaken in the following stages:

- **Identifying themes or patterns**—Based on the analysis of the sources, common themes, patterns or relationships are identified that emerge across the research and evidence base that was explored.
- **Organising the evidence**—Your aim is to combine ideas from a range of sources in order to group together related information or ideas into subtopics, identifying key concepts or theories or establishing connections and relationships between different ideas or arguments.
- **Making connections and drawing conclusions**—Next, you connect the synthesised evidence to form a coherent argument or conclusion. Consider how the various sources or ideas relate to each other and contribute to a deeper understanding of the topic. Here, you can also highlight gaps or unresolved issues in the literature, develop recommendations and connect your practice to the research.
- **Integrating with your own views**—Here, you integrate the synthesised information with your own analysis, interpretation or perspective. You can present your own informed viewpoint and support it with evidence from the literature.

PIT STOP!

What does the literature that you have appraised tell you about the concept of AP you have identified and raised from the first pitstop in this chapter? Does it provide clarity? Does it provide a deeper level of understanding? Does it provide conflicting thoughts? How does this relate to other work? How does it relate to practice?

Critical Writing

Writing is not a linear process, rather an ongoing process that involves editing as you read critically and widely. Some initial key messages to hold are:

- Do not be scared!
- Hold your own thoughts to take from the research into practice. There will always be a practical value to your reading and critical thoughts, and this

process should not be seen as just an academic exercise for assignments. The implications of this process are real and tangible for your ongoing careers.

- Have confidence and belief that it is okay if you do not initially understand what you are reading or the purpose of the exercise is not clear.

Before you begin writing, and during your search, reading phase and appraisal, you will have used keywords and kept notes. You may have also prepared a critical synopsis of the papers you have read, or your critical appraisal. These notes will inform your critical writing, describing, evaluating and offering informed judgements about the theories, research or texts you have read. In your writing, like your critical thinking, you will question assumptions, and consider alternative viewpoints, drawing on the breadth of literature you have explored presenting both supporting and opposing literature.

A key aspect of critical writing is the development of an argument that is supported by evidence and logical reasoning. During the planning phase, you would have thought about how you can group points and arguments together to support or develop your own ideas. When synthesising these arguments, you will construct your paragraphs in ways that draw out the main point or theme, from your reading and analysis. The 'writing roadmap' at the end of the chapter will help further support this direction and structure. This helps assemble your arguments with evidence from multiple references, and the synthesis is the collaboration of these ideas in a way that presents your own views supported by the literature.

PIT STOP!

Now try and write a paragraph from your critical reading and thinking about the concept of AP you have identified and raised in the first pitstop of this chapter.

It is important when starting to write that you make it clear what you aim to cover and use appropriate language. Sword (2012) deems this to be 'stylish' writing that contains the following:

- Express complex ideas clearly and precisely.
- Use elegant, carefully crafted sentences.
- Convey energy, commitment and passion.
- Engage and hold the attention of the reader.
- Tell a story.
- Avoid jargon if possible.
- Write with originality, imagination and creativity.

When faced with an academic assignment or piece of critical writing, it is often too easy to use overcomplicated language to make it sound more critical. A good piece of academic and critical writing is one that flows, is easy to read and is well structured. Some key pointers here are to keep prose academic, in a formal tone. Avoid colloquialisms (quote—'the NHS is on its knees'; well, actually, the NHS does not have knees!), slang or contractions such as 'don't' and 'can't'. Aim for precise and concise writing and consider your sentence length; ideally, this should be no longer than three lines approximately. Consider your use of connector words; these are words that draw and link sentences together and can be used successfully to build up your analysis and its valuation, thereby increasing your synthesis of the literature into your work. Avoid informal vocabulary, and as you read around your subject, look at how the authors have used language in that field of work. A useful resource here is the Manchester Academic Phrasebank (https://www.phrasebank. manchester.ac.uk), and this will help meet these pointers and allow you to find your academic voice (The University of Manchester, 2023).

The goal to make critical writing pertinent, useful and real is to cultivate your voice as a writer and aim for your own arguments and analysis to be centred. At times, you may need to draw this academic voice out in the editing phase of writing; however, throughout, ensure that you make the analysis explicit and not implicit. All too often, we run the risk of jumping from the reading stage to the writing stage. The inherent risk here is that you jeopardise the flow of your writing by trying to 'pigeonhole' a usable text into writing.

Critical Editing

The hard work starts here!!!

Editing may take a majority of your time allocated to a piece of critical writing. Multiple rounds of revision may be necessary to refine the synthesis and improve its clarity, coherence and persuasiveness. Honing your choice of words and ensuring succinct paraphrasing of your text to ensure that your synthesised, critical arguments are clear and obvious are essential.

The temptation is to write your work and believe it is good enough after the first draft. In fact, this rarely happens.

- Flow—Read out loud. Use the read aloud function on Microsoft Word or ask a critical friend to assess it for readability, not necessarily content, but how easy it is to read. Once we are very familiar with our writings, as we read, our brains will tell us what we think it should say, rather that reading the words on the page. So, allowing others to read it before completion is essential.

- Work on finding and allowing your own voice to come through. Using language effectively can help how you strengthen your analysis and synthesis in your writing. You of course need to reference the facts, but explanation, interpretation and application of the facts to your own practice situation are where your own voice comes in.

- Have you used third- or first-person tense and been consistent in this? It is often difficult to achieve the level of criticality required if you write in the first person. Remaining objective and personally distant from the themes you raise will automatically provide you with the scope to be more analytical about the research you have read and your synthesis of this into your work will be easier.

Use of Artificial Intelligence in Assessed Work

Artificial intelligence (AI) is advancing rapidly and is increasingly integrated into our daily digital experiences, featuring in many academic and professional workplaces. It is recognised that its use may be of benefit to a number of individuals, to enhance the learning process; however, it can also be limiting, diminishing opportunities to hone your own writing, and can also provide misleading or incorrect information.

There is significant ongoing discourse regarding the utilisation of AI within academic studies, and the implications on assessments. Many universities hold the view that AI has significant potential as a valuable resource for enhancing learning and using it to help with aspects like idea generation or planning may be appropriate. Nevertheless, it must be used responsibly in a manner that aligns with the principles of academic integrity and it is never acceptable to use AI tools to write your assignment.

Remember that AI is a tool to assist your learning, but it should not replace the essential skills of critical thinking, analysis, synthesis and creativity, all of which are pivotal in both your academic journey and career in AP.

Your university will provide you with advice and guidance on using AI in learning and assessment to help you maintain best practices. This will ensure that you are well informed about the latest advice before incorporating AI into your assignments. If lecturers have made clear that you may use AI sources in your assessed work, then you should acknowledge and properly reference their inclusion.

Academic Writing Roadmap

Fig. 9.1 is a roadmap designed to provide you with direction and structure when considering your critical writing, to help navigate your way through the steps detailed earlier. Use it to weave your different arguments together from your critical reading, thinking, appraisal and synthesis stages, so that commonalities can be established and used together to create a theme or subject throughout the piece. This will enable you to draw together conclusions and recommendations for your practice.

Summary

You will see that criticality is and should be inherently unique to you, especially as you move into the master's level education required for AP. Your process and formula for this will become unique and bespoke to you as you develop your own skills. Through critical analysis, you show your understanding; however, to get there, you need to deconstruct or unpick other people's theories. This is more than just explaining their arguments but clarifying in what context they make their arguments and how they use their evidence, thus demonstrating your own argument is front and centre, highlighting your own position and your own thoughts. As you weave

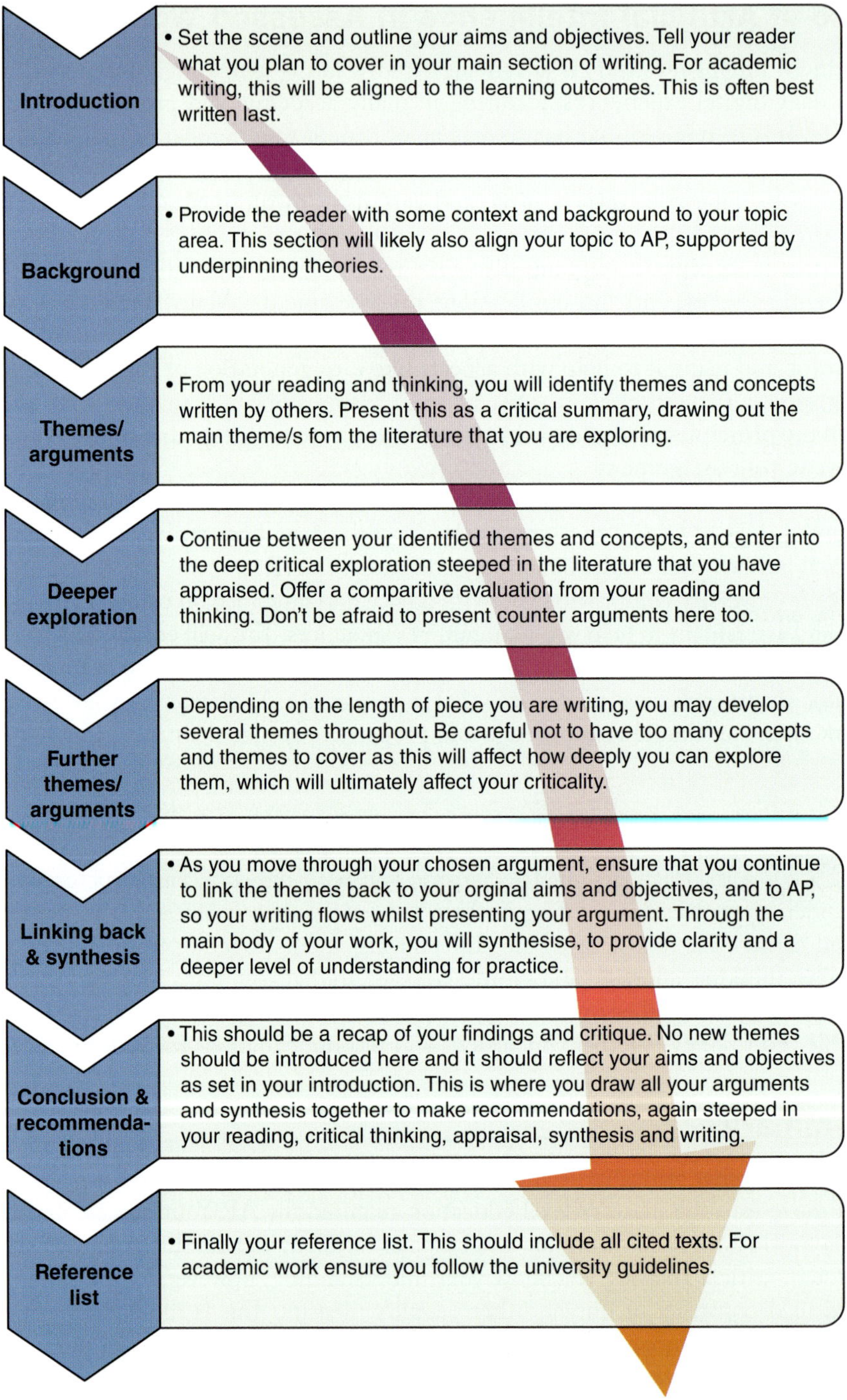

Introduction	• Set the scene and outline your aims and objectives. Tell your reader what you plan to cover in your main section of writing. For academic writing, this will be aligned to the learning outcomes. This is often best written last.
Background	• Provide the reader with some context and background to your topic area. This section will likely also align your topic to AP, supported by underpinning theories.
Themes/ arguments	• From your reading and thinking, you will identify themes and concepts written by others. Present this as a critical summary, drawing out the main theme/s fom the literature that you are exploring.
Deeper exploration	• Continue between your identified themes and concepts, and enter into the deep critical exploration steeped in the literature that you have appraised. Offer a comparitive evaluation from your reading and thinking. Don't be afraid to present counter arguments here too.
Further themes/ arguments	• Depending on the length of piece you are writing, you may develop several themes throughout. Be careful not to have too many concepts and themes to cover as this will affect how deeply you can explore them, which will ultimately affect your criticality.
Linking back & synthesis	• As you move through your chosen argument, ensure that you continue to link the themes back to your orginal aims and objectives, and to AP, so your writing flows whilst presenting your argument. Through the main body of your work, you will synthesise, to provide clarity and a deeper level of understanding for practice.
Conclusion & recommenda-tions	• This should be a recap of your findings and critique. No new themes should be introduced here and it should reflect your aims and objectives as set in your introduction. This is where you draw all your arguments and synthesis together to make recommendations, again steeped in your reading, critical thinking, appraisal, synthesis and writing.
Reference list	• Finally your reference list. This should include all cited texts. For academic work ensure you follow the university guidelines.

Fig 9.1   Roadmap to consider for critical writing. *AP*, Advanced practice.

and draw together the best different viewpoints you have established, combining these together may present a new, overall perspective for your own area of AP.

Conclusion

To conclude, this chapter has introduced the key themes and concepts that underpin critical reading, thinking and writing. Following a step-by-step approach, and the development of an academic writing roadmap, will support you on your journey through the navigation of the academic skills needed at master's level. With explanation and guidance, key stages are discussed along each step which are core to the criticality and synthesis that underpin master's level study. Often, these skills will not be formally taught within a master's programme but need to be developed independently through the resources offered by the university/HEI. Furthermore, it has been highlighted that criticality and synthesis skills are transferable throughout all the pillars of AP, so mastering and developing these key skills at an early stage will lay the foundations for you as an advanced practitioner.

References

Aveyard, H., Sharp, P., & Woolliams, M. (2011). *A beginner's guide to critical thinking and writing in health and social care*. London: Open University Press.

Cottrell, S. (2013). *The study skills handbook*. Basingstoke: Palgrave Macmillan.

Critical Appraisal Skills Programme (CASP). (2023). *Critical appraisal skills programme*. https://casp-uk.net/

Stillwell, S. B., Fineout-Overholt, E., Melnyk, B., & Williamson, K. (2010). 'Evidence-based practice, step by step: Asking the clinical question: A key step in evidence-based practice'. *AJN, American Journal of Nursing, 110*(3), 58–61. doi:10.1097/01.NAJ.0000368959.11129.79

Sword, H. (2012). *Stylish academic writing*. Cambridge, MA: Harvard University Press.

The University of Manchester. (2023). *Academic phrasebank*. https://www.phrasebank.manchester.ac.uk/

Wallace, M., & Wray, A. (2021). *Critical reading and writing for postgraduates* (4th ed). London: SAGE.

CHAPTER 10

Professional and Ethical Issues in Advanced Practice

Julie-Ann Hayes ■ Andrew Martin ■ Sarah Fisher

CHAPTER OUTLINE

Within this chapter, we will explore some ethical and professional considerations in relation to advanced practice. The chapter will begin by exploring what is ethics and how this is applied to the advanced practitioner. The four principles of ethics will be explored, and some ethical considerations will be discussed. The second part of this chapter will review the professional aspects of advanced practice, through a review of being accountable as an advanced practitioner. The chapter will conclude with a section around statement writing, and a scenario is presented which is based on a consultation where the patient sought legal action against the advanced practitioner. The aim of this chapter is to provide a foundation of some key ethical and professional considerations that need to be developed as the trainee advanced practitioner's educational training progresses, and it can be used as a 'refresh' for those advanced practitioners working in practice.

Introduction

Advanced practitioners are expected to act ethically and professionally and to '*do the right thing*'. Being both ethical and professional is not just about working within your own professional boundaries. The professional, statutory and regulatory bodies (Nursing and Midwifery Council (NMC), General Pharmaceutical Council (GPhC) and Health and Care Professions Council (HCPC)) do not provide a set of rules that will assist the advanced practitioner to resolve every ethical or professional dilemma that can be encountered within their practice.

This chapter will examine the process of being ethical, working within professional boundaries and what that means in terms of professional accountability and advanced practice (AP). We will consider when things go wrong and how advanced practitioners can manage in these circumstances.

What Is Ethics?

Ethics in the simplistic form is focussing on our morals and how these influence our behaviours and decisions. Beauchamp and Childress (2019, p. 1) state:

'ethics is a generic term covering several different ways of examining and interpreting the moral life.'

The Medical Protection Society (2024) notes that ethics drives the behaviour, and the law reflects the ethics. Fox (2024) recognises that healthcare is challenging and can present the advanced practitioner with many ethical decisions, hence the importance of ethical awareness to support safe and ethical care. Ethics is core to all healthcare registrants, and this starts with individuals' professional regulators and their published standards which map out expected behaviours and conduct for practice. Clinicians can face many ethical dilemmas within practice, such as around consent, confidentiality and withholding of treatment as just a few examples (Beauchamp & Childress, 2019). It is beyond the scope of this chapter to provide a detailed analysis of ethics and the ethical dilemmas that can occur within clinical practice; however, the focus will set to explore the underlying principles of ethics.

Being Ethical in AP

PIT STOP!

What does being ethical mean to you as a practitioner?

WHY DO WE, AS ADVANCED PRACTITIONERS, NEED TO INVOLVE OURSELVES IN ETHICS?

As highlighted throughout the various chapters within this book, the four nations of the United Kingdom (UK) have their own AP frameworks (Advanced Nursing Practice Framework, Department of Health, Social Services and Public Safety (DHSSPS), 2016; Health Education and Improvement Wales, 2023; National Health Service England (NHSE) 2025; Scottish Government, 2021); however, these only mention ethics on a few occasions. Ethics is not a new debate in healthcare and can be traced back to ancient Greek times (Lategan & van Zyl, 2017). However, the context in which the debates are taking place is becoming more and more complex. These are due, in part, to a number of evolving constructs that impact on all elements of not only our patients' lives but also the healthcare practitioner.

Technology has changed healthcare dramatically, for example, with the introduction of new drugs and treatments to new innovative imaging that helps to treat and diagnose illness more quickly (Morilla et al., 2017). Thimbleby (2013) identified that despite the positive outcomes of the advancements in technology, this often created a false hope that technology can keep people alive for longer, when previously this may not have been the case. People are living longer, partly as a result of better technology; however, they can also develop more comorbidities as they age and this can negatively impact on the quality of life (Rayman et al., 2022). Multimorbidity and complexity in long-term conditions continue to increase and advanced practitioners have a recognised role in the long-term management of these patient groups (Bales et al., 2023).

It could be argued that medicine is or has become an industry, particularly within the pharmaceutical side (Henry, 2023). The aim of an industry does not always align; in some cases, it can directly contradict the aims of healthcare. Industry can bring great economic benefits to the companies and people affiliated to the companies, but the question of what is being developed, the companies' profits or better healthcare outcomes needs to be asked (Lategan & van Zyl, 2017).

The other compounding factor that makes ethics important in healthcare and for advanced practitioners is around health inequalities and being able to manage this challenge. In The King's Fund report produced by Williams et al. (2022), it was highlighted that health inequalities continue to exist and impact upon people's life expectancy, access to care services, the quality of care service and the quality of housing, to name a few. These inequalities vary across the world, and this has been recognised by the World Health Organization (2023) and United Nations (2023). Chapter 15 provides further discussion around the role that advanced practitioners can play in the achievement of universal health coverage.

WHY DO ADVANCED PRACTITIONERS NEED TO BE MINDFUL OF THESE CONSTRUCTS?

Advanced practitioners are now employed across most health and social care settings (Hardy et al., 2021) and as such will be exposed to services that can only offer certain technology to aid with diagnosis, despite this not reflecting the most up-to-date evidenced-based approaches. The different bodies that approve the use of medication across the UK, such as local Clinical Commissioning Groups in England, may only support the use of certain drugs for a disease that do not represent the guidance suggested by the evidence. The examples given earlier may be affected by financial constraints and it could be argued that if you do not have access to certain diagnostic tools or medications, it is easier to decide. However, like the development of technology, the evidence base changes recommending new tools and treatments that carry less side effects and better outcomes. We are encouraged as practitioners to practice evidence-based medicine, when sometimes factors around us prevent us from doing this.

All of these factors influence how advanced practitioners make decisions in certain situations. This is even before you come across the dilemmas that are faced by advanced practitioners in practice. These can range from seemingly simple decisions like deciding what is right (Rasoal et al., 2017) to engaging in conversations that involve conflicting interests between the practitioner, their patient and next of kin (NoK) (Beauchamp & Childress, 2019). Power hierarchies also play a significant part in decision-making, whether that is between the advanced practitioner and their patient or between other medical professionals involved in a patients, care (Heath, 2018). Historically, there has been an attitude that healthcare providers should provide the guidance that the patient should adhere to; however, contemporary thinking now centres around making joint decisions with the patient around their care, even if that goes against the advice of the healthcare provider (Heath, 2018).

There is evidence to suggest that practitioners experience distress as a result of making ethical issues in healthcare (Pauly et al., 2009). Despite this, some would argue that training providers do not focus on ethics enough to prepare practitioners, and that actually practitioners are being encouraged to consult on highly complex cases more commonly than dealing with ethical dilemmas that are far more prevalent (Madden, 2022). Chapter 14 explores the emotional and spiritual well-being of the advanced practitioner.

HOW CAN WE INTRODUCE ETHICS INTO AP?

Most healthcare courses will incorporate some kind of ethics teaching, even if this is informal. Some are going further by integrating ethics training into their programmes, albeit being seen as a very different subjective subject (Knight & Papanikitas, 2021).

The literature does not identify a preferred model of ethical teaching (Machin & Proctor, 2021), although it is not unusual to introduce ethical frameworks for practitioners to use to help them make sense and resolve some of their dilemmas.

One of the established and utilised frameworks for practitioners to consider in healthcare is that offered by Beauchamp and Childress (2019). They offer a list of four moral principles which can be used as framework when faced with ethical decisions. They consist of:

1. *Respect for autonomy*
2. *Nonmaleficence*
3. *Beneficence*
4. *Justice*

(Beauchamp & Childress, 2019, p. 13)

The principles are broadly based on a set of ethical norms; for example, it is generally regarded that we should all respect an individual's autonomy, and to disregard this would be seen as ethically wrong (Beauchamp & Childress, 2019). In practice, an advanced practitioner may consider each of these principles to aid them with their decision-making.

Autonomy is the right of the individual and respecting this right. Fox (2024) highlights that autonomy within healthcare is around informed choices, with the practitioner providing appropriate information to make an informed decision. Risks versus benefits about any intervention clearly need to be explained in a manner for the patient to understand and decide. The Medical Protection Society (2024) recognises consent within autonomy but also the patient's right to privacy and maintaining confidentiality. Furthermore, they recognise age as a factor within autonomy and draw upon the 'Gillick' competence.

Nonmaleficence is the principle to cause no harm to the patient. However, there can often be unintentional harm caused to the patient, such as the iatrogenic effects of prescribing. For example, an advanced practitioner might prescribe an antihypertensive medication to control blood pressure, but that medication impacts upon the patient's renal function. Advanced practitioners need to weigh the benefits versus the risk of any intervention with involvement of the patient in any decision-making.

Beneficence is acting within the patient's best interest. For example, an advanced practitioner would be acting in the patient's best interest through managing a hypoglycaemic event. In this scenario, the patient would have impaired consciousness due to the hypoglycaemia and would be unable to reverse this situation themselves.

Justice is recognised as a set of norms distributing benefits, risks and cost (Beauchamp & Childress, 2019). Discrimination is an important concept applicable to this concept with decisions not to discriminate against race, religion as examples; however, the Medical Protection Society (2024) recognises that there are certain grounds to refuse treatment, such as lifestyle choices (smokers). Justice is around balancing the patient's right versus need versus the availability of resources.

The Medical Protection Society (2024) highlights how the law reflects these principles, which is captured in Box 10.1.

Reflecting on the types of decisions that an advanced practitioner may make for example, 'what is right?' may be answered by 'does my decision respect the individual's autonomy?', for example, allowing the patient to be involved in any decisions made about or for them. 'Does my decision avoid any causes of harm (nonmaleficence), whilst actively seeking to prevent or lessen harm whilst also being cost effective (beneficence/justice)?'. Finally, considering justice, 'does my decision consider the distribution of benefits, risks and costs?' If the advanced practitioner has considered all these principles and the balance falls positively, then they could argue that their decision is 'right'. It can also be observed when an ethical principle has not been applied and where the law will be involved (Box 10.1).

Engaging in conversations that involve conflicting interest between the practitioner, their patient and the NoK/carer may involve a completely different balance of views. However, using the same four principles offered by Beauchamp and Childress (2019) may allow the advanced practitioner to take more of a balanced approach to decision-making. Reflecting on the earlier example and presuming the patient has consented to allowing the NoK/carer to be present, many questions can be posed, such as,

Is the advanced practitioner allowing the patient and their NoK/carer the opportunity to be involved in any decision-making?

Is the balance of those decisions being led by any one individual in that relationship?

BOX 10.1 ■ How the Law Reflects the Ethical Principles (Medical Protection Society, 2024)

Autonomy
Consent
Confidentiality/privacy
Access to records

Beneficence
Negligence law

Nonmaleficence
Criminal law
Negligence law regulation

Justice
Antidiscrimination law

Is this something that has been agreed (lasting power of attorney) or assumed (patient lacks capacity)?

Is this having an impact on allowing the patient to make autonomous decisions?

The advanced practitioner may decide to think of strategies to address this imbalance. To the extreme, the advanced practitioner may not know the motivation of the NoK's/carer's views, and they may stand to benefit or lose out from a decision made about the patient. Although the principles are based on general norms, decisions made that appear to go against those norms, for example, the patient decides to make a decision not to proceed with an invasive procedure or treatment because of the side effects, do need to be critiqued but respected, despite best efforts to facilitate an informed decision of risks versus benefits. If the advanced practitioner then feels that the patient has made an autonomous decision, even if this on balance goes against the views of those around them, the advanced practitioner can be assured that they have respected their patient's autonomy.

The framework of Beauchamp and Childress (2019) may help advanced practitioners explore decisions in clinical practice, but it has to be acknowledged that some decisions stretch beyond the day-to-day ethical dilemmas. Each clinical setting is likely to have access to an ethics committee that will consist of a panel of clinical experts, those trained in ethics and often legal representation (Rasoal et al., 2017).

Ethical practice can be challenging, and as discussed, can cause lasting stress to individuals who are making those decisions (Pauly et al., 2009). It is anticipated that this provides an introduction and further thought about these ethical considerations that will be needed within practice. Ethics is embedded into daily practice from decision-making, to consent and maintaining confidentiality, as some examples. Beauchamp and Childress (2019) draw upon the importance of the professional–patient relationship being underpinned by 'truth telling', being honest and transparent. The next section examines the duty of candour.

Duty of Candour

The Francis Inquiry into the failing at the Mid-Staffordshire NHS Foundation Trust in 2013 led to the recommendations of the introduction of a duty of candour both at statutory and professional levels. Up until this point, there was no legal requirement for care providers to share information to those harmed (Care Quality Commission, 2022). The duty of candour is about being open and transparent for those users of a service that is being provided to them. In relation to the statutory duty of candour, this also carries the requirement for notifiable safety incidents. Throughout the four nations of the UK, statutory regulation is upheld and monitored through various bodies. Within the Mid-Staffordshire NHS Foundation Trust, when things were going wrong, there should have been the application of a statutory duty of candour as well as the notifiable safety incidents; however, this did not happen (Francis Inquiry; Francis, 2013).

In relation to professional duty of candour, this is overseen by the professional bodies, NMC, HCPC and GPhC. In a joint guidance by the NMC and General Medical Council (GMC), healthcare professionals must:

Tell the person (or, where appropriate, their advocate, carer or family) when something has gone wrong.
Apologise to the person (or, where appropriate, their advocate, carer or family).
Offer an appropriate remedy or support to put matters right (if possible).
Explain fully to the person (or, where appropriate, their advocate, carer or family) the short- and long-term effects of what has happened.

(GMC & NMC, 2022, p. 3)

Saying sorry is recognised as being a central feature within the duty of candour when mistakes have happened and acknowledging error, but saying sorry is not an admission of guilt (Care Quality Commission, 2022). As registrants, we need to be open and honest with our patients.

PIT STOP!

NHS Resolution has produced guidance on saying sorry; please follow the web link to access this resource.
https://resolution.nhs.uk/resources/saying-sorry/

Consent

PIT STOP!

The Medical Protection Society has produced an overview of consent and capacity which can be accessed via this web link:
https://www.medicalprotection.org/uk/articles/essential-learning-consent-and-capacity

Being open and honest underpin the principles of consent when communicating risks versus benefits to support the patient to make an informed choice. Fox (2024) recognises that consent is both a legal and an ethical principle. For example, if a patient is not given relevant information to make an informed decision and this leads to an intervention being performed that they did not understand or fully consent to, then this can lead to legal action (Box 10.1). The openness and transparency are core to providing accurate information to allow the patient with capacity to make an informed decision. It is not intended for this chapter to explore consent and the many facets this brings to healthcare practice, but to highlight that consent is an ethical principle.

What Is Accountability?

Often, healthcare practitioners will define accountability through language such as responsibility. Responsibility is task orientated; every person in a team, for example,

---

> **BOX 10.2** ■ **Four Main Fields of Accountability by Griffith and Dowie (2019)**
>
> **Public**—Criminal law, criminal courts
> **Patient**—Civil law and civil courts
> **Profession**—Code of professional conduct, regulatory body (NMC/GPhC/HCPC), Conduct and
>   Competence committee
> **Employer**—Contract of employment, employment tribunals

---

may be responsible for a given task. Accountability is what happens after a situation has occurred. Cornock (2017, p. 18) articulates this difference well and clearly defines accountability by referring

'to the practice of holding healthcare practitioners accountable for their actions, whether or not a mistake occurred in their practice.'

An important distinction to make is the scope of accountability, and this is achieved by considering to whom we are accountable. Griffith and Dowie (2019) suggest four main fields of accountability for healthcare professionals. These four main fields are illustrated in the Box 10.2.

This perspective captures the broad scope of accountability across all professions within the healthcare field. Each field of practice may provide more specific focus relating to the profession demands. For example, from a nursing perspective, these four main fields of accountability are reflected in guidance provided by the Royal College of Nursing (RCN) (2023) that identifies accountability to the employer through a contract of employment and the profession through codes of conduct and in addition articulates accountability in the form of a duty of care and in the NMC (2020) guidance which defines accountability in these terms:

'Being accountable means being open to challenge. It means being held to account for your actions, being able to confidently explain how you used your professional judgement to make decisions – even in complex situations.'

What Is a Duty of Care?

There is no universal duty of care in the UK. However, in certain situations, called duty situations, the nature of the relationship gives rise to a duty of care. The relationship between the healthcare practitioner across all fields of AP and the patient is recognised in English Law as giving rise to a duty situation. This is a duty to be careful, to take care of and not to harm the patient through careless acts or omissions and significantly to deliver the agreed standard of care. Advanced practitioners are generally expected to meet the standard of care set by the profession, employer and the law. In law, the professional standard of care is determined by the case

Hunter v Hanley (1955). This case resulted in the legal test for standard of care in Scotland and which is referred to in Bolam v Friern Hospital Management Committee (HMC) (1957) and resulted in the 'Bolam test'. Both tests are consistent with the skill and care test. We will explore these legal tests later in this chapter. To understand the standards required of healthcare professionals, we must consider how these professionals are regulated, and regulatory bodies set the standards that are expected of them.

Regulation

Within Chapter 1, it was highlighted how the AP frameworks were introduced and discussed across the four nations of the UK. It also highlighted that AP is currently not regulated; however, the plans are in motion for the NMC to lead on this work to regulate advanced level practice within the nursing and midwifery profession. Chapter 1 also highlighted the development of medical associate profession roles and how some of these are currently unregulated, such as the physician associate. Advanced practitioners are regulated through their professional qualification via their regulatory body, for example, a physiotherapist is regulated via the HCPC, but the level of practice (advanced) is not (at least at present). The Department of Health and Social Care (DHSC, 2019) recognises the need for regulation for healthcare professions as this will

'ensure that they have the skills, competence, health and attitudes to deliver safe, high quality care that commands public trust and patient confidence.'

(DHSC, 2019, p. 9)

There are three professional regulators within the UK that regulate various different healthcare professions, which include the NMC, GPhC and HCPC.

NURSING AND THE NURSING AND MIDWIFERY COUNCIL

In the UK the nursing profession is regulated by the NMC. This body has both regulatory and statutory powers and came into force in 2002. This body has multiple functions ranging from setting standards for practice and education, maintaining the register, advising the government regarding changes in the profession, conducting research and investigating issues surrounding fitness to practise. The NMC provides a code of conduct which outlines professional standards that nurses, midwives and nursing associates (in England) must uphold to be registered to practice in the UK. The code is structured around four themes—prioritise people, practise effectively, preserve safety and promote professionalism and trust. Each theme contains a series of statements that taken together signify the standards required for nursing and midwifery practice. Chapter 1 provides an outline of the current NMC work around proposed plans for regulating AP.

PIT STOP!

NMC code of conduct: this link includes the code of conduct that applies to nursing, midwifery and nursing associates.

https://www.nmc.org.uk/standards/code/

This link includes a broad definition of accountability for nursing, midwifery and nursing associates. There is a short, animated film.

https://www.nmc.org.uk/standards/code/code-in-action/accountability/

PHARMACY AND GENERAL PHARMACEUTICAL COUNCIL

The GPhC regulates pharmacists, pharmacy technicians and pharmacies across the UK. The GPhC is a statutory body set up by the UK and Scottish parliament. The Health Act 1999, as amended by the Health and Social Care Act 2008, is the primary legislation which enabled the GPhC to be established via the Pharmacy Order 2010. The Pharmacy Order 2010 (Statutory Instrument 2010, No. 231) awards the GPhC the powers and responsibilities for registration of pharmacy premises and for enforcing provisions under the Medicines Act 1968 and the Poisons Act 1972. The GPhC (2017) provides standards for pharmacy professionals which contribute to delivering and improving health, safety and well-being of patients and the public. These include:

1. Provide person-centred care.
2. Work in partnership with others.
3. Communicate effectively.
4. Maintain, develop and use their professional knowledge and skills.
5. Use professional judgement.
6. Behave in a professional manner.
7. Respect and maintain the person's confidentiality and privacy.
8. Speak up when they have concerns or when things go wrong.
9. Demonstrate leadership.

ALLIED HEALTH AND THE HEALTH AND CARE PROFESSIONS COUNCIL

In the UK, there are varied and diverse groups of professions that are considered allied health. The HCPC is a regulatory body for 15 professions, which are highlighted in Box 10.3.

As noted in Box 10.3, the regulation of professions within the HCPC is both diverse and large. Similarly to the NMC and the GPhC, this body has regulatory and statutory powers, and it came into force in 2003. It was formerly the Health Professions Council (HPC). Its purpose is to protect the public and it does this through setting and maintaining standards of proficiency and conduct, approving education and training, maintaining a register of professionals and investigating issues surrounding fitness to practice. Due to the diversity of the professions, HCPC has standards of proficiency for each of the 15 professions. Each standard

---

BOX 10.3 ■ Professions and Protected Titles Regulated by the HCPC

Art therapists	Orthoptists
Biomedical scientists	Paramedics
Chiropodists/podiatrists	Physiotherapists
Clinical scientists	Practitioner psychologists
Dieticians	Prosthetists/orthotists
Hearing aid dispensers	Radiographers
Occupational therapists	Speech and language therapists
Operating department practitioners	

---

has a set of core principles which apply to all professional groups and then profession-specific standards.

PIT STOP!

The standards of proficiency produced for each of the 15 professions can be found in this web link:

https://www.hcpc-uk.org/standards/standards-of-proficiency/

Review some of the standards even if this is not your profession to develop an understanding of these professional groups.

The NMC, GPhC and HCPC are themselves regulated by the Professional Standards Authority for Health and Social Care (PSA). This independent standards body oversees the nine statutory bodies that regulate health professionals in the UK and social care in England. The PSA is crucial as it assesses the performance of each regulator, scrutinising their decisions and processes. This is a key issue to consider in AP. As previously noted, advanced practitioners will be required to transform and modernise pathways of care which will enable the safe and effective sharing of skills across traditional professional boundaries; therefore, an understanding of each profession's decision-making relating to standards of practice and conduct is crucial.

What Happens When Things Go Wrong?

NEGLIGENCE

NHS Resolution (2023) in their annual review reports the figures for new claims of negligence within the NHS. In 2021–22, there were a reported 15,078 new claims. In 2022–23, there were a reported 13,511 new claims. This decrease of 1567 cases on the previous year figure is a positive statistic; however, caution needs to be applied to this figure as there might be underreporting. With the increased scope of practice, the risk of litigation is significant; therefore, it is essential for advanced practitioners to understand how to deal with things when they go wrong and the issues surrounding negligence.

Negligence is a civil wrong or tort and is best defined as actionable harm (Bolam v Friern HMC, 1957). Negligence has developed in UK law under the common law by judges setting rules through decided cases. McNair J described several tests for negligence, but one test has become known as the 'Bolam test'. There is significant development in the field of negligence since the period of Hunter v Hanley (1955) and Bolam v Friern HMC (1957). Cases such as Maynard v West Midlands RHA (1984) 1 WLR 634, Sidaway v Bethlem and Maudsley Hospitals (1985) AC 871, Bolitho v City Hackney HA (1999) 4 Med LR 381 and, more recently, Montgomery v Lanarkshire (2015) UKSC11 have offered challenges in different ways to this judicial test. However, what is consistent is that these cases have established three key elements for a successful negligence action, namely, that:

- The patient was owed a **duty of care** by the practitioner;
- There was a breach of that duty of care; and
- The breach of duty caused loss or **harm** recognised by the courts (Whitehouse v Jordan, 1981).

Earlier in the chapter, we discussed the concept of duty of care and that a crucial aspect of the duty of care is to deliver the agreed standard of care. If the advanced practitioner falls short of the agreed standard of care, this is potentially a breach of the advanced practitioner's duty of care. Following accepted practice is normally enough when considering the standard of care. This can be established through adhering to guidelines and protocols. It is also important for advanced practitioners to be up to date with their knowledge by applying evidence-based practice. Legally, the standard of care utilises the 'Bolam test', which derives from the case Bolam v Friern HMC (1957). Ellis and Ellis (2021) outline this test and states that it determines and sets the precedent of what the appropriate standard of care and degree of skill is and what can be expected from a reasonable member of that profession. AP has transformed healthcare delivery, with advanced practitioners undertaking a wide range of clinical skills and roles. Cornock (2017) captures the potential of advanced practitioners by highlighting that there is almost no limit to how healthcare practitioners can advance their practice if they are competent in those areas. The central issue is competence, and this reflects the advanced practitioner meeting the agreed standard. It is possible for the advanced practitioner to fail in their duty of care to the patient and for the patient to suffer harm. The process of establishing that the harm occurred because of falling short of the standard is complex (Griffith & Dowie, 2019).

PIT STOP!

Take this opportunity to review your clinical practice. Have you encountered any issues with concerns or complaints? How were the patient/families supported through that process? What support were you offered?

THE IMPORTANCE OF DOCUMENTATION

Maintaining a good standard of record keeping is an essential aspect of professional practice and the advanced practitioner's duty of care and plays an important role in supporting the advanced practitioner when things go wrong in clinical practice.

The NMC (2018), GPhC (2017) and HCPC (2021) all provide guidance regarding the responsibility of nurses, pharmacists and allied health professionals to keep full, clear and accurate records. The HCPC (2021) states that this will ensure service users receive appropriate treatment that is in their best interests, meets the legal requirements of record keeping and will be evidence of decision-making processes if latter queried or investigated. APs need to understand the legislation that underpins how they keep and store records. This includes the Data Protection Act (2018) and the Freedom of Information Act (2000).

> **PIT STOP!**
>
> Review your own professional body's guidance around documentation.

The requirement to keep effective records is clear, but what does this mean? The key principles of effective record keeping are outlined in Box 10.4.

AP presents some distinctive challenges for effective record keeping. With AP spanning several clinical professions, team working and effective communication are pivotal to effective record keeping. Stein et al. (2022) explored the unique communication challenges including navigating team dynamics and goals of care planning. The importance of communication within the clinical pillar is discussed within Chapter 4. Frain (2018) recognises that communication in healthcare is multifactorial, but when this is done poorly, the consequences are significant, ranging from patient safety through to malpractice risks.

STATEMENT WRITING

When things do go wrong, there are many occasions when statements are required. It is important to consider the purpose of the statement. The purpose of the statement will affect the detail and style and content of what is required. It is not necessary to wait until you have received a request for a statement before you make your own record of events. You should establish the purpose of writing the statement before sharing to ensure there is no danger of incrimination. Table 10.1 outlines how statements can be used when the purpose differs.

BOX 10.4 ■ Principles of Effective Record Keeping

- Accuracy—Set out the facts of what took place.
- Factual—Keeping to the facts.
- Avoid hearsay.
- Conciseness.
- Relevance—Ensure the content is relevant to the patient, incident.
- Legibility—When records are handwritten, it should be legible.
- Store safely—This is to ensure confidentiality and privacy.
- Use of abbreviations—the NMC (2018), GPhC (2017) and HCPC (2021) provide guidance regarding the use of abbreviations.

TABLE 10.1 ■ **Purpose of Statements Relating to Incidents**

Incidents	How the Statement Could Be Used
Statement to the police re: criminal act by patient/employee	• Could be used as formal evidence. • The person making the statement could be questioned on the statement.
Statement to police re: criminal act by self	• Could be used as formal evidence. • The person making the statement could be questioned on the statement.
Statement to senior staff re: incident concerning patient	• Could be used as formal evidence. • Could potentially be criminal or civil case—this will depend on the nature of the incident.
Statement to senior staff re: conduct of colleague	• Could be used as formal evidence. • Could potentially be criminal or civil case—this will depend on the nature of the incident. • This could be escalated to the regulatory body—NMC/GPhC/HCPC. • The person making the statement could be questioned on the statement.
Statement to senior staff re: conduct of self	• Could be used as formal evidence. • Could potentially be criminal or civil case—this will depend on the nature of the incident. • This could be escalated to the regulatory body—NMC/GPhC/HCPC. • The person making statement could be questioned on the statement.
Statement re: accident to self or colleague	• Could be used as formal evidence. • Could potentially be criminal or civil case—this will depend on the nature of the incident.

GPhC, General Pharmaceutical Council; *HCPC,* Health and Care Professions Council; *NMC,* Nursing and Midwifery Council.

The principles for effective record keeping apply to the process of statement writing. It is essential that advanced practitioners include the following key information:

- Date/time of incident
- Full name of the statement writer, role and location
- Full name of all persons involved in the incident
- Date/time of the statement
- A detailed account of the incident
- Signature
- Additional information such as supporting statement, photographs and evidence

PIT STOP!

The RCN has produced advice regarding statement writing; this is found in the following link address.

https://www.rcn.org.uk/Get-Help/RCN-advice/statements

Dealing with complaints and concerns requires accurate record keeping of the incident or issues. Take this opportunity to review the following scenario.

In this scenario, an advanced practitioner is involved in the assessment of a patient who presents at a primary care setting; concerns are raised regarding decisions the advanced practitioner made during this assessment.

Scenario

A 32-year-old married woman presented to a primary care setting and consulted with an advanced practitioner.

Presenting complaint: 2-week history of lower abdominal pain.

History of presenting complaint: The patient reports gradual onset of a dull ache in her lower abdomen with the occasional stabbing pain. This symptom had been reported to a general practitioner (GP) 1 week earlier and it was deemed that no action was required at that time and safety netting advice was given.

The patient returned due to the persistence and worsening of the pain. The patient denied any loss of consciousness, no dyspnoea, no chest pain, no palpitations and no fevers/chills. The pain was located in the hypogastric region; there were no aggravating or relieving factors. Pain score given was 7/10. There was no radiation of pain, no shoulder tip pain. The patient reported normal bowel motions and no urinary symptoms. The patient stated her periods were irregular and this was a normal pattern for her. She had not previously had any gynaecological history or investigations. However, her last bleed was 1 week ago. She is currently sexually active and doesn't believe she is pregnant. There were no reports of nausea and vomiting and she was eating and drinking normally. Cervical smears are all up to date.

Treatment tried: Paracetamol and ibuprofen with some effect, as per manufacturer dosing instructions.

Past medical history: Nil significant.

Medications: Not taking any regular prescribed medication, including any oral contraception.

Allergies: None known.

Social history: The patient lives with her husband. Works as a teacher. Non-smoker. Drinks minimal alcohol.

Examination: The patient has good colour and is alert and orientated. Blood pressure 134/83 mmHg, pulse 80 bpm and regular, temperature 37.0°C, oxygen saturations 99%, respiration rate 14 bpm and capillary refill time less than 2 seconds. Pregnancy test negative. Urinalysis showed no abnormality. No clubbing observed. Abdomen—no scars or striae visible. Not distended. Bowel sounds normoactive in all four quadrants and the abdomen was tympanic on percussion. Abdomen soft, slight tenderness over the suprapubic region. No rebound tenderness, no guarding. No organomegaly. Liver not palpable, no costovertebral angle tenderness. Vaginal examination declined despite chaperone offered.

Plan: Reassurance given to the patient. Advised that blood samples would be taken to investigate the cause and booked into the next available phlebotomy clinic appointment in 2 days' time. Review appointment given. Recommended taking analgesia regularly.

Outcome: Two months later, the surgery receives a letter from a solicitor advising that their client was suing the practitioner for negligence. The patient attended the emergency department 2 days after the consultation with the advanced practitioner. It was confirmed that the patient had suffered a ruptured ectopic pregnancy and required surgery to remove a fallopian tube. The patient was claiming that if the advanced practitioner had referred her to hospital that same day and told her what worsening symptoms to observe for, she could have received quicker treatment and avoided the surgery.

PIT STOP!

Do you feel the patient has a case for negligence?

Would you have done anything different from the advanced practitioner in this scenario?

The advanced practitioner was requested to write a statement for their employers to share with the appointed solicitor. The advanced practitioner was a member of a nursing union who was able to provide support with the writing of this statement. The advanced practitioner also received support from the AP lead and the medical protection union that the practice was a member of.

PIT STOP!

Could you write a statement surrounding this incident? Give it a try.

It was agreed following a significant event review and discussion at the primary care's quality meeting that the advanced practitioner had covered in their documentation a full history and examination and the outcome was appropriate to the clinical findings at that time. However, the advanced practitioner had failed to document and advise the patient of specific worsening symptoms to observe for and what action to take if they occurred—safety netting.

The advanced practitioner, despite not being at fault, still learnt from this situation and implemented teaching to colleagues within their clinical environment to highlight and remind of the importance of not relying on a negative pregnancy test to exclude ectopic pregnancy.

PIT STOP!

Ectopic pregnancy is a common differential diagnosis and based on an accumulation of clinical findings which normally includes a negative pregnancy test. However, 2% of all ectopic pregnancies have a negative pregnancy test and often present with abdominal pain or vaginal bleeding (Hughes et al., 2017, https://doi.org/10.1080/08998280.2017.11929547).

Conclusion

This chapter has focussed on professional and ethical issues of AP. It has not been possible to cover every aspect of the NMC, GPhC and HCPC guidance, but this chapter provides an overview of some areas of complexities that advanced practitioners are faced with in practice. It has been highlighted that the advanced practitioner will have to make ethical decisions in their practice, and the four principles of ethics (Beauchamp & Childress, 2019) have been highlighted and discussed as framework to support this. With advancing a level of practice, this will bring a greater degree of autonomy and increased risk of legal or civil action. The legal aspects of practice are applicable to all registrants; however, this increases as an individual's practice advances.

References

Case Law:
Bolam v Friern Hospital Management Committee [1957] 2 All ER 11
Bolitho v City Hackney HA [1999] 4 Med LR 381
Hunter v Hanley [1955] ScotCS CSIH-2
Maynard v West Midlands RHA [1984] 1 WLR 634
Montgomery v Lanarkshire [2015] UKSC11
Sidaway v Bethlem and Maudsley Hospitals [1985] AC 871
Whitehouse v Jordan [1981] 1 All ER 267

Legislation:
Data Protection Act (2018)
https://www.legislation.gov.uk/ukpga/2018/12/contents/enacted
Freedom of Information Act (2000)
https://www.legislation.gov.uk/ukpga/2000/36/contents
Medicines Act (1968)
https://www.legislation.gov.uk/ukpga/1968/67
Poisons Act (1972)
https://www.legislation.gov.uk/ukpga/1972/66
Bales, G., Hasemann, W., Kressig, R. W., & Mayer, H. (2023). Impact, scope of practice and competencies of advanced practice nurses within APN-led models of care for young and middle-aged adult patients with multimorbidity and/or complex chronic conditions in hospital settings: A scoping review protocol. *BMJ Open.* 13(10), e077335. https://doi.org/10.1136/bmjopen-2023-077335
Beauchamp, T. L., & Childress, J. F. (2019). *Principles of biomedical ethics* (8th ed.). Oxford: Oxford University Press.
Care Quality Commission. (2022). *Regulation 20: Duty of candour.* https://www.cqc.org.uk/guidance-providers/regulations-enforcement/regulation-20-duty-of-candour#:~:text=Registered%20persons%20must%20act%20in,carrying%20on%20a%20regulated%20activity.&text=provide%20reasonable%20support%20to%20the,including%20when%20giving%20such%20notification
Cornock, M. (2017). Advancing professional health care practice and the issue of accountability. *EWMA Journal, 18*(2), 15–19.
Department of Health and Social Care. (2019). *Promoting professionalism, reforming regulation. Government response to the consultation.* https://assets.publishing.service.gov.uk/media/5d386abfed915d0d0446885f/Promoting_professionalism_reforming_regulation_consultation_reponse.pdf#page=10&zoom=100,72,109 (Accessed January 10, 2024)
Department of Health, Social Services and Public Safety (DHSSPS). (2016). *Advanced nursing practice framework.* Belfast: Northern Ireland Practice and Education Council for Nursing and Midwifery.
Ellis, P., & Ellis, H. (2021). Ethical and legal concepts: Legal aspects of a duty of care. *Journal of Kidney Care, 6*(3).

Fox, N. (2024). Ethics and legal principles. In S. Diamond-Fox, B. Hill, S. Stone, C. McCrea, N. Gardner, A. Roberts, et al. (Eds.), *The advanced practitioner in acute, emergency and critical care* (pp. 37–49). Sussex: Wiley Blackwell.

Frain, J. (2018). Why communication matters. In N. Cooper & J. Frain (Eds.). *ABC of clinical communication* (pp. 1–6). Sussex: Wiley Blackwell.

Francis, R. (2013). Report of the Mid Staffordshire NHS Trust Public Inquiry-Executive Summary. https://www.gov.uk/government/publications/report-of-the-mid-staffordshire-nhs-foundation-trust-public-inquiry (Accessed December 12, 2023)

General Medical Council and Nursing and Midwifery Council. (2022). *Openness and honesty when things go wrong: The professional duty of candour*. https://www.nmc.org.uk/globalassets/sitedocuments/nmc-publications/openness-and-honesty-professional-duty-of-candour.pdf (Accessed April 20, 2024)

General Pharmaceutical Council. (2017). *Standards and guidance for pharmacy professionals*. https://www.pharmacyregulation.org/standards/standards-for-pharmacy-professionals (Accessed April 22, 2024)

Griffith, R., & Dowie, I. (2019). *Dimond's legal aspects of nursing: A definitive guide to law for nurses* (8th ed.). Pearson.

Hardy, M., Snaith, B., Edwards, L., Baxter, J., Millington, P., & Harris, M. (2021). *Advanced practice: Research report*. https://www.hcpc-uk.org/globalassets/resources/policy/independent-research-report-advanced-practice-27th-january-2021.pdf?v=637483937140000000 (Accessed April 7, 2024)

Health and Care Professions Council. (2021). *Record keeping*. https://www.hcpc-uk.org/standards/meeting-our-standards/record-keeping/ (Accessed April 25, 2024)

Health Education and Improvement Wales (HEIW). (2023). *Professional framework for enhanced, advanced and consultant clinical practice in Wales*. https://heiw.nhs.wales/files/enhanced-advanced-and-consultant-framework/ (Accessed April 7, 2024)

Heath, S. (2018). *Understanding the power hierarchy in patient-provider relationships*. Patient Engagement. https://patientengagementhit.com/news/understanding-the-power-hierarchy-in-patient-provider-relationships (Accessed April 29, 2024)

Henry, B. (2023). *Medicines manufacturing has the potential to drive UK growth over the next 10 years*. https://www.abpi.org.uk/media/news/2023/january/medicines-manufacturing-has-the-potential-to-drive-uk-growth-over-the-next-10-years/ (Accessed April 27, 2024)

Hughes, M., Lupo, A., & Adrianne, B. (2017). Ruptured ectopic pregnancy with a negative urine pregnancy test. *Baylor University Medical Center Proceedings, 30*(1), 97–98. https://doi.org/10.1080/08998280.2017.11929547

Knight, S., & Papanikitas, A. (2021). Teaching and learning ethics in healthcare. In D. Nestel, G. Reedy, L. McKenna, & S. Gough (Eds.), *Clinical education for the health professions* (pp. 587–606). Singapore: Springer.

Lategan, L., & van Zyl, G. (2017). *Healthcare ethics for healthcare practitioners*. Johannesburg: UJ Press.

Machin, L. L., & Proctor, R. D. (2021). Engaging tomorrow's doctors in clinical ethics: Implications for healthcare organisations. *Health Care Analysis, 29*(4), 319–342. doi:10.1007/s10728-020-00403-z

Madden, J. T. (2022). Medical students' exposure to ethically complex realities of medicine is inadequate. *BMJ, 378*, o1900. https://doi.org/10.1136/bmj.o1900

Medical Protection Society. (2024). *The four principles of medical ethics*. https://www.medicalprotection.org/uk/articles/essential-learning-law-and-ethics (Accessed April 20, 2024)

Morilla, M. D. R., Sans, M., Casasa, A., & Giménez, N. (2017). Implementing technology in healthcare: Insights from physicians. *BMC Medical informatics and Decision Making, 17*(1), 92. doi:10.1186/s12911-017-0489-2

HS England (2025); *Multi-professional framework for advanced Practice in England*. Birmingham: Centre for Advancing Practice.

NHS Resolution. (2023). *Collaboration continues to cut costs and resolve cases without need for litigation*. https://resolution.nhs.uk/2023/07/13/collaboration-continues-to-cut-costs-and-resolve-cases-without-need-for-litigation/#:~:text=In%20line%20with%20NHS%20Resolution's,over%20the%20past%20six%20years (Accessed January 10, 2024)

Nursing and Midwifery Council. (2018). *The Code*. https://www.nmc.org.uk/standards/code/ (Accessed April 25, 2024)

Nursing and Midwifery Council. (2020). *Accountability. Caring with confidence: The Code in action*. Accountability—The Nursing and Midwifery Council. Available at: https://www.nmc.org.uk/news/news-and-updates/code-in-action/ (Accessed January 10, 2024)

Pauly, B. (2009). Registered nurses' perceptions of moral distress and ethical climate. *Nursing Ethics*. 16(5), 561–573.

Rasoal, D., Skovdahl, K., Gifford, M., & Kihlgren, A. (2017). Clinical ethics support for healthcare personnel: An integrative literature review. *HEC Forum, 29*(4), 313–346.

Rayman, G., Akpan, A., Cowie, M., Evans, R., Patel, M., Posporelis, S., & Walsh, K. (2022). Managing patients with comorbidities: Future models of care. *Future Healthcare Journal, 9*(2), 101–105.

Royal College of Nursing. (2023). *Accountability and delegation: Your pocket guide*. https://www.rcn.org.uk/ Professional-Development/Accountability-and-delegation (Accessed April 20, 2024)

Scottish Government. (2021). *Advanced nursing practice – Transforming nursing roles: Phase two*. https://www. gov.scot/publications/transforming-nursing-roles-advanced-nursing-practice-phase-ii/ (Accessed March 31, 2023)

Stein, D., Cannity, K., Weiner, R., Hichenburg, S., Leon-Nastasi, A., Banerjee, S., & Parker, P. (2022). General and unique communication skills challenges for advanced practice providers: A mixed methods study. *Journal of the Advanced Practitioners in Oncology, 13*(1), 32–43.

Thimbleby, H. (2013). Technology and the future of healthcare. *Journal of Public health Research, 2*(3), e28. doi:10.4081/jphr.2013.e28

United Nations. (2023). *Take action for the sustainable development goals*. https://www.un.org/sustainabledevel-opment/sustainable-development-goals/ (Accessed April 22, 2024)

Williams, E., Buck, D., Babalola, G., David Maguirem D. (2022). *What are health inequalities?* The King's fund. https://www.kingsfund.org.uk/insight-and-analysis/long-reads/what-are-health-inequalities#what-are-health-inequalities? (Accessed February 3, 2024)

World Health Organization. (2023). *Universal health coverage (UHC)*. https://www.who.int/news-room/fact-sheets/detail/universal-health-coverage-(uhc) (Accessed April 22, 2024).

CHAPTER 11

Surviving as a Trainee Advanced Practitioner

Marianne Jenkins　■　Claire Manderson　■　Nicola Assassa　■　Sandie Haigh
■　Gillian Morris　■　Rebecca Britton　■　Caz Crossland　■　Jonathan Drury

CHAPTER OUTLINE

This chapter has been written for students by students. It provides a narrative of their own experiences and the lessons learnt which can be shared with future aspiring advanced practitioners. Building on the themes of personal identity, imposter syndrome and supervision, experiences and perspectives are discussed and explored. This has allowed for the creation of the top 10 tips to surviving as a trainee advanced practitioner.

Introduction

The move from a traditional professional role into the advanced practice (AP) professional space is not easy. It reflects a shift from an expert level of professional practice that brings with it confidence and comfort in your professional abilities to a novice level which causes a lack of confidence and a lot of discomfort. Working through the training process with the tensions of academic requirements, work-based pressures and a personal life will leave you feeling overwhelmed. The aim of this chapter is to reassure you that these transitional challenges reflect the AP journey, and it is an experience that most, if not all, go through regardless of foundation profession. Moran and Naim (2018) identified six themes associated with the transition from existing role into advanced clinical practitioner (ACP) role:

1. Experience of change in work environment
2. Orientation to role, environment, new colleagues and culture
3. Appropriate mentorship
4. Supported development of clinical skills
5. Clinical supervision
6. Appropriate education at master's level

Themes 2, 3 and 5 will be discussed further in this chapter under the concept headings of:

- Professional identity
- Imposter syndrome
- Supervision

This chapter will discuss current evidence regarding this transitional experience as well relating it back to the experience of seven trainee ACPs from across the UK. These ACPs also have a variety of professional backgrounds—nurses (primary care, emergency medicine, paediatrics and mental health), physiotherapist, dietician and orthoptist. This diversity captures the same themes from across the UK and across the professional groups.

There is a list of the top 10 tips from those who have survived the trainee advanced practitioner stage and are now establishing themselves in their ACP roles. During the transition from trainee to qualified advanced practitioner, there are personal and practical considerations that you need to be mindful of and plan to manage them to support your success (and survival).

Professional Identity

Professional identity reflects not only what others perceive you are in a professional role but also what you as a professional recognise and own as your identity. It is formed by aligning your values, morals, knowledge and skills with your profession through socialisation and role modelling (Kidner, 2022). The challenge as a trainee advanced practitioner is reconciling a new professional identity with your existing one. The identity you develop in your foundation profession is developed from working with your professional group—nursing, physiotherapy, paramedic, occupational therapist, dietician, pharmacist or any other allied health professional. Once you have been appointed to a trainee advanced practitioner role, then you will start changing the way you approach patient assessment and care; this, combined with an increasing responsibility and autonomy, is more challenging than anticipated. Kluijtmans et al. (2017) describe this initial phase of developing a new professional identity as duality, where both identities are visible. Over time, a meta-identity develops, and this facilitates a new professional identity that can successfully work across the previous and new professional spaces (Kluijtmans et al., 2017). For advanced practitioner roles, the new professional identity has shared skills with medicine, so having good support and supervision from medical colleagues is vital. Role modelling and socialisation with the medical team allow you to develop aspects of the advanced practitioner's identity that can only be developed this way. Clinical decision-making and diagnosis have long been the purview of medicine, and with this being a key responsibility of an advanced practitioner, then learning these skills from medical colleagues will support your development.

Trainee ACP (physiotherapist) Claire Manderson describes her experience of this transition.

'Life as a trainee ACP is unique and challenging, so being prepared for it will undoubtedly stand you in good stead. You will have been told how hard the course is and how much of a challenge it is—but you can take action to not only survive but thrive as a trainee. Firstly, this is not a brand-new role for you; to even be considered for the training, you have been identified as an experienced and skilled healthcare professional

and so you bring with you a battery of talent that you can use every day. Things that some people might call "the basics" but I would argue are the things that make the biggest difference to our patients and their families: communication, teamwork, leadership, role model behaviour, compassion, self-awareness and a strong professional identity. There have been times in my training when I have felt like an absolute novice, and this is an uncomfortable sensation to experience too often. However, I can always call upon my existing skills and, in so doing, can remind myself that whilst a learner, I am definitely not a novice. I'm a physiotherapist with 25 years' experience of assessing patients, formulating treatment plans, delegating where appropriate, using outcome measures, reassessing and ultimately discharging patients. As a trainee ACP, I am learning to add layer upon layer of knowledge and skills to that existing rock-solid foundation. At least 20 years of my career was spent working in elderly medicine and rehabilitation services and my apprenticeship is with the acute frailty and elderly medicine teams at my employing organisation. Most days involve at least one "Eureka moment" as something I have always wondered about gets answered!

My second point is the value of a strong professional identity, and indeed that is an emerging dual identity for me. I am a physiotherapist, and I am an ACP. Each identity enhances the other, and often when new colleagues find out that I am a physiotherapist, they realise they have been noticing a different skill set and qualities to the trainee ACPs from other professions. Don't lose sight of who you are, and what has brought you to this position. In the first year of my training, I made some very strong professional alliances with the Foundation Year doctors in the hospital; there was no doubt that I needed to lean on their clinical skills and medical training, but my contribution was invaluable to them where communication was challenging, the families were in need of additional emotional support or where moving and handling was complex. The mutual learning opportunities from these working relationships are unique.'

It is a key survival skill to find the right role model and support when developing this new professional identity, and developing relationships not only with doctors but also with other advanced practitioners will provide the support when you become unsure of who you are. Losing sight of your professional identity during this transitional period is not uncommon; however, remembering the experience and professional background that you brought to the role should provide you with the grounding to keep you on track. As the first dietician to train as an ACP in her organisation, Nicola Assassa drew on her previous experience to remind herself of the skills she already had:

'I am a dietitian by profession with 30 years' experience and the first dietitian in my Trust to be an apprentice ACP and the first dietitian on an advanced clinical practitioners course at Huddersfield University. There are less than 10 dietetic ACPs training in the Yorkshire region and this may be because they think the role is not for them; however, I am now nearing the end of my third year of training and am thoroughly enjoying the experience and I can honestly say it is the best decision I have ever made in my career, and I would encourage more dietitians to train.

Although the role is far removed from dietetics, I feel my previous experience in three of the pillars has been helpful—previous leadership and management experience as a dietetic manager; the teaching of dietetic students, nursing and medical staff; and having some audit experience. The clinical role, however, was more of a challenge for me. Dietetics is very much a hands-off profession with our main skills being in communication and counselling; the thought of clinical examination was rather daunting. But working on a same day emergency care department with experienced ACPs and medical consultants has given me opportunities to practice clinical examination with support and guidance and I now feel competent in this area and teach medical students how to do clinical examination.'

As part of professional identity development, there is a need to know and understand what the role is and where it sits within the wider professional arena. Understanding who you are and where you fit is a key aspect of the transition from foundation profession to advanced practitioner. As an experienced nurse, Sandie Haigh describes how she reconciled this:

'In 2020, I started my journey as a trainee ACP. I had nearly 20 years' experience in various settings as a staff nurse, clinical educator and later a resuscitation officer (RO). I was ready for a change and a new challenge; however, what I wasn't ready for was the complete change in mind set that I had to learn.
One of the other challenges I came up against was that of "who am I", "Where do I fit", since the ACP role within the emergency department was a new concept in the National Health Service (NHS) Trust I was employed at. We didn't quite fit into the nursing side but also were not doctors. The doctors would treat us as junior doctors as they knew we had the core skills and capabilities, but what we didn't have is the same approach to patient care, or the 5 years in medical school to gain the theory. As a nurse, I feel we take a much more holistic approach to patient care and take the time to unpick the problems, whereas I found doctors tend to approach in a different way; this form of thinking took a long time to develop, not that I wasn't being holistic but more that rapid system thinking and decision-making, such as, did I need to treat now, what is the presentation today?
Over time, and practice, this started to become second nature and the ability to then join the two ways of working (nursing and medicine) together meant I was able to sit on both sides and provide a much more holistic, all-in-one patient care.'

Challenges with developing this new professional identity are noted where there is a lack of understanding of the advanced practitioner role, which is made more challenging when training and supervision are not adequately organised. As an experienced nurse with significant clinical and teaching background, Gillian Morris experienced challenges with training and professional identity development:

'It took me a few weeks to become familiar with the new clinical area. There were issues relating to staff vacancies and sickness. This often meant that I was expected to

undertake the role of a staff nurse because there was nobody else there to do this for the patients. I also did not have a designated practice assessor. It took some time to be allocated a medical colleague who worked in the area 1 day per week. There were other trainees in the area, and we quickly formed a support network. I was surprised that amongst both nursing and medical colleagues, the role and function of an advanced practitioner was misunderstood. This led to a strong lack of role identity which was uncomfortable. I felt like I did not fit into a nursing or medical role. I realised that in order to receive the support and training required to prepare me for becoming a qualified advanced practitioner, I would have to be more assertive in seeking out learning opportunities and not gravitating to the comfortable duties of a staff nurse. It took a number of meetings within the area to begin to establish what my needs were in relation to developing skills in advanced clinical assessment. Within the cohort that commenced the MSc AP, it was reassuring to hear that others were in similar situations, where the training requirements of the role were not well understood and that this sometimes led to conflict and stress. It was sometimes difficult to get the chance to practice skills such as chest auscultation, abdominal examination and cardiovascular assessment. However, once the presence of the trainee advanced nurse practitioners became more established, the medical staff tried hard to make sure there were opportunities to develop these skills through practice. An interesting part of this was making sense of the clinical skills we had been taught and what the medical team thought we needed to know. This led to interesting discussion and debate. It was also a challenge to get study time. The areas were very busy and there was no agreed plan for time allocated for this. However, this was common in the cohort and the support from the academic team and fellow students helped keep morale high and motivation maintained.'

Support and good supervision from medical colleagues are a great enabler and choosing the right practice supervisor is important.

Imposter Syndrome

The initial feelings of uncertainty about role and identity often feed into the deeper worries about being 'found out'. There is increasing awareness and recognition regarding the concept of imposter syndrome, and the challenges relating to developing a new professional identity also create feelings associated with imposter syndrome. Imposter syndrome describes the feeling of being a fraud in your professional role (Burkeman, 2013), this feeling of not being good enough and that personal success is related to luck and not ability or talent, which can lead you to believe you have 'tricked' others into thinking you are more competent than you are (Bannatyne, 2015). This was first acknowledged as a phenomenon in the 1970s by Clance and Imes, who researched the experiences of high-achieving women. It was identified that despite evidence of their abilities, they could not acknowledge their achievements and felt undeserving of their success and were concerned about being exposed as frauds (Clance & Imes, 1978). It is recognised that the transition from expert to novice that occurs as part of the transition to advanced practitioner contributes to the imposter feelings (Murphy & Mortimer, 2020). Completing your training to become a safe and competent advanced practitioner is a significant achievement; therefore, developing a strategy to accept and acknowledge your achievements and minimise the feeling of being an imposter is important.

Rebecca Britton is a trainee ACP with a background as a mental health nurse, and she describes her experience and advice regarding imposter syndrome:

> 'You will feel like an imposter; a fraud, like you don't belong or shouldn't be on the course...this is completely normal; and I guarantee that if you speak to other trainee colleagues at sometime within their training, they will have felt the same way. Normalise feeling an imposter, use it to your advantage; you are in a privileged position; upon qualifying, you will never again get to spend time with colleagues of different specialties, immersing yourself in all the different experiences and the various ways of working of other practitioners. Yes, you feel like an imposter but when else are you actually "protected" to undertake these opportunities?'

Using reflective practice to support your personal and professional development will provide a quantifiable record of how you are developing in the role. This can be helpful when imposter syndrome makes you doubt your skills, abilities and worthiness to do the role. Your portfolio will provide the reassurance that you are not a fraud and that you do know what you are doing. As you mature into the role, these feelings lessen as you become more comfortable and confident in your role.

Good supervision (academic and practice) and support can also help reconcile the imposter syndrome feelings, and the following section explores this further.

Supervisor

A pivotal relationship to support, guide and help you survive the transition is that with your clinical supervisor—choose them wisely. Traditionally, this would have been a medical consultant; however, with the expansion of AP roles, there are an increasing number of senior or lead advanced practitioners who can fulfil the supervisor role. Moran and Naim (2018) identified the supervisor role as being key to the successful transition to an advanced practitioner role. Take some time to reflect not only on how you learn and what works to keep you on track but also on whose approval will provide you with the validation that will give you confidence. This relationship is important in ensuring you develop not only the clinical skills to fulfil your role but also the confidence to use them. Medical colleagues with experience of working with or supervising advanced practitioners positively endorsed the benefits of the role (Hooks & Walker, 2020). Being honest with your supervisor about your learning needs is important, so choosing someone who you feel comfortable having this conversation with is beneficial:

> 'I have found being honest about what I don't know and making my clinical supervisor, the university and other ACPs aware have enabled me to address my

areas of weakness and get more experience and support, so I am now a competent practitioner.'

(Nicola Assassa, trainee ACP, dietician)

The mentoring support from medical consultants has been identified as an overwhelmingly positive experience (Mannix & Jones, 2020). Fothergill et al. (2022) noted inconsistency in supervision provision in a wider study, but for those who had supervision, it was a positive experience. There are growing numbers of experienced advanced practitioners who can support your supervision also. Gillian Morris (trainee ACP, nurse) recognised the benefit of an advanced practitioner as a practice assessor:

'I was placed in a general practice setting and my practice assessor was an advanced nurse practitioner. Again, I encountered a steep learning curve but found my time in acute medicine helped me identify unwell patients. I enjoyed the more focused and structured model of supervision from my practice assessor and wider medical team. I was able to identify my own learning opportunities in both primary and secondary care and felt more autonomous.'

With the growing numbers of experienced and senior or lead advanced practitioners within teams, there are opportunities for both medical and advanced practitioner supervisors to support you. Caz Crossland, a trainee ACP in paediatrics, found the support of senior advanced practitioner colleagues invaluable:

'I completed my MSc during the COVID-19 pandemic. Learning online was different and tricky on times—it took a while to get used to. There were fewer opportunities to ask questions/bounce ideas off fellow students; the teaching and practicing of clinical skills were diminished as we were not meeting face to face. This meant that time in clinical practice became even more important, utilising every opportunity to develop necessary skills and working closely with senior advanced nurse practitioners. I was lucky to have such experienced colleagues who were able to offer me guidance. I am still constantly learning from them as I continue to develop across the four pillars of advanced practice.'

The medical supervisor can also be the one that provides validation within the team, so choosing a supervisor who not only understands AP but also values it can be helpful in gaining acceptance. There is a growing body of evidence regarding the benefits of good supervision as part of the role transition and also for ongoing development and support (Murphy & Mortimer, 2020). Wood et al. (2021) identified the wider options for supervision and support through peer and informal support sessions, as well as looking outside the organisation for regional and national groups.

The supervisor's role is not only to support and guide but also to assess and identify areas for improvement; this role is separate from a mentorship role

(Murphy & Mortimer, 2020). Therefore, being clear as to who you want for what aspect of your training and development is important.

In summary, these three concepts of the transition process are key considerations to be addressed to ease you through this challenging time. Recognising and developing your new professional identity will minimise the feelings associated with imposter syndrome. A good practice supervisor and support network will facilitate this transition and ensure you start your qualified advanced practitioner phase with confidence and competence. The following are 10 practical tips compiled from advice tendered by current and recently qualified ACPs.

Top Tips for Surviving as a Trainee Advanced Clinical Practitioner

1—ELEPHANT EATING

Plan small, manageable goals and keep working to achieve these. The workload within an MSc AP programme might appear daunting at first; however, if you keep working at it, piece by piece, this will stop the work from piling up and becoming overwhelming and unmanageable. You cannot leave any academic work or practice supervision hours until the last minute as this will be unachievable, for example with assignments, exam revision or the development of a portfolio. Remember the answer to 'how do you eat an elephant?' is 'one bite at a time.'

Sandie Haigh (trainee ACP in emergency medicine) used this approach when finding the breadth of learning for the clinical conditions that could present in an emergency department:

'Another problem I had was the huge variety of patients which came through the doors. I found it very difficult to know where to start, what subject to read about, what did I need to know; this was another challenge to overcome. The broad spectrum of conditions, injuries, illnesses, presentation and ages of patients was overwhelming. With this, I found that I needed to break it down and have some self-discipline. I would select a system (initially whatever I was learning on the clinical patient assessment module at the time) and focus on only seeing patients who presented with that area of concern, e.g., chest pain—cardiorespiratory. Once I had gained the basics of applying the theory to practice, such as auscultation, I built on the differential diagnosis and achieved a few tickets (evidence for my practice portfolio); I then moved to the next system. For me, this was the easiest way to reduce the horror of where to start in the huge field of emergency medicine. I also decided to set myself goals to have,* *say, five tickets (pieces of evidence) by x date. That way, I was able to manage my portfolio and not discover near the end that I had lots to do.'*

All the trainees have recommended developing the habit of collecting evidence constantly, little and often means that you do not slip behind. Sandie Haigh also recognised the challenge of asking for the required assessments for the practice portfolio, so-called 'tickets':

'The tickets! This is the key, lots of tickets. It took me a while to feel comfortable in sending (and resending!) these as it wasn't something I have ever needed to do before. The tickets needed time to complete. Some of them were straightforward, but others required a bit of thought, case-based discussions (CBDs) and mini clinical evaluation exercise (mini-CEX). The best way to get the evidence which covers multiple aspects of the portfolio is to put the effort into the tickets; this I did find pretty early on, which was a huge help later down the line.'

PIT STOP!

Chapter 13 explores the portfolio for practice and the evidence that can be gathered to develop this piece of work.

2—WORK SMART

The value of digital solutions to support practice cannot be underestimated, but know the good ones. Use available apps to work smart, especially formulary and clinical guidelines. You do not need to know everything all the time, but knowing where to find relevant information and how to use it in your practice is helpful. There are well-recognised websites with quality information and guidelines to support your practice that can be easily accessed. Speak to colleagues to see what they use, especially the foundation doctors who are often in the similar position of knowing how to work smart.

Another aspect of working smart is recognising the learning opportunities available to you as a trainee advanced practitioner. Attending other clinical environments and spending time with different specialities are invaluable in expanding your knowledge and skills. This was noted by Jonathan Drury, who is a trainee ACP in ophthalmology with a background as an orthoptist:

'I am in quite a unique position in that my training has not followed one of the ACP pathways in ophthalmology available in the country. I joined the generic MSc AP programme as it was felt that this would further my holistic development and at the end of the training, I would be a more complete, well-rounded practitioner. Is this what I was expecting when I took on my new role? No. Has it so far been worthwhile? Absolutely!
My first year was spent working on an acute ward assessing patients with a whole manner of systemic complications. In fact, I barely saw an eye for 12 months,

and when there was anyone with a visual symptom, I was very popular, as you would be surprised how little experience trained professionals on the wards have using an ophthalmoscope. But what I did learn with the acute team and with the tutors at the university has changed the way I approach and manage a patient forever.'

Remember also that a single encounter with a patient can evidence your learning and development across more than just the clinical pillar. Think about what you learnt; turn it into a teaching session for colleagues (education pillar). Explore the evidence base behind your clinical decision-making and identify if there are guidelines to support or not, and if not, write them (leadership and research). Present an article at journal club on the condition it provides evidence for both the education and research pillars, so work smart.

3—STUDY SMART

Develop an academic timetable for your learning and stick to it, but make sure there is rest time in the timetable. Be creative about your learning; as an adult learner, find what works for you to be efficient with your learning. Anatomy and physiology colouring books are great for learning and revising (as well as relaxing). Practice your clinical skills with friends and family, not just at work. Use online videos to revise, but make sure they are suitable for your course; some of the Royal Colleges have Objective Structured Clinical Examination (OSCE) practice videos that are high quality and worth watching. Treat every clinical assessment as if it is under examination conditions so you develop a confident and practiced approach. This works particularly well for the challenging system assessments such as a neurological examination. Nicola Assassa recognised the importance of identifying learning needs, areas for development and asking for help:

'The hardest area for me as a trainee has been looking after the acutely ill patient as I had no prior experience, and I made the university teaching team aware of this personal challenge. In Year 2 the programme teaching team organised a day on caring for the patient with sepsis. This day alleviated my fears and I now feel more confident. I have found the university programme teaching team very flexible if you make them aware of the areas you are finding more challenging.
I have found being honest about what I don't know and making my clinical supervisor, the university teaching team and other ACPs aware have enabled me to address my areas of weakness and get more experience and support, so I am now a competent practitioner.'

Podcasts are great for bitesize learning, many produced by the Royal Colleges and by other reputable organisations which cover all topics applicable to the four pillars of AP. Speak to your colleagues about the ones they use; you will be surprised about the number of high-quality ones available. Writing a structured reflection on your learning and then adding to it when you apply it in practice or in teaching provides evidence of your learning and development. This is a good practice to develop and maintain at the start of your AP journey, as you will need to maintain an AP portfolio when working as an advanced practitioner.

4—ASK FOR HELP

You are learning, so do not expect to know everything; remember no one knows everything. Your medical colleagues will have gone through these assessments and can help support and guide you. Speak to advanced practitioners and your peers who are training with you and learn from their experiences. Speak to your university programme teaching team about measures to address personal learning needs that are unmet. During this transition stage, it is a safe time to ask for help and expect to be helped; do not try to do this alone and do not think you are alone. Caz Crossland (trainee advanced paediatric nurse practitioner) noted the need to ask for help:

> 'take the time you need around exams and OSCEs. It's ok to have time away from clinical practice when the academic load is great. Set small, achievable goals when the end goal seems too much.'

5—BE REFLECTIVE

Take time to think about yourself, your learning, your achievements and challenges, then capture this through reflection within your portfolio. It is helpful to look back on these reflections as you progress through your training as they mark your development in both a personal and a professional way.

Rebecca Britton (trainee ACP, mental health nurse) found it an invaluable process and highly recommends it:

> 'Reflections will become your ally; not only do they provide great learning opportunities to reflect on clinical practice, they also allow for a platform whereby you can measure your own progress and development. Personal reflective accounts I have found invaluable; reading back through these has taught me so much about my development as a trainee ACP, my progress as a clinical practitioner; but most importantly, they have taught me so much about myself as a person when in a place of uncertainty.'

6—UNDERSTAND WHAT YOUR ROLE IS, BE PREPARED TO EXPLAIN IT OFTEN AND KNOW YOUR LIMITS

Despite the increasing body of knowledge regarding the advanced practitioner role, it remains a 'new' role to many and you will be asked who you are and what you are on multiple occasions, so be prepared! To do this, you need to be clear about your role and scope of practice so you can clearly communicate it to others. While the advanced practitioner role is generic in nature, it is fulfilled by a variety of healthcare professionals. This brings with it differing scopes and permissions to practice, so understanding both your professional responsibilities is important. Nicola Assassa (trainee ACP, dietician) recommends:

> *'People don't understand what I do. Be prepared for doctors, patients and other health professionals to not understand the ACP roles. Many healthcare professionals do not realise you are a senior member of staff because you are not a manager. Doctors may not want the role as they feel their job should not be done by ACPs. Be prepared to explain the role and justify the work you do.'*

Knowing your role and its limits is particularly helpful when being asked to work outside your scope or skills. Jonathan Drury (ACP, ophthalmology) reported challenges with their role transition, notably associated with independent prescribing and being a healthcare professional without permissions to prescribe.

> *'As a registered orthoptist, I am not eligible to prescribe. This is my biggest challenge with the role of an ACP. I don't practice as an orthoptist on a day-to-day basis; I am more likened to a nurse practitioner. But despite my change in role, this doesn't change my ability to prescribe. I am the only trainee in the class who is unable prescribe or take the prescribing module, so I have had to take on additional modules to compensate. I hope one day this will be rectified as it is the one thing holding myself and other orthoptists back from fully embracing the ACP role. For now, PGDs will have to suffice.'*

Nicola Assassa also gives advice for other dieticians undertaking this role transition that would apply for other healthcare professionals who need some foundation skills in place to help them in their training:

> *'Dietitians must have an extended role approved by their organisation to deliver medicines. This is a Health Care Professions Council (HCPC) requirement. I would therefore encourage dietitians who want to be ACPs to get this approved before starting the role as this has been quite time consuming to achieve while doing the training. I had no nursing practical skills prior to training, and these are required, and I recommend contacting the clinical skills team at your organisation to learn cannulation and venepuncture.*
>
> *Prescribing has been the most frustrating part of the course for me. I completed my independent and supplementary prescribing course in year 2, but as a dietitian, I can only be awarded supplementary prescribing rights, which is a regulation by HCPC. This does hinder my role as an ACP, and I would encourage more dietitians to train as ACPs for there to be a stronger voice for dietitians to become independent prescribers.'*

7—LEARN THE ART OF SAYING YES

As a trainee advanced practitioner, you are in a unique position to learn. This is a singular time in your career where you are permitted to actively seek out learning opportunities and experience. Claire Manderson (ACP, physiotherapist) advises:

> *'My final suggestion is one that I have committed to since the start of my training, and it is the art of saying yes. Being unchained from the workplace and caseload demands of being a senior physiotherapist and stepping into a role where my aim is learning and development have been nothing short of a revolution in thinking. The learning needs ahead of me at any point can feel like an ocean to cross, but with every experience that I can say yes to, I dip my toe in just that little bit more. This applies firmly across all four pillars of AP and as often is the case the clinical opportunities are maybe the most obvious; I have taken all and every offer of work-shadowing and observation, from cardiac physiology to palliative care and so much more. If anyone has asked "would you like to see x, y, z...", I have said yes. I have seen and experienced more variety in the past 18 months than in the preceding quarter century, and every opportunity has helped me to put together another piece of the jigsaw. It really is a gift to be able to step back and be curious; I have formed new friendships across the hospital and have an ever-growing network of people I have worked alongside, any one of whom may prove to be an essential contact at some point in my future career. I have also presented myself as somewhat of an evangelist for AP on these occasions as awareness of the diversity of the role can be lacking.*
>
> *Of course, AP goes well beyond the clinical pillar, and since starting my training, I have been able to attend webinars, meetings and special interest groups not open to me before. I have spoken with the vice chancellor of the university and to groups of aspiring ACPs about my experiences; I have got involved in teaching undergraduate physiotherapy students on frailty and care of the older person, and on every occasion the daunted feelings give way to a feeling of achievement. All these small wins add to the confidence that will be needed when I am a qualified ACP to walk into a clinical situation and handle it with skill, grace and professionalism.*
>
> *So be bold, say yes and take every opportunity. You may even find yourself contributing to a chapter of a book!'*

8—LOOK AFTER YOURSELF

This is a 3-year minimum training process which will impact on your life significantly. Get your family and friends on board with supporting you and not distracting you. Life will challenge you throughout the process, so use your support networks to help you. Looking after yourself does not just happen outside of work, but also within practice. Learning the art of a clinical consultation and taking on greater responsibility for patients is challenging. As highlighted in Chapter 4, with Neighbour's (1987) Inner Consultation and the housekeeping stage which focuses on the practitioner's own needs post a consultation.

Jonathan Drury (trainee ACP, orthoptist) is mindful of this:

'One piece of advice. The patient in the room with you is the most important person and deserves your attention. Patients waiting outside will have their time and will expect the same level of attention from you. So never feel the need to rush under pressure. You are learning and it is expected you will take a little longer.
What about when the patient leaves the room? Well then you are the only person in the room and therefore the most important. It is essential that you acknowledge this and take a moment for yourself. You may need a drink of water, a bathroom break or time to reflect on your last consultation. You may have broken bad news and need a moment to process what was said and consolidate your own feelings surrounding often difficult conversations. This is crucial and should be encouraged because the moment you call the next patient into the room, they become the most important person. After all, they deserve your full attention and the expertise of a compassionate practitioner with a clear, focused mind, ready to deliver high standards of care and a few moments to take stock will help you achieve this.'

9—PEER NETWORK

Reach out and find your AP family. There are growing networks within organisations and across regions; find them (social media is good for this). You do not have to wait until you are qualified until you join in with the wider AP community. Everyone was a trainee at some point, so participating in a network that can support you through the challenges of transition is helpful.

Caz Crossland noted the benefit of peer and senior support:

'utilising every opportunity to develop necessary skills and working closely with senior advanced nurse practitioners. I was lucky to have such experienced colleagues who were able to offer me guidance. I am still constantly learning from them as I continue to develop across the four pillars of AP.'

10—ENJOY IT!

Although it is recognised as a challenging time and rite of passage, all the trainees who contributed advised to take the time to enjoy the learning and widen your professional circle of colleagues and peers. Remember when it is overwhelming that this is the role you have been drawn to do and your motivation and desire to achieve will get you through this. The benefits at the end of the training and transitioning far outweigh the challenges; the expanded scope and the autonomous practice that improves patient care and services are worth it.

Conclusion

This chapter has brought together the views and perspectives of those training to become an advanced practitioner. This offers a unique opportunity as it draws from practitioners across the UK and from different professional and specialist backgrounds. Common themes have emerged around professional identity and that feeling of being an imposter syndrome. The recognition of robust practice supervision has been identified as an important factor within the AP journey. The top 10 tips for the aspiring advanced practitioner have provided a valuable foundation for reflection for development.

References

Bannatyne, A. J. (2015). When will my cover be blown? The experience of imposter syndrome in emerging and early career academics/educators [online]. pdfs.semanticscholar.org/5378/f1d26d9c2b065945fdaef-c777e98abccffa3.pdf (Accessed April 14, 2024)

Burkeman, O. (2013). This column will change your life: Do you feel like a fraud? www.theguardian.com/lifeandstyle/2013/nov/09/impostor-syndrome-oliver-burkeman (Accessed April 14, 2024)

Clance, P., R., & Imes, S., A. (1978). The imposter phenomenon in high achieving women: Dynamics and therapeutic intervention. *Psychotherapy: Theory, Research & Practice, 15*(3), 241–247.

Fothergill, L. J., Al-Oraibi, A., Houdmont, J., Conway, J., Evans, C., Timmons, S., et al. (2022). Nationwide evaluation of the advanced clinical practitioner role in England: A cross-sectional survey. *BMJ Open 12*(1), e055475. doi:10.1136/bmjopen-2021-055475

Hooks, C., & Walker, S. (2020). An exploration of the role of advanced clinical practitioners in the East of England. *British Journal of Nursing, 29*(15), 864–869.

Kidner, M. (2022). *Successful advanced practice nurse role transition: A structured process to developing professional identity through role transition.* Switzerland: Springer.

Kluijtmans, M., de Haan, E., Akkerman, S., & van Tartwijk, J. (2017). Professional identity in clinician-scientists: Brokers between care and science. *Medical Education 51*, 645–655.

Mannix, K., & Jones, C. (2020). Nurses' experiences of transitioning into advanced practice roles. *Nursing Times, 116*(3), 35–38.

Moran, G., M., & Naim, S. (2018). How does role transition affect the experience of trainee advanced clinical practitioners: Qualitative evidence synthesis. *Journal of Advanced Nursing, 74*(2), 251–262.

Murphy, K., & Mortimore, G. (2020). Overcoming the challenges of role transition for trainee advanced clinical practitioners. *Gastrointestinal Nursing, 18*(5), 35–41.

Neighbour, R. (1987). *The inner consultation.* Oxford: Radcliffe Medical Press.

Wood, E., King, R., Robertson, S., Senek, M., Tod, A., & Ryan, T. (2021). Sources of satisfaction, dissatisfaction and well-being for UK advanced practice nurses: A qualitative study. *Journal of Nursing Management, 29*(5), 1073–1080.

CHAPTER 12

Supervision and Assessment in Advanced Practice

Deborah Harding ■ Colette Henderson

CHAPTER OUTLINE

In this chapter, we share some key concepts and ideas about both supervision and assessment in advanced practice (AP) which can support you with developing clear expectations for your own AP development. We aim to try and demystify some of the key terminology utilised around supervision and assessment. The regulatory context for supervision and assessment is considered and what this means for advanced practice. We continue this chapter by thinking about supervision, including its relationship with assessment, and then move on to consider education and practice assessment in more detail.

Introduction

As an experienced registered professional embarking on becoming an advanced level practitioner, you might already feel that supervision and assessment are familiar concepts. The standards of proficiency for registration bodies such as the Nursing and Midwifery Council (NMC, 2018), the Health and Care Professions Council (HCPC, 2023) and the General Pharmaceutical Council (2017) encourage registrants to engage in continuing professional development (CPD) activities such as supervision both as recipients and as supervisors and educators for others. However, we hear from our colleagues and our students that supervision and assessment in advanced practice (AP) can feel quite unfamiliar. We also know that the transition from experienced practitioner to advanced practitioner can be unsettling and that supervision plays an important part in supporting that progression (Moran & Nairn, 2018; Murphy & Mortimore, 2020). Reflecting on your existing experiences and associated understanding of both supervision and assessment can be a helpful part of the preparation for this developmental journey. In this chapter, we share some key concepts and ideas about both supervision and assessment in AP which can support you with that reflection and help you to develop clearer expectations for your own AP development. We begin by thinking about supervision, including its relationship with assessment, and then move on to consider education and practice assessment in more detail. You will notice that there are ways in which both supervision and assessment intertwine during the progression to AP.

Expectations and Assumptions About Supervision and Assessment

PIT STOP!

Before we proceed, we encourage you to pause and think about your current understanding of both supervision and assessment. You might capture your thoughts in writing, add them to your CPD portfolio and revisit these from time to time during your AP journey. Here are some questions which might help you with this:

- What sorts of assumptions do you have about supervision and assessment and how do these influence your definitions? Individual supervision experiences, a familiar definition, professional body or regulator guidance might be among the things which influence your definitions.
- What is your definition of supervision?
- How would you define assessment?
- What similarities and differences do you notice about supervision and assessment?
- In what ways might supervision and assessment be similar or different in your AP journey?

For many health professionals, our expectations about supervision and assessment will be based on assumptions we have developed through our prior experiences. While access to career-long supervision varies across professions and practice settings, it is possible that as you begin your AP development you have some recent supervisor and/or supervisee experiences. However, it might be some time since you feel you were assessed in practice. Your supervision expectations may be informed by profession-specific guidance from your professional body and or regulator in combination with any local policies and guidance your employer might have in place. You may have a range of supervision experiences from both supervisee and supervisor perspectives, some highly supportive and facilitative while others may have been less comfortable and, perhaps, as some have described, feeling rather like surveillance (Gilbert, 2001). Inevitably, because each of us will have our own unique and varied experiences of supervision and assessment, our assumptions and expectations also differ.

The Regulatory Context for Supervision

Regulatory bodies provide standards of proficiency to guide registrants about their scope of practice. This refers to the area or areas of a specified profession in which the registrant can demonstrate the necessary knowledge, skills and experience to practice effectively ensuring both registrant and public safety. Regarding supervision, the NMC Standards of Proficiency state a need to 'contribute to supervision and team reflection activities to promote improvements in practice and services...' (NMC, 2018, p. 20), and the HCPC refers to the need to 'understand the importance of active participation in training, supervision and mentoring' (HCPC, 2023).

Employers have legal responsibilities for ensuring registered professionals and other staff have 'the support, training, professional development, supervision and appraisals that are necessary for them to carry out their role and responsibilities' (Health and Social Care Act, 2008, 2014 Regulation 18), responsibilities which are increasingly recognised in guidance to employer organisations (NHS Employers, 2022; Scottish Government (SG), 2023).

As you develop to an advanced level of practice, you will want to look after your hard-won professional registration. Through your AP education and beyond, you will remain registered in your original qualifying profession. Registration renewal requires registrants to sign a declaration indicating that they continue to meet the standards for proficiency for the relevant scope of practice. The NMC has recently completed a review of AP which has resulted in the NMC Council agreeing to regulate AP (NMC, 2024). However, further work is required to enact this regulation, and the position regarding supervision for registrants in nursing and other professions meantime is discussed in detail here.

As AP is not regulated within the UK currently, the regulatory guidance does not refer explicitly to AP; however, guidance to registrants about safety and scope of practice provides some indication of how supervision is an integral part of registrants' training not just as a way to support learning but also as a professional responsibility. For example, the HCPC states:

> 'As long as you make sure that you are practising safely and effectively within your given scope of practice and do not practise in the areas where you are not proficient to do so, this will not be a problem. If you want to move outside of your scope of practice, you should be certain that you are capable of working lawfully, safely and effectively. This means that you need to exercise personal judgement by undertaking any necessary training or gaining experience, before moving into a new area of practice.'
>
> (HCPC, 2023)

Similarly, the NMC (2018, p. 4) indicates

> 'The professions we regulate have different knowledge and skills, set out in three distinct standards of proficiency. They can work in diverse contexts and have different levels of autonomy and responsibility. However, all of the professions we regulate exercise professional judgement and are accountable for their work.'

As you develop to an advanced level of practice, both supervision and assessment are fundamental for ensuring your ongoing professional safety and by implication, the safety of the public.

Defining Supervision

A published definition can provide a good starting point for a discussion about supervision assumptions, expectations and purpose. As you develop in AP, you will be encouraged to apply your critical thinking and appraisal at master's level. The search for a definition of supervision is a good illustration of why this critical awareness is so valuable because you will quickly discover a variety of perspectives about this aspect of practice. Consider, for example, this popular definition by Bernard and Goodyear (2004, p. 8), which describes supervision as:

'...an intervention provided by a more senior member of a profession to a more junior member or members of that same profession. This relationship is evaluative, extends over time, and has the simultaneous purposes of enhancing the professional functioning of the more junior person(s), monitoring the quality of professional services offered to the clients, she, he, or they see, and serving as a gatekeeper for those who are to enter the particular profession.'

Bernard and Goodyear's (2004) definition is often cited, but new definitions continue to be shared. The following definition from Snowdon et al. (2017, p. 787) draws on three sources: Lyth (2000), Kilminster et al. (2007) and Milne (2007), to suggest that clinical supervision is:

'... a professional development activity where the less experienced clinician can utilise the knowledge and experience of their supervisor, to address any gaps in knowledge or skill set and thereby improve their own clinical performance and patient quality of care.'

Comparing these two definitions, we can see some similarities and differences. Both indicate that a supervisor is a more experienced colleague, but what might that mean for peer supervision? For Bernard and Goodyear (2004), supervision is an enduring relationship and there is something about the supervisor's role in deciding whether the supervisee has met a threshold for professional practice which implies an assessment function. For Snowdon et al. (2017), there is something about addressing gaps in knowledge and improving the practitioner's performance. Both definitions link supervision with the quality of care for patients or clients. Snowdon et al. (2017) state that their definition is about clinical supervision. AP involves not only clinical advancement but also developing across the pillars of practice, which may mean that clinical supervision is relevant for clinical capabilities but not others. It is also often the case that supervision happens with experienced colleagues from other professions and not always as Bernard and Goodyear (2004) describe, with colleagues from the same profession. As you begin to explore the supervision literature, you will find a variety of other prefixes and descriptors: education supervision, professional supervision, managerial supervision, practice supervision, restorative supervision, associate supervision, peer supervision and research supervision, for example, as well as concepts which seem to overlap with supervision, like mentoring and coaching. The HCPC acknowledges this ambiguity on their website and state:

TABLE 12.1 ■ **Ten Indicators of Effective Supervision Drawing**

- Mutual trust and respect
- Matching supervisor with supervisee (expertise, personal and cultural factors)
- Shared understanding of purpose of supervisory encounter
- Focus on sharing and enhancing knowledge and skills to support professional development and service improvement
- Regular and based on supervisee needs—ad hoc as necessary
- Supervisory models (e.g., one-to-one, group) based on individual needs
- Protected time supported by employer
- Feedback and training for supervisors
- Flexible timetable to ensure accessibility to supervision
- Access to different types of supervision and supervisors

From: Rothwell, C., Kehoe, A., Farook, S. F., & Illing, J. (2021). Enablers and barriers to effective clinical supervision in the workplace: A rapid evidence review. BMJ Open.

'While there is no single or agreed definition of supervision, at its core, supervision is a process of professional learning and development that enables individuals to reflect on and develop their knowledge, skills, and competence, through agreed and regular support with another professional.'

(HCPC, 2021)

As you begin your AP development, it will be important to recognise that you will encounter different definitions, interpretations and assumptions about supervision. Supervision will be most effective when supervisors and supervisees discuss and establish a shared understanding about supervision and its purpose (Rothwell et al., 2021). It is valuable therefore, at an early stage, for supervisors and supervisees to share and discuss their assumptions and expectations about supervision and its purpose. Drawing on the work of Rothwell et al. (2021), 10 indicators of effective supervision are set out in Table 12.1.

The Relationship Between Supervision and Assessment

The definitions considered earlier provided a hint of the relationship between supervision and assessment. Bernard and Goodyear (2004, p. 8) referred to monitoring the quality of professional services and to a gatekeeping role in supervision, while Snowdon et al. (2017, p. 787) refer to addressing knowledge and skills gaps. The NHS England Centre for Advancing Practice recognises this relationship between supervision and assessment in their guidance for supervisor learning and development (NHS, 2023a). They propose 10 dimensions of supervisor capability (Fig. 12.1), one of which is 'fair, valid and reliable assessment'.

Arguably, this assessment dimension of supervisor capability is relevant for supervisors of the regulated and unregulated healthcare workforce at all levels as it

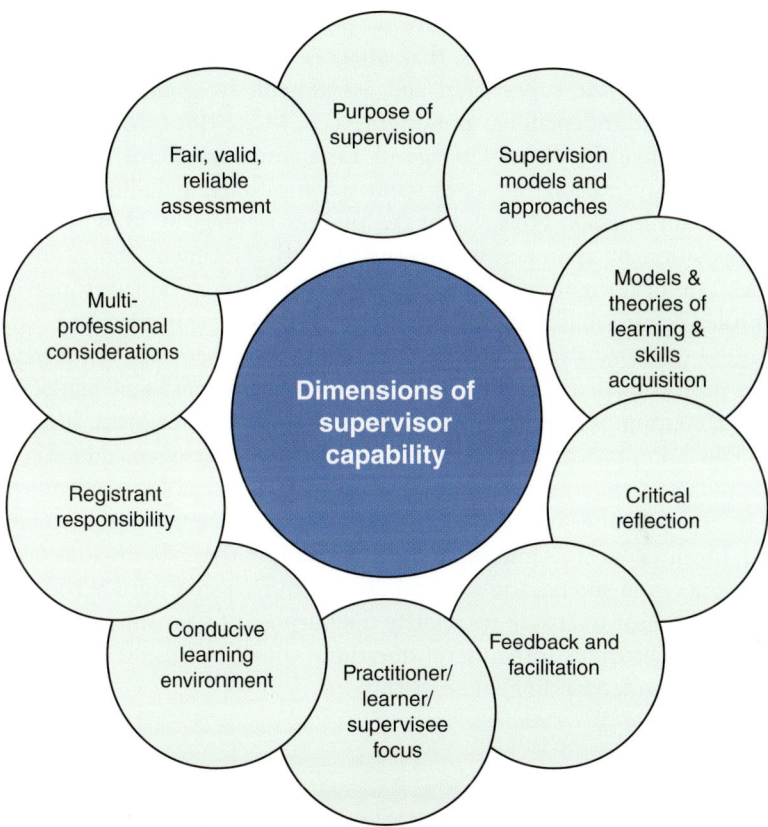

Fig. 12.1 NHS England Centre for Advancing Practice dimensions of supervisor capability. *(From NHS. (2023a). Advanced practice supervisor capabilities. Guiding principles for supervisor learning and development. https:// advanced-practice.hee.nhs.uk/our-work/supervision/advanced-practice-supervisor-capabilities/)*

underpins judgements about supervisee competence, safety and, where necessary, decisions about fitness to practice. The need for supervisors who are capable of fair, valid and reliable assessment will be more prominent when supervisees are actively learning and developing. Examples might include supervision during preregistration training or at times when a registered practitioner is acquiring new knowledge and skills, such as prescribing or other aspects of advanced level practice. Given that we are not always engaged in structured acquisition of new knowledge and skills, it is unsurprising that the assessment aspects of AP and the relationship with supervision can feel less familiar and more novel than other dimensions of supervision.

PIT STOP!

Reflect on your practice supervisors who supported you in practice when you were undertaking your preregistration training and what qualities made them good practice supervisors for you.

For many, progression to AP will involve both structured academic learning and workplace learning. In most cases, this entails a combination of university-based learning and workplace supervision and assessment. In some instances, such as supplementary and independent prescribing (HCPC, 2019; NMC, 2023) or specialty curricula, like the Royal College of Emergency Medicine (RCEM, 2022), there are clear supervision and assessment specifications, including who can be a supervisor or an assessor. However, at the time of writing, in 2024, there is not a universal position or approach to supervision and assessment across all AP and specialties. An ideal situation might see the separation of workplace supervisor and assessor roles, but in smaller specialty areas or workplaces, this may not be practical. It is also the case that supervisors, assessors and supervisees will not always share the same professional registration. Given this rather inconsistent landscape, it is vital that a common understanding of supervision and assessment is established between education providers, workplace supervisors and assessors and AP trainees from the outset of the trainee's development. It is also valuable to schedule regular points in the training when these tripartite arrangements are discussed and reviewed. Ideally, educators and supervisors will ensure these discussions take place, but as a trainee, you should also feel empowered to have and initiate conversations with your supervisor to ensure you clarify the purpose of your supervision encounters. Table 12.2 provides some useful questions which can facilitate the development of shared understanding and expectations.

TABLE 12.2 ■ Questions and Considerations to Establish a Common Understanding of Supervision and Assessment

Supervision and Assessment Checklist

The following questions might be useful to help guide conversations. Consider:

- Is this about guiding acquisition of skills?
- Will supervision be about critical reflection away from practice?
- Will supervision involve working with my supervisor in practice and being observed?
- How often will supervision take place?
- Is this an activity guiding understanding (formative)?
- Is this an activity for verification or sign-off (summative)?
- Will the supervisor and the assessor be the same person?
- Is this about knowledge and skills development?
- Is this about protocol or governance?
- Is this about supporting aspects of practitioner well-being?
- Is this about professional transition to an advanced level of practice?
- Which pillar is this specific to?

Share terms you are used to using and what you understand and expect from them, for example, if you have a specific understanding of clinical supervision or restorative supervision.

As someone embarking on your AP development, you will already be a very experienced registered practitioner in your own right and this can mean that much of your more recent supervision experiences have been **on** practice rather than **in** practice. In other words, you are probably less often observed in practice by your supervisor at this point in your career and instead use supervision as a time for critical reflection away from practice. The distinction is akin to reflection in and on action (Schön, 1983), which may be familiar. It is a distinction between learning through reflection *on* events after they have concluded while reflection *in* action is where an experienced practitioner reflects during a practice encounter, potentially adjusting their actions in real time. Rolfe (2011) draws on this distinction and the way in which it has been applied as live supervision in the training for novice family therapists (Montalvo, 1973) to suggest that there are aspects of wider healthcare practice where live workplace supervision can be valuable. Live supervision, while not explicitly labelled as such, will be familiar to medical doctors in training who often work side-by-side in practice with a designated clinical supervisor who is a more experienced colleague such as a general practice trainer or specialty consultant. Episodes of supervised practice may be combined with structured evaluation and formative assessment which provide supervised learning for the trainee (COPMed, 2022) and/or form the basis of later reflection on practice. This formative learning aspect of supervision provides important preparation for but is distinct from summative assessment and the verification or sign-off which indicates that the required level of practice has been achieved. In areas of AP where there is a strong overlap between the capabilities and curriculum for medical specialty trainees and those of AP trainees, workplace supervision arrangements for both sets of trainees are often similar. In these settings, trainee advanced practitioners can certainly expect a combination of workplace supervision *in* and *on* practice. However, live supervision will feature in other settings too. Working together with a supervisor in practice is a feature of AP supervision which is sometimes uncomfortable for experienced practitioners. However, it is a vital aspect of development, ensuring the AP trainee develops within the relevant scope of practice and professional code of conduct so that both practitioner and public safety is maintained. If the supervisor has grown up professionally with live supervision, then it can also be a surprise to the supervisor that this is unfamiliar for the trainee. We will return to this idea later in the chapter when we will explore the different supervisory needs of professionals with different registrations and in our discussion about workplace assessment of capability.

Supervision and Assessment Roles

Across the UK, a range of terminology reflecting supervision and assessment and role requirements exists. The UK multiprofessional focus of AP (Department of Health (DoH), 2016, 2019; National Health Service England (NHSE) 2025; SG, 2017, 2021; Welsh Government (WG), 2020) has no doubt increased the variety of terms used relating to supervision and assessment and what is understood on a profession-to-profession basis about what these terms actually mean. We need to spend a little time *demystifying*, reviewing and considering the various different terms that you may come across relating to supervision and assessment. However, as approaches to AP education and training continue to evolve and mature, it is not possible to provide a definitive list of the terms and roles you might encounter. Once again, our advice is to clarify the academic and workplace educator, supervisor and assessor titles and roles in the setting where you are advancing your practice. In the context of a programme of education, supervision and assessment may relate to either academic work or clinical practice learning.

Some of the commonly encountered roles include clinical supervisor, practice supervisor (PS), practice educator (PE), practice assessor (PA), academic assessor (AA), designated prescribing practitioner (DPP), coordinating education supervisor, associate workplace supervision and mentor. You may encounter others.

PE, PS, PA, DPP and AA all relate to regulatory bodies' terminology (NMC, 2023; HCPC, 2019; Royal Pharmaceutical Society (RPS), 2021). These terms are used within a supervision and assessment context when trainees undertake a regulatory body-approved module such as prescribing.

> **PIT STOP!**
>
> It would be useful for you to refer to your own professional guidance and clarify your understanding of the terms used by your regulator.

From the discussion earlier, the (clinical) supervisor tends to support and facilitate trainees' clinical development but is not necessarily involved in a summative assessment of a trainee's practice or the supervision of capabilities in the other pillars of practice.

Another factor that needs consideration is the requirement for a clinician who is not necessarily from the same professional group as the trainee to undertake an assessment of a trainee's clinical practice. This is clearly challenging as initial understandings about role requirements may vary between the trainee and the clinician in practice. In addition, it is not always clear what development the clinician in practice has undertaken to support their ability to undertake an assessment of competence. Practitioners have professional requirements to ensure they work within their scope of practice. It might be useful to consider the support you needed to develop the knowledge and skills required to practice clinically. Similarly, supervision of trainees requires practitioners to develop knowledge and skills to support robust supervisory capability.

Formative, Normative and Restorative Supervision and Assessment in Advanced Practice

A widely cited model of supervision, often attributed to Proctor (2008, p. 7), proposes three overlapping dimensions: formative, normative and restorative. The formative dimension of supervision is about supporting the learning and development of knowledge and skills, the normative refers to the maintenance of standards and the restorative aspect supports professional well-being as the practitioner navigates practice. Within AP, the formative dimension of supervision can support the augmentation of knowledge and skills acquisition which is required for the practitioner to progress from competent to capable, not just in clinical practice but also in the education, leadership and research pillars. A useful differentiation of competence and capability (Skills for Health, 2020, p. 9) describes competence as consistently performing to defined standards in stable environments with familiar problems. Within AP, encounters across the pillars of practice are more complex and problems less familiar, requiring advanced level capabilities, where capability can be thought of as being competent and beyond. This augmentation of knowledge and skills is accompanied by becoming familiar with relevant practice standards and protocols, along with the need to retain critical awareness of one's own registrant responsibilities. These are aspects of professional development which are consistent with the normative functions of supervision. As indicated in the opening paragraphs of this chapter, this transition from competent, experienced practitioner to capable advanced practitioner can be unsettling (Moran & Nairn, 2018; Murphy & Mortimore, 2020). AP trainees often describe something similar to the transition shock which has been identified in newly qualified nurses (Duchscher, 2009) and a sense of reverting from intuitive expert to rule-bound novice (Benner, 1984). These socioprofessional uncertainties can be felt very acutely when in a training role in a specialty where the practitioner has worked for some time and is already an established, experienced team member. This is when restorative aspects of supervision can be especially valuable.

Harding (2019) has suggested that supervision provides a safe place to share uncertainties (sanctuary) and an opportunity to explore ways to resolve practitioner uncertainties, in other words, a practice-based opportunity to think about practice (meta-practice). Harding's (2019) sanctuary function is not uniquely restorative; it is also about feeling safe to share formative and normative uncertainties. While some uncertainties can be resolved in supervision, supervisors will not have all the answers. Meta-practice in supervision refers not to solving an uncertainty but to the supervisor and supervisee exploring the sources of practice uncertainties and how these might be resolved or tolerated. This might mean being signposted to other formative activities like training or working with another supervisor around a specific capability, reviewing the trainee's progress against the required advanced capabilities (normative) or accessing psychological or staff support when necessary. Fig. 12.2 draws on Proctor's (2008, p. 7) ideas to demonstrate how supervision can entail both formative learning and assessment, summative verification that a required normative standard is met or restorative navigation of a professional transition.

Enablers and Helpful Behaviours and Characteristics for Supervisors and Supervisees

Harding (2019) also identified that practitioners only use supervision as a place of sanctuary and meta-practice when they perceive that there are conducive conditions

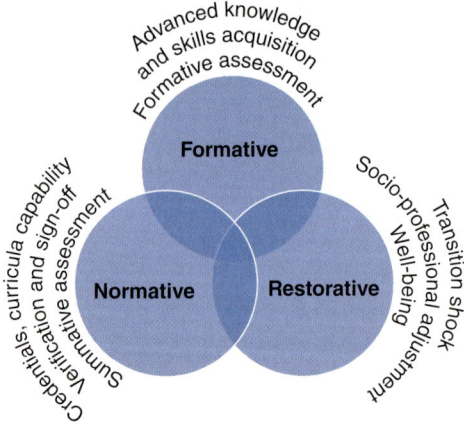

Fig. 12.2 Using Proctor's (2008, p. 7) dimensions to understand supervision and assessment in advanced practice. *(From Proctor, B. (2008).* Group supervision: A guide to creative practice. *(2nd Ed). London: Sage.)*

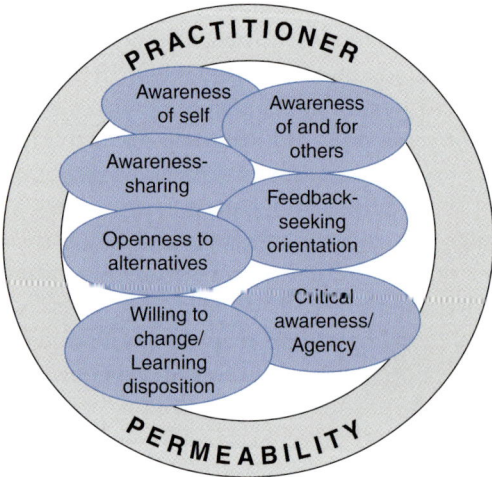

Fig. 12.3 Dimensions of practitioner permeability. *(From Harding, D. (2019).* Practitioner permeability and the resolution of practice uncertainties: A grounded theoretical perspective of supervision for allied health professionals *(PhD thesis). St George's, University of London. Available at: https://eprints.kingston.ac.uk/id/eprint/43854/ (Accessed 28.03.2023).)*

such as trust, a focus on the needs of the supervisee and a collaborative approach between supervisor and supervisee, enablers which are consistent with those identified across the supervision literature (Rothwell et al., 2021). Harding (2019) identified a cluster of practitioner behaviours and characteristics which are useful in identifying, learning from and resolving uncertainties. These behaviours and characteristics—self-awareness, awareness of and for others, awareness-sharing, feedback-seeking, open to alternatives, critical awareness and willingness to change—can be thought of in combination as 'practitioner permeability', as illustrated in Fig. 12.3.

TABLE 12.3 ■ **Preparing for Supervision: Being a Permeable Practitioner**

- **Self-awareness:** What aspects of your advanced practice development are creating uncertainties for you?

- **Awareness of others:** How might the ways you think others view you influence your uncertainties?

- **Awareness for others:** What are the implications of the uncertainties you are currently aware of for others: patients, colleagues, outside of work?

- **Awareness-sharing:** How are you going to present this uncertainty in supervision? Are there specific aspects of the uncertainty you want to explore with the supervisor?

- **Feedback-seeking:** Are you willing to receive feedback about the uncertainty?

- **Open to alternatives:** Are you prepared to have feedback and discuss alternative ways of addressing your uncertainty which might not have occurred to you or may be challenging?

- **Critical awareness:** How will you appraise any feedback and alternatives to explore a helpful way forward with your uncertainty?

- **Willingness to change:** How will you apply any new learning to your practice?

Table 12.3 provides some guidance to support thinking about how your own permeability can help you to make the most of supervision as suggested in Fig. 12.3.

Permeability is also important for supervisors as described in Table 12.4.

Practitioner permeability is a varying spectrum, and in any given day, inside and outside of practice, there will be times when we feel the need to be more impermeable, to stick to our position and others when we feel more porous and are seeking more support. Remaining at one or other extreme tends not to serve us so well, making us fragile because we are stuck in our ways and unwilling to change or because our insecurity is making us highly dependent on the support of others. However, if we pay attention to our permeability, we can adjust it to help us find the learning in the practice events we are navigating.

TABLE 12.4 ■ **Being a Permeable Supervisor**

- **Self-awareness:** Recognises own uncertainties. Recognises own position and experience.

- **Awareness of self:** Recognises own visibility to others and seeks to provide a positive role model for others.

- **Awareness of and for others:** Uses own position and experience thoughtfully and skilfully for the supervisee's benefit with an eye on public and professional safety.

- **Awareness-sharing:** Shares concerns and celebrates successes with supervisee—identifying how to build on what is going well.

- **Feedback-seeking:** Welcomes feedback about self as a supervisor and educator.

- **Open to alternatives:** Explores and is open to other ways of learning and doing—recognising other ways of learning and doing may be safe.

- **Critical awareness:** Weighs up what is working well and what is safe.

- **Willingness to change:** Continues to engage in own professional development, including in the education pillar.

> **PIT STOP!**
>
> A permeability self-assessment checklist is available to download (Harding, 2023). Please review this checklist and consider your practice.

Understanding Assessment in Advanced Practice

EDUCATIONAL ASSESSMENT

Assessment is an essential component in programmes of education. Higher education institutes (HEIs) are required to develop and administer robust assessments to evaluate student learning. The UK Quality Code details the mandatory expectations and practice for UK higher education in terms of consistency, comparability and credibility (Quality Assurance Agency (QAA), 2018). To support this, appropriately qualified staff design and deliver high-quality programmes that align learning outcomes with teaching and assessment strategies. Programmes and assessment strategies are reviewed by external examiners and student feedback is requested to ensure transparency, validity, reliability, benchmarking and, importantly, application to practice (QAA, 2018). Additionally, postqualification educational programmes may be subject to specific professional, statutory and regulatory body (PSRB) requirements. PSRBs are external bodies who approve programmes of education that may lead to a professional qualification. One example of this is prescribing programmes which may be a core requirement within AP MSc programmes (NMC, 2023).

Assessment is a vital component of student learning where individual performance is examined, and a determination made about whether students have met the required learning outcomes and standards (QAA, 2018). Quality assurance processes ensure that assessments used are fair, valid and reliable indicators of performance (QAA, 2018). In addition to summative assessment, which is used to identify if the learner has met the assessment criteria, formative assessments can be utilised to support development by providing feedback on performance (QAA, 2018). There are many examples of innovative assessment strategies utilised within educational programmes; some assessment strategies such as objective structured clinical examinations (OSCEs) will be familiar to AP students UK wide and internationally. In some countries such as Canada, for example, OSCE assessment is also required for revalidation purposes.

Assessment used in these circumstances indicates an assessment *of* learning. More recently, we have witnessed a move towards assessment *for* learning, reflecting a more student-centred empowering approach to learning (Pitt & Quinlan, 2022). Pitt and Quinlan (2022) undertook a global literature review which revealed the importance of authentic and compassionate assessment practice. Pitt and Quinlan (2022) argue for more focused group assessments which would promote the requirement for teamwork, thus demonstrating the value and importance of this key aspect of contemporary practice. Teamwork is particularly relevant within healthcare and for advanced practitioner students. Demonstrating teamwork is relevant and required (Pitt & Quinlan, 2022). It is worth considering the impact of contemporary assessment practices. It may be that an experienced practitioner developing in AP could encounter approaches to assessment which are less familiar. Spendlove and Best (2018) report on the addition of innovative assessments to undergraduate midwifery curricula. Spendlove and Best (2018) found that whilst students both enjoyed and felt benefit from the new approaches to assessment, student preparation was crucial to ensure trust and belief in these different assessments. In addition, this variation in approach may be challenging for supervisors in practice. This reflects the need for supervisors to ensure currency of knowledge and understanding of AP programme assessment strategies. Recent and as yet unpublished original research identified the importance of induction and support for AP supervisors to ensure adequate preparation for this key supportive role.

Collier-Sewell et al. (2023) concur with Pitt and Quinlan (2022), proposing that to develop autonomous practitioners who are adept at critical and analytical thinking, a move away from the ubiquitous competency-based approach to assessment is needed. They opine that a reductionist tick-box approach to competence development favours a task-orientated approach. Although their discussion is focused on undergraduate nurse education, there are similarities across professions and within postgraduate education. The challenge with this type of approach to education, Collier-Sewell et al. (2023) contend, is the development of practitioners who may be fixated on standards and competency requirements. In contrast, Collier-Sewell et al. (2023) indicate that the development of an autonomous holistic practitioner requires an approach that would promote curious, imaginative, reflexive practitioners who embrace uncertainty and complexity. Pitt and Quinlan (2022) promote peer assessment and feedback as one method of fostering enquiring practitioners. Peer assessment, Stančić (2021) states, is an important component of assessment for learning (formative). Peer assessment involves students assessing and providing feedback on the quality of each other's work. Currently, Finland integrates peer assessment into approved prescribing programmes as an assessment strategy. Feedback from colleagues in Finland indicates that this is a welcomed approach to formative assessment. Pitt and Quinlan (2022) argue that peer assessment is often more beneficial for the peer providing feedback as it encourages a commitment to assessment criteria where practitioners begin to observe and understand what constitutes good quality. This observation, Pitt and Quinlan (2022) indicate, can then be applied to the peer reviewer's practice encouraging reflection and supporting improvement in their practice. This is an important consideration for advanced practitioners. Peer assessment offers an opportunity to progress personal development, gaining skills and experience through providing peer assessment feedback, and would align with demonstration of development across the education pillar.

ASSESSMENT EXPECTATION

PIT STOP!

Reflect now on what you have just read about assessment strategies and consider:
- What impact have the assessments you have undertaken to date had on your practice?
- How would you feel about providing peer assessment?
- What might support you to provide robust peer feedback?
- How do you see the relationship now between supervision and assessment?

CONSIDERATIONS FOR DEVELOPMENT

In Chapter 1, we introduced the background to AP developments within the UK and identified the multiprofessional UK-wide focus on four pillars of practice. Pharmacy colleagues have indicated slight divergence from this approach with concentration on what is identified as five domains of practice. These domains are articulated in the RPS Core Advanced Pharmacist Curriculum, which was published in 2021. The variation lies with the clinical practice pillar that requires both *person-centred care and collaboration* and *professional practice*. Internationally, there is variation in terminology but similarity of focus across individual countries (International Council of Nurses (ICN), 2020) in terms of emphasis on clinical practice, leadership, research and education. It is useful to note that, generally, internationally, AP is limited to nursing, whilst within the UK, a multiprofessional approach is evident across the four UK countries (DoH, 2016, 2019; NHSE 2025, SG, 2017, 2021; WG, 2020); for an international perspective, please see Chapter 15.

Another variation of note to mention discussed in Chapter 1, are the regulatory requirements for AP. The UK currently has no regulatory requirements for AP beyond initial registration except for prescribing programmes, which are regulated and require PSRB approval. However, this has created an anomaly within AP programmes where prescribing necessitates this additional regulation and approval from the regulators. Whilst prescribing is a core component for many advanced practitioners, there are some HCPC registrants, for example, for whom prescribing is not currently within their scope of practice. These practitioners working at an AP level will have access to medicines through other routes such as *patient group directions*, otherwise known as *PGDs*. PGDs are written instructions to supply or administer medicines for planned episodes of care that only qualified, named and authorised healthcare professionals can use. Individual HEIs can develop their own MSc programmes with their own standards set with the exception of prescribing which requires regulatory body approval; this adds a level of complexity and potentially confusion as professionals supporting trainee advanced practitioners in practice may be referred to using a variety of titles, such as supervisor, PE and PA, for example. NHS England has adopted a credential and assurance process. This involves the development of credential specifications and a quality assurance process (NHS, 2023b). The aim of this is to provide some standardisation across AP programmes within England; this work is further discussed in Chapter 2. However, the NMC approved plans to regulate AP with work to do this commencing in April 2024. The main aim of this is for public protection and to provide consistency across the four UK countries. Whilst all professional regulators are involved in collaborating with the NMC in this work, the NMC can only regulate AP for nurses and midwives. The implications of this NMC regulatory approach for other professionals have, at the time of writing, yet to be clarified.

The focus of AP often is on clinical practice. However, to demonstrate knowledge and understanding required as an advanced practitioner, you should integrate all four pillars into your practice (Henderson, 2021). In achieving this, you should ensure you do not employ a reductionist tick-box approach and make certain you fully consider and embed the complex nature of AP throughout. Methods you might take to achieve this include those which enable interaction such as peer review and feedback or case-based discussion and reflection with colleagues. Chapter 13 explores methods to capture knowledge and understanding via a portfolio.

Currently within the UK, Scotland is the only country to have included requirements for dedicated nonclinical pillar time into a policy document. Transforming Roles Programme Paper 7 stipulates that 10% working time pro rata should be spent on developmental work towards the nonclinical pillars (SG, 2021). The impact of this has yet to be seen as COVID-19 prevented complete incorporation of this requirement initially. However, you should consider at an early stage how you might measure the impact that you have as an advanced practitioner as this is a relevant requirement to support continuance of these roles in practice areas.

PIT STOP!

Paper 7 (SG, 2021) provides detail about the metrics that may be used to measure impact. You may be interested in reviewing these metrics as these will provide useful guidance irrelevant of the country you work in.

ASSESSMENT FOR PRACTICE

Your MSc AP programme will include several different assessment elements that provide an opportunity for you to demonstrate your developing knowledge and capability across the four pillars. You may be asked, for example, to submit a portfolio of evidence (see Chapter 13) or a written critical discussion or undertake a pharmacology exam or an OSCE assessment. Assessments within AP programmes tend to require demonstration of application to practice and consequently you must clearly detail your learning in practice. There are regulatory requirements specific to some modules as discussed earlier with reference to prescribing. Often, theory can seem to be an abstract concept in relation to practice learning and students will need guidance and support to integrate concepts into practice (Stančić, 2021). Having access to a variety of supervisors can support this integration (HEE, 2020).

Academic assessment strategies for AP programmes require a measurement of impact of the learning. This measurement normally occurs with both an academic and a practice perspective. Often, this is achieved through a tripartite approach to assessment with the supervisor in practice and the AA working with the student to achieve outcomes or to intervene and offer more comprehensive support if this is required. For regulated and accredited programmes, this is specifically detailed through the approval, but for modules unique to individual HEIs, the approach may vary but will be underpinned by QAA requirements (QAA, 2018). What is similar across institutions is the commitment to support student learning and achievement and this takes a variety of forms such as having an identified and named AA and opportunities for contact with your AA, as some examples of this support.

Montgomery et al. (2021) advise that AP programmes of education supporting incorporation of critical thinking and clinical and research knowledge to apply evidence-based practice are a crucial requirement for quality person-centred care. The authors report several factors that prevent qualified practitioners from fully achieving this beyond completion of education programmes. Montgomery et al. (2021) cite issues such as lack of resources, skills or opportunities. This aligns with recent research from the North of Scotland Advanced Practice academy who reviewed AP nurses' engagement with research activity. The findings demonstrate that in the areas reviewed, clinical practice continues to be the main focus for advanced practitioners and infrastructure is needed to support engagement with research activity. This will undoubtedly have an impact on the ability for some of these staff to supervise and support trainee development across all pillars. As discussed earlier in the chapter, you may need to consider multiple supervisors to ensure robust support to enable your knowledge and skill development.

Students face challenges with gaining and maintaining knowledge and skills for practice, and we know that these challenges have grown considering COVID-19 impact. Attrition and redeployment of staff have impacted on the support available. The positive impact of advanced practitioners during the recent pandemic on the health and care of patients cannot be underestimated (Rosa et al., 2021), and this has supported recommendations for investment in AP (Lopes-Júnior, 2021).

Supervisors can have a key role in preparing students for assessment in practice settings. This workplace-based assessment gives the supervisor an opportunity to undertake a live assessment at varied points (HEE, 2020; NHSE 2025). If the supervisor also has an assessor role, trainees need to be clear when the assessment is formative and when it will be summative. These formative and summative assessment occasions enable authentic assessment. Authentic assessment has been described as a contextualised assessment that is realistic and meaningful (Villarroel et al., 2018). There are, however, a number of considerations that relate to a workplace-based assessment.

As discussed earlier, AP curricula require theoretical preparation supported by practical application in clinical practice areas. In reference to a discussion about nursing education, Immonen et al., (2019) identify the essential role that supervisors in practice play. Immonen et al., (2019) indicate that workplace-based learning is vital, arguing for strengthened collaborations between stakeholders, organisations and HEIs, advising that inconsistencies and variation in supervision support have long been a problem. A recent evaluation of assessment processes for advanced practitioners in one county in England found that supervisory engagement with assessment processes is vital (Wallis et al., 2021). Quality education which includes robust supervision in practice is the basis for quality care (Immonen et al., 2019), and this has been alluded to in the narrative earlier. The expansion in AP developments has led to consideration of the requirements for supervision in practice and it is known that there is variation in relation to preparation of supervisors. Except for prescribing modules, there is no statutory regulation standardising supervision for assessment in practice, and across the UK, there are known variations (Wallis et al., 2021). This is a challenge for AP students, but there are opportunities for students to choose their own supervisor. This might be appealing as any choice would ensure consideration of areas such as knowledge and understanding of the assessment and professional respect that is supportive for learning. This respect often emanates from having worked with colleagues and knowing that they are supportive. However, being able to choose your supervisor is not without difficulty. Supervisors are required to maintain objectivity in their assessment. This may be challenging at times if corrective advice is needed or in cases where the assessment leads to a failed outcome and this may adversely impact the future working relationship with your supervisor (Immonen et al., 2019).

PIT STOP!

What qualities would you want in a practice supervisor?
Are there any benefits or challenges for choosing a supervisor who you know and are friendly with?

Often, workplace-based assessment will involve more than two people, the supervisor and the trainee, and normally a patient will be present. Arguably, this too creates a level of uncertainty for trainees. Any area of correction might be considered a criticism and cause additional anxiety for the trainee. McGuire (2018) speaks of the power that supervisors hold and suggests that early and continued discussions about relationships will promote a supportive and successful rapport. Having open and frank discussions about the assessment being undertaken and maintaining a focus on assessment *for* learning aim to ensure supportive development of trainees (Pitt & Quinlan, 2022). Opportunities for reflection with your supervisor can support continuous learning and development of self-awareness (Marshall, 2019). Marshall (2019) advises that reflection is a cognitive process that can be used to make sense of complex problems which clearly aligns to the complex decision-making required in AP. In a scoping review of the literature, Torrens et al., (2020) identified concerns from advanced nurse practitioners (ANPs) who expressed self-doubt about their own competence and capabilities for the role. This was accompanied by concern from medical staff who lacked knowledge about the educational programmes for ANPs and questioned ANPs' competence for the advanced role. This is concerning both from a governance and a patient safety perspective for a few reasons. Trainee advanced practitioners require constructive feedback about their progress in order to achieve a competent level of practice (HEE, 2020; NHSE 2025). A more concerning issue is that the lack of knowledge and understanding of the advanced practitioner role requirements identified in Torrens et al.'s (2020) scoping review may lead to an assessor who fails to fail. Immonen et al., (2019) identified inconsistency and variation in reliable assessment in practice, supporting Torrens et al.'s (2020) concerns regarding the reliability of practice assessments and potential for infallible assessment practices. Ultimately, this means the practitioner would be failing in their duty of care for the trainee and in their duty of care for the public, arguably putting their own hard-won registration at risk by judging unsafe practice to be adequate.

In their systematic review, Immonen et al., (2019) reflect on the challenge of clinical competence assessment. Immonen et al., (2019) propose clarity in terms of assessment content and processes that are required at the outset, a point that Wallis et al., (2021) concur with. Systematic approaches with valid assessment tools are vital (Immonen et al., 2019). One such validated assessment process is that of the OSCE. OSCE assessment originated in 1979 in Dundee, Scotland (Stirling and Henderson, 2021). This assessment is extensively utilised internationally as a form of assessment in AP curricula. OSCE assessment requires several stations that students will revolve through, completing the requirements of each station. Capability is assessed by a variety of assessors using a structured preprepared marking guide (Pinson, 2023). This aims to reduce bias and ensure consistency of marking. The requirement for several varied stations enables a robust assessment of individual capability. The challenge with the application of this assessment is the variation in approaches across countries in terms of the numbers of stations a trainee must undertake and successfully pass and concerns about reliability as a result (Pinson, 2023). For example, one university might require students to complete three OSCE stations, once in an MSc programme. Another university may require students to complete OSCE assessments every year of the programme. In 2011, a meta-analysis was undertaken to establish the reliability of OSCE assessment. Brannick et al., (2011) reported from this meta-analysis that a higher number of OSCE stations increased the reliability of this form of assessment. An increased number of OSCE stations raises concerns about the feasibility of applying this form of assessment in terms of the capacity of staff (Stirling & Henderson, 2021).

This assessment strategy was originally applied to undergraduate medical students (Harden & Gleeson, 1979). It is worth considering, therefore, the validity of applying this assessment strategy to different professional groups such as advanced practitioners who will be practicing at a different level of practice. Arguably, this assessment can be seen to be a very scientific approach to capability assessment that is perhaps reductionist and tick-box in approach and perhaps not reflective of the current complexity of presentations that trainee advanced practitioners face. Adaptations to OSCE assessment have occurred because of the COVID-19 pandemic; in one area, this assessment was moved to be a workplace-based assessment (Stirling & Henderson, 2021). Anecdotal feedback from students who have consequently undertaken this assessment in workplace settings has indicated that this has enabled assessment *for* learning and they have reported it to be a valued and supportive assessment strategy.

More recently, QAA Scotland (2020) has led enhancement work that considered the concept of compassionate assessment. The QAA Scotland forms part of a UK-wide agency for higher education. Their role is to safeguard standards and quality in UK higher education. QAA Scotland has an enhancement-led process within the Scottish higher education sector and promotes enhancement themes as a method of improving the student experience of higher education. This work formed part of the 2020–2023 enhancement theme 'Resilient Learning Communities' and promoted an evaluation of assessment. The ensuing work suggested the need to consider stressful assessment practices and develop assessments that are authentic and inclusive and support practice reflection. This aligns with the benefit of workplace-based assessment and supports reconsideration of OSCE assessment practice.

Strategies to support effective and robust workplace-based assessment have been identified in the narrative earlier. In addition to these, collaborative multiprofessional networks will further enable individual learning and development of capability in AP.

Being Supervision and Assessment Ready

Tuning in to your own practitioner permeability (Harding, 2019) will be helpful for your AP supervision. It will prepare you to work with multiple supervisors and assessors, identifying your advanced level learning needs and priorities, matching your supervision with those needs and appointing a supervisor before you begin your training.

IDENTIFYING YOUR LEARNING NEEDS

AP is at different stages of maturity in different specialties, professions and across nations. For some specialties, the AP trainee curriculum is clearly set out (RCEM, 2022), while in other emerging areas of AP, there may be a locally agreed curriculum. Either way, it is crucial to identify from the outset the advanced level capabilities you are working towards across the pillars of practice as these will guide your learning needs analysis and in turn the supervision you will need to support these learning needs. Specialty curricula may be restricted to specified professions which have been identified as being able to develop to the required advanced level within the scope of professional practice. For example, in emergency medicine, the 2017 Emergency Care Advanced Clinical Practice (ACP) curriculum (RCEM, 2022) is open to registered nurses, pharmacists, physiotherapists and paramedics. In a multiprofessional cohort of emergency medicine ACP trainees, there will be different starting points and learning needs for trainees from different professions. A nurse and paramedic might be close to or beyond advanced level in wound care for example, while the physiotherapist and the pharmacist might need closer supervision in this regard. In contrast the physiotherapist might be at advanced level in musculoskeletal assessment and the pharmacist well advanced in polypharmacy considerations. It is frequently the case that a trainee in AP has been working in a practice setting for some time already. A nurse training in AP might find themselves working on similar capabilities to medical colleagues in training but the supervision that each needs to maintain professional and public safety may differ. Take endotracheal intubation for example; having assisted in the procedure many times before, the nurse may have lots of practical insights but feel less secure about the theory, while the medical colleague might be stronger on the theory and have less practical know-how.

APPOINTING A SUPERVISOR BEFORE YOU BEGIN AND HAVING A SUPERVISION AGREEMENT

It is vital to identify a supervisor from the beginning of AP training. Ideally, the supervisor and trainee will meet in advance to discuss and agree on the approach to supervision and assessment. Earlier in the chapter, establishing a shared understanding about the purpose between supervisor and supervisee was described as a feature of effective supervision, as were enablers such as trust, collaboration and supervisee focus (Rothwell et al., 2021). Rothwell and colleagues also identified the importance of regular, protected time for supervision and the value of a private space. Reaching an agreement about these ahead of commencing training ensures that supervision begins on secure foundations and points of assessment are understood. It is valuable to include in this agreement the course of action in case of unanticipated difficulties and in the event that the supervisor has a lengthy period of leave. It is wise to build in regular points when the supervision agreement is reviewed along the AP developmental pathway to ensure supervision and assessment arrangements remain fit for purpose and matched to the trainee's progress towards advanced level practice.

MULTIPLE SUPERVISORS AND ASSESSORS

Increasingly in the UK, the route to AP involves a combination of workplace learning and academic learning at master's level through completion of an MSc and/or integrated degree apprenticeship. The HEIs or universities which offer AP MSc courses will have much in common, but programmes are not identical and there may be variations in expectations about academic and workplace supervision and assessment. What you can expect is more than one supervisor. Where guidance exists, the supervisors' roles and responsibilities may be defined; for example, the Centre for Advancing Practice in England (NHSE, 2025) recommends that each trainee have a coordinating education supervisor who provides a consistent supervisory relationship for the duration of the practitioner's training in combination with access to associate workplace supervisors who are experienced practice-based educators or supervisors supporting the development of a specific capability or aspect of advanced level practice. In addition, depending on the trainee's role or programme of study, there may also be academic or research supervision.

Conclusion

This chapter has considered supervision and assessment for advanced practitioners and the ways in which both may be similar to or different from your previous experiences as a registered health professional. The interrelationship between supervision, formative and summative assessment has been explored. There has been discussion of the ways in which supervision can support your knowledge and skills development as well as helping you to be prepared for the challenges and uncertainties which can accompany the transition from experienced health professional to advanced level practitioner. The behaviour and characteristics which can support both supervisor and supervisee to get the most out of supervision and to navigate assessment have also been highlighted. Workplace-based assessment is an integral component of AP curricula. This assessment strategy requires robust supportive supervision from a workplace supervisor alongside an appropriate academic-based assessor.

The next chapter will explore portfolio assessment.

References

Benner, P. (1984). *From novice to expert: Excellence and power in clinical nursing practice.* Pearson.

Bernard, J. M., & Goodyear, R. K. (2004). *Fundamentals of clinical supervision* (3rd ed.). Boston: Allyn & Bacon.

Brannick, M. T., Erol-Korkmaz, H. T., & Prewett, M. (2011). A systematic review of the reliability of objective structured clinical examination scores. *Medical Educcation, 45*(12), 1181–1189. https://doi.org/10.1111/j.1365-2923.2011.04075.x

Collier-Sewell, F., Atherton, I., Mahoney, C., Kyle, R., Hughes, E., & Lasater, K. (2023). Competencies and standards in nurse education: The irresolvable tensions *Nurse Education Today, 125*, 105782. https://doi.org/10.1016/j.nedt.2023.105782

COPMed. (2022). *The gold guide: A reference guide for postgraduate foundation and specialty training in the UK* (9th ed.). Available at: https://www.copmed.org.uk/publications/gold-guide/gold-guide-9th-edition

Department of Health. (2016). *Advanced nursing practice framework.* https://www.health-ni.gov.uk/publications/advanced-nursing-practice-framework (Accessed November 27, 2023)

Department of Health. (2019). *Advanced AHP Framework.* Advanced AHP Practice Framework | Department of Health. Available at: https://www.health-ni.gov.uk/publications/advanced-ahp-practice-framework (Accessed November 27, 2023)

Duchscher, J. E. B. (2009). Transition shock: The initial stage of role adaptation for newly graduated registered nurses. *Journal of Advanced Nursing, 65*, 1103–1113. https://doi.org/10.1111/j.1365-2648.2008.04898.x

General Pharmaceutical Council. (2017). *Standards for pharmacy professionals.* Available at: https://www.pharmacyregulation.org/pharmacists/standards-and-guidance-pharmacy-professionals/standards-pharmacy-professionals

Gilbert, T. (2001). Reflective practice and clinical supervision: Meticulous rituals of the confessional. *Journal of Advanced Nursing, 36*, 199–205.

Harden, R. M., & Gleeson, F. A. (1979). Assessment of clinical competence using an objective structured clinical examination (OSCE). *Medical Education, 13*(1), 39–54. https://doi.org/10.1111/j.1365-2923.1979.tb00918.x

Harding, D. (2019). Practitioner permeability and the resolution of practice uncertainties: A grounded theoretical perspective of supervision for allied health professionals. (PhD thesis). St George's, University of London. Available at: https://eprints.kingston.ac.uk/id/eprint/43854/

Harding, D. (2023). *Working with the idea of practitioner permeability.* The Permeable practitioner. Available at: https://thepermeablepractitioner.com/ideas-and-resources/working-with-the-idea-of-practitioner-permeability/

HCPC. (2019). *Standards for prescribing.* https://www.hcpc-uk.org/standards/standards-relevant-to-education-and-training/standards-for-prescribing/

HCPC. (2021). *What is supervision?* Available at: https://www.hcpc-uk.org/standards/meeting-our-standards/supervision-leadership-and-culture/supervision/what-is-supervision/

HCPC. (2023). *Standards of proficiency.* (hcpc-uk.org) (Accessed March 28, 2023)

Health and Social Care Act. (2008). *(Regulated Activities) Regulations 2014 Section 2 (18).* Available at: https://www.legislation.gov.uk/ukdsi/2014/9780111117613/contents

Health Education England (2024). *Multi-professional framework for advanced clinical practice in England.* Available at: https://www.hee.nhs.uk/sites/default/files/documents/multi-professionalframeworkforadvancedclinicalpracticeinengland.pdf

Health Education England. (2020). *Workplace supervision for advanced clinical practice.* Available at: https://advanced-practice.hee.nhs.uk/workplace-supervision-for-advanced-clinical-practice-2/

Henderson, C. (2021). Advanced practice education and development. *Practice Nursing, 32*(11), 84–88.

ICN. (2020). *Guidelines on advanced practice nursing.* https://www.icn.ch/system/files/documents/2020-04/ICN_APN%20Report_EN_WEB.pdf (Accessed March 27, 2023)

Immonen, K., Oikarainen, A., Tomietto, M., Kääriäinen, M., Tuomikoski, A.M., Miha Kaučič, B., et al. (2019). Assessment of nursing students' competence in clinical practice: A systematic review of reviews. *International Journal of Nursing Studies, 100*, 103414. https://doi.org/10.1016/j.ijnurstu.2019.103414

Kilminster, S., Cottrell, D., Grant, J., & Jolly, B. (2007). AMEE Guide no. 27: Effective educational and clinical supervision. *Medical Teacher, 29*, 2–19.

Lopes-Júnior, L. C. (2021). Advanced practice nursing and the expansion of the role of nurses in primary health care in the Americas. *SAGE Open Nursing, 7*, 23779608211019491. https://doi.org/10.1177/23779608211019491

Lyth, G. M. (2000). Clinical supervision: A concept analysis. *Journal of Advanced Nursing, 31*, 722–729. https://doi.org/10.1046/j.1365-2648.2000.01329.x

Marshall, T. (2019). The concept of reflection: A systematic review and thematic synthesis across professional contexts. *Reflective Practice, 20*(3), 396–415. doi:10.1080/14623943.2019.1622520

McGuire, M. J. S. (2018). *How does supervisor power influence clinical supervision from the perspective of the supervisor? An interpretative phenomenological analysis* (PhD Thesis). University of Limerick.

Milne, D. (2007). An empirical definition of clinical supervision. *British Journal of Clinical Psychology, 46,* 437–447.

Montalvo, B. (1973). Aspects of live supervision. *Family Process, 12*(4), 343–359.

Montgomery, K. E., Ward, J., Raybin, J. L., Baylian, C., Gilger, E. A., & Smith, C. (2021). Building capacity through integration of advanced practice nurses in research. *Nursing Outlook, 69*(6), 1030–1038. https://doi.org/10.1016/j.outlook.2021.06.013

Moran, G. M., & Nairn, S. (2018). How does role transition affect the experience of trainee advanced clinical practitioners: Qualitative evidence synthesis? *Journal of Advanced Nursing, 74*(2), 251–262.

Murphy, K., & Mortimore, G. (2020). Overcoming the challenges of role transition for trainee advanced clinical practitioners. *Gastrointestinal Nursing, 18*(5), 1–17.

HS England (2025). *Multi-professional framework for advanced Practice in England.* Birmingham: Centre for Advancing Practice.

NHS. (2023a). *Advanced practice supervisor capabilities: Guiding principles for supervisor learning and development.* https://advanced-practice.hee.nhs.uk/our-work/supervision/advanced-practice-supervisor-capabilities/ (Accessed August 4, 2024)

NHS. (2023b). *NHS England centre for advancing practice credentials.* https://advanced-practice.hee.nhs.uk/our-work/credentials/ (Accessed August 7, 2024).

NHS England (2025). *Workplace Supervision for Advanced Practice.* Birmingham: Centre for Advancing Practice.

NHS Employers. (2022). *Clinical supervision models for registered professionals.* Available at: https://www.nhsemployers.org/articles/clinical-supervision-models

NMC. (2018). *Future nurse: Standards of proficiency for registered nurses.* Available at: https://www.nmc.org.uk/globalassets/sitedocuments/education-standards/future-nurse-proficiencies.pdf

NMC. (2023). *Standards for prescribing programmes.* Available at: https://www.nmc.org.uk/standards/standards-for-post-registration/standards-for-prescribers/standards-for-prescribing-programmes/

NMC. (2024). *Advanced practice review.* https://www.nmc.org.uk/about-us/our-role/advanced-practice-review/ (Accessed March 29, 2024)

Pinson, S. (2023). Desired OSCE competency levels for advanced clinical practice students. *Nursing Times, 119,* 4.

Pitt, E., & Quinlan, K. M. (2022). *Impacts of higher education assessment and feedback policy and practice on students: A review of the literature 2016–2021.* Advance HE.

Proctor, B. (2008). *Group supervision: A guide to creative practice* (2nd ed.). London: Sage.

Quality Assurance Agency. (2018). *The UK quality code, advice and guidance: Assessment.* https://www.qaa.ac.uk/the-quality-code/advice-and-guidance/assessment (Accessed March 27, 2023)

Quality Assurance Agency Scotland. (2020). *Compassionate assessment post COVID19: Improving assessment long term.* Available at: https://www.bing.com/search?q=Quality+Assurance+Agency+Scotland+(2020).Compassionate+assessment+post+COVID19%3A+Improving+assessment+long+term.+Available+at%3A+https%3A%2F%2Fwww.enhancementthemes.ac.uk%2Fexplore-the-enhancement-themes%2Fevidencefor-+enhancement%2Fstudent-engagement-and-demographics%2Fstudent-mental-wellbeing+(Accessed+06.04.2023).&cvid=ec1346abc38c4bebbb820eb56b36af7e&gs_lcrp=EgRlZGdlKgYIABBFGDkyBggAEE UYOTIICAEQ6QcY_FXSAQsxOTk0MTUwajBqOagCALACAA&FORM=ANAB01&DAF0=1&PC=U531

Rolfe, G. (2011). Reflection-in-action. In G. Rolfe, M. Jasper, & D. Freshwater (Eds.), *Critical reflection in practice: Generating knowledge for care* (2nd ed.). London: Springer, 160–182.

Rosa, W. E., Fitzgerald, M., Davis, S., Farley, J. E., Khanyola, J., Kwong, J., et al. (2020). Leveraging nurse practitioner capacities to achieve global health for all: COVID-19 and beyond. *International Nursing Review, 67*(4), 554–559. doi:10.1111/inr.12632

Rothwell, C., Kehoe, A., Farook, S. F., & Illing, J. (2021). Enablers and barriers to effective clinical supervision in the workplace: A rapid evidence review. *BMJ Open, 11*(9). http://dx.doi.org/10.1136/bmjopen-2021-052929

Royal College of Emergency Medicine. (2022). *Advanced clinical practitioner curriculum.* https://rcem.ac.uk/acp-curriculum/ (Accessed August 8, 2024)

Royal Pharmaceutical Society. (2021). *RPS Core Advanced Pharmacist Curriculum.* https://www.rpharms.com/development/credentialing/core-advanced-pharmacist-curriculum (Accessed March 27, 2023)

Schön, D. A. (1983). *The reflective practitioner: How professionals think in action.* New York: Basic Books.

Scottish Government. (2017). *Transforming nursing midwifery and health professions' roles: Paper 2 advanced nursing practice.* Available at: https://www.gov.scot/publications/transforming-nursing-midwifery-health-professions-roles-advance-nursing-practice/

Scottish Government. (2021). *Advanced nursing practice – Transforming nursing roles: Phase two.* https://www.gov.scot/publications/transforming-nursing-roles-advanced-nursing-practice-phase-ii/ (Accessed March 27, 2023)

Scottish Government. (2023). *Health and care (staffing) (Scotland) Act 2019: Statutory guidance.* https://tinyurl.com/57e5jfu7 (Accessed March 1, 2024)

Skills for Health. (2020). *Core capabilities framework for advanced clinical practice (nurses) working in general practice/primary care in England.* Available at: https://www.skillsforhealth.org.uk/wp-content/uploads/2021/01/Portfolio-Guidance.pdf

Snowdon, D. A., Leggat, S. G., & Taylor, N. F. (2017). Does clinical supervision of healthcare professionals improve effectiveness of care and patient experience? A systematic review. *BMC Health Services Research, 17,* 786. https://doi.org/10.1186/s12913-017-2739-5

Spendlove, Z., & Best, R. (2018). Innovation in assessment: Building student confidence in preparation for unfamiliar assessment methods. *British Journal of Midwifery, 26,* 3. https://doi.org/10.12968/bjom.2018.26.3.180

Stančić, M. (2021). Peer assessment as a learning and self-assessment tool: A look inside the black box. *Assessment & Evaluation in Higher Education, 46*(6), 852-864. doi:10.1080/02602938.2020.1828267

Stirling, K., & Henderson, C. (2021). The reliability and validity of the OSCE as an assessment of capability within advanced practice curricula. *British Journal of Nursing, 30,* 2–3.

Torrens, C., Campbell, P., Hoskins, G., Strachan, H., Wells, M., Cunningham, M., et al (2020). Barriers and facilitators to the implementation of the advanced nurse practitioner role in primary care settings: A scoping review. *International Journal of Nursing Studies. 104,* 103443. https://doi.org/10.1016/j.ijnurstu.2019.103443

Villarroel, V., Bloxham, S., Bruna, D., Bruna, C., & Herrera-Seda, C. (2018). Authentic assessment: Creating a blueprint for course design. *Assessment & Evaluation in Higher Education, 43*(5), 840–854. doi:10.1080/02602938.2017.1412396

Wallis, L., Locke, R., Sutherland, C., & Harden, B. (2021). Assessment of advanced clinical practitioners. *Journal of Interprofessional Care, 36,* 946–950. https://doi.org/10.1080/13561820.2021.1997950

Welsh Government. (2020). *Allied health professions framework for Wales.* Available at: https://heiw.nhs.wales/our-work/allied-health-professions-ahps/

CHAPTER 13

Portfolio Development

Angie Banks ■ Geinor Bean ■ Melanie Clarkson ■ Sarah Fisher

CHAPTER OUTLINE

Portfolios are required at every level of practice to evidence continuing professional development (CPD). However, within advanced practice (AP), an individual's portfolio provides so much more than a collection of CPD activities (although these are still important to reflect upon and include). This portfolio chapter will guide you through the practicalities of the different types of portfolios, the platforms used and the educational curricula that may be associated with them.

Developing your portfolio will allow your own knowledge and skills to be evidenced as they develop. Recognising your development needs through individual learning plans will increase self-awareness of your abilities and allows you, as practitioners, to be proactive in your development. This will strengthen your competencies and capabilities and support clinical decision-making and autonomous practice. Workplace-based assessments can be a useful tool in reflecting and developing your professional skills, and inclusion of a variety of assessments as outlined in this chapter provides you with a well-rounded portfolio of evidence of your education and training.

This chapter highlights the importance of critical reflection to support critical thinking and development, rather than providing just a description of the task that is completed. It will consider how all four pillars of practice may be evidenced, providing examples to encourage you to consider the wider work you complete within your AP role. Guidance within this chapter will allow you to evidence your personal and professional development, competency and capability and, ultimately, currency within your AP role.

Introduction

This chapter focuses on the development of your advanced practice (AP) portfolio, which may be needed for academic award or a requirement of your training and ongoing continuing professional development (CPD) by your employer. As authors, we have drawn on our experience of using portfolios as a means of capturing evidence of competencies and capabilities to work at an AP level across the four pillars of practice, as discussed in other chapters of this book.

It is recognised that portfolios are an excellent way to collate evidence of knowledge and skills (Hamilton et al., 2023), and it is important to acknowledge that the development and governance of AP across the four countries of the United Kingdom differs. However, all four nations state that there is a clear expectation that people working at this level are required to operate at master's level, to have the ability to make sound judgements in the absence of full information and to manage varying levels of risk when there is complex, competing or ambiguous information or uncertainty (Department of Health Northern Ireland (DHNI) 2019; Health Education and Improvement Wales (HEIW), 2023a; NHS England (NHSE), 2025); The Scottish Government, 2017).

Why Are Portfolio and Specialism Frameworks Required?

HEIW (2023b), NHSE (2025), NHS Education Scotland (NES) (2018) and DHNI (2019) highlight that individuals working towards AP or those who are already advanced practitioners should align their knowledge, skills and behaviours to their area of practice, competency frameworks and national standard frameworks such as the multiprofessional framework (NHSE, 2025). See Chapter 1 for further information. The competency frameworks and national standard frameworks enable standardisation of education and training, improving quality of patient care whilst allowing opportunity for individuals to align with defined competencies (DHNI, 2019; NHSE, 2025; HEIW, 2023a; NES, 2018). To note, from Chapters 1 and 2, the use of the title advanced practitioner is not currently regulated and what is termed 'advanced level practice' is practised across a variety of role settings. Therefore, it is imperative that those using the title appropriately should align to a relevant set of competencies or capabilities. A professional portfolio provides structure to do this and can be used by all healthcare professionals as a way of gathering and collating appropriate evidence of knowledge, skills and behaviours across the four pillars of practice at an advanced level.

Often, practitioners are fearful of the electronic portfolio (commonly referred to as an e-portfolio) platforms, due to low digital literacy (Janssens et al., 2022). For educators and employers, consideration of what support practitioners require in the implementation of e-portfolios is necessary to improve engagement (Hamilton et al., 2023). However, electronic platforms are not foolproof, and it is suggested that all of your work is saved and backed up in other formats.

Many organisations, professional bodies and Royal Colleges have developed their own capabilities, competencies and frameworks, for example, the Multi Professional Framework (HEE, 2017), Faculty of Intensive Care Medicine (FICM, 2023) for advanced critical care practitioners (ACCPs) and the Royal College of Emergency Medicine (RCEM, 2022) competencies for advanced clinical practitioners. These frameworks allow practitioners to develop a portfolio of evidence highlighting their advanced level of knowledge and skills across the four pillars of practice within a specialism. Based on the variety of frameworks available, there may be a need to demonstrate knowledge, skills and behaviours in different ways, depending on the nature of the scope and context of practice, role and profession (HEE, 2017). This is an opportunity to uniquely showcase abilities and evidence of knowledge and skills. A portfolio should therefore be specific to the individual and their specialty and no two will look the same, even when mapping against the same frameworks (Eddy et al., 2015).

Overview of the Types of Portfolios

Supervision and assessment of competence and capability are of paramount importance to ensure patient and practitioner safety (NHSE, 2025). Currently, there are various portfolios, templates and platforms which aim to guide the practitioner in documenting evidence of their education and training. There are specialty-specific portfolios which are used in emergency medicine, paediatrics (Royal College of Paediatrics and Child Health (RCPCH), 2023) and critical and emergency care settings (FICM, 2023; RCEM, 2022). However, for most advanced practitioners, there isn't a defined, or recommended, portfolio.

Advanced practitioners work across a variety of clinical areas such as primary care, mental health, community, learning disabilities and prison health, and professionals regularly cross boundaries with their transferable skills into other specialties (Kennedy et al., 2015). There is a requirement for a purposeful and adaptable portfolio that is clear and specific in enabling trainee and qualified advanced practitioners to document evidence in relation to national frameworks and their respective clinical frameworks and credentials.

Advanced practitioner roles can be multiprofessional, and advanced practitioners are accountable to their parent profession (Department of Health and Social Care (DHSC), 2021). The Nursing and Midwifery Council (NMC, 2021), for example, stipulates that all registered nurses and midwives must maintain their registration via revalidation and have a portfolio of evidence available. This revalidation process occurs every 3 years and evidence such as professional feedback, clinical hours, educational/CPD hours and a professional discussion form part of this portfolio. The NMC portfolio consists of identified resources/templates that must be completed. However, should the process of revalidation not be undertaken thoroughly by individuals who, for example, are not conversant with the AP role, there is a potential that satisfactory ongoing competence and capability are not assessed accurately, impacting on the currency and validity of revalidation. Furthermore, different professions have differing requirements for revalidation, which, due to the multiprofessional nature of AP, creates an argument for an AP-specific portfolio. Often, speciality frameworks are highly focussed on the clinical pillar; however, it is important to remember that the other three pillars require detailed attention, and many workplace-based learning and assessments can, and should, be applied to the three other pillars of AP (NHSE, 2025).

The use of an electronic portfolio is normally a safe way to add and maintain evidence in a protected format that is robust and easily accessible (Bridge & Eddy, 2006). It can safeguard against the loss of quality evidence that the advanced practitioner has spent time and effort in producing. An electronic portfolio can be kept up to date in a timely manner and provide ease of access (Eddy et al., 2015), for cross-referencing high-quality workplace-based learning and evaluations which span across clinical specialities, professions and frameworks.

PIT STOP!

The FICM ACCP curriculum can be found here. This is a portfolio that some practitioners use in the speciality emergency medicine.

https://www.ficm.ac.uk/careersworkforceaccps/accp-curriculum

Currently, trainee and qualified advanced practitioners have the freedom to choose which portfolio format they adopt. Some may be guided by their employers' requirements, but this is an individual choice. It was previously recognised that paper portfolios were the main mode for practitioners to collect and reflect on their practice (Orland-Barak, 2005). This method can give rise to the potential of lack of structure and alignment to relevant frameworks (Murray et al., 2006). However, it is recognised that practice has since developed and Professional, Statutory and Regulatory Bodies (PSRBs) can provide guidance, e.g., NMC (2021). Nevertheless, the paper portfolio is easy to use, and those who experience challenges with technology may prefer this low-cost method.

Electronic portfolios are increasing in availability and provide an opportunity for practitioners to choose a model that meets their clinical needs. An e-portfolio generally offers the user the ability to clearly document their learning and reflections and allow easy access to the supervisor. The benefit includes easy access in the clinical environment without the need for remembering the paper portfolio (Forte et al., 2013).

Within some areas in England, trainees are encouraged to participate in an annual review of competence (NHS England, 2022). This review is known locally by varying nomenclature, but you may hear the term 'CASP' (Clinical Assessment Support Panel) (NHS England, 2022). This review focuses on the current knowledge, skills and behaviours of the trainee and assigns them an indicative score which demonstrates level of progression. The advanced practitioner is required to ensure they have a portfolio of evidence available which demonstrates their capability against national documents and any relevant speciality frameworks.

PIT STOP!

Review your employer's guidance/requirements for evidencing AP via a portfolio and how this is monitored.

The type of evidence captured within a portfolio is variable and can be dependent upon the requirements of the employer, university or college board and/or professional or speciality body. The crucial element is that the evidence written within a portfolio has depth, critical analysis, synthesis and reflection (Langridge et al., 2023). The evidence should meet recognised learning outcomes or evidence of ongoing CPD. The quality of the evidence is important, but equally, if the portfolio is being used as part of a programme of learning and academic award, it must meet the learning outcomes of the module and/or course.

How to Collect and Demonstrate Competency and Capability in a Portfolio

As evidence is collected, it is important that each capability, competency and pillar is not viewed in isolation; often, there is a crossover of knowledge, skill and behaviour that can be used to evidence more widely. An example of this is completion of a service improvement project (see Chapter 6), which demonstrates the research pillar; however, for the portfolio, consider how leading the project can be evidenced by the advanced practitioner (leadership pillar), the education of others about the change (education pillar), as well as impact upon clinical practice (clinical practice pillar) to expand and maximise the synthesis of the evidence.

A portfolio should be inclusive of evidence which is indirect and direct.

- *Indirect—Information about you (for example, colleague feedback)*
- *Direct—Information from you (for example, case studies, critical reflections)*

(Eddy et al., 2015)

How to Start a Portfolio of Evidence

At the commencement of portfolio development, it is important to self-reflect on the transferable skills a practitioner currently has so they are used as a foundation to build upon existing skills and develop new skills. Often, practitioners may have moved into a new clinical speciality and are therefore developing and evidencing speciality knowledge, progressing professional judgement to aid clinical decision-making at this level of practice. In addition, for those in training, they are developing a new and different level of practice, where additional knowledge, skills and behaviours are expected to be evidenced at master's level (NHSE, 2025; HEIW, 2023a). Some evidence can be collated using self-assessment tools (many of which are easily available online), to provide evidence of baseline skills at the start of training or portfolio development. At this level of practice, simply adding the scores of these tools is not sufficient. It is expected that as an advanced practitioner, critical reflection on the feedback and results and consideration of further development are necessary, further exploring the key skill of critical thinking. Some of the results may be surprising and empowering, and other results may be dependent on the environment; for example, leadership may be affected by context and situation, with the advanced practitioner demonstrating an authoritarian style necessary in an emergency compared to compassionate style for supporting colleagues and peers. Recognising and reflecting on the results will allow the practitioner to establish a baseline that can be further measured at intervals throughout training and continuing practice as an AP to demonstrate progression. Examples of areas to consider are:

- Communication
- Teamworking
- Leadership
- Research

- Learning skills
- Emotional intelligence
- Compassion
- Wellbeing
- Digital literacy skills
- Mapping against the current competency standards

With all the information collated, a practitioner can then develop an individual learning plan (ILP), also known as a personal development plan (PDP). This is a personal and a live document that can be added to throughout the practitioner's learning, in training and beyond. It is recommended that a first copy of the ILP/PDP and any results are saved as a separate document, to show development throughout education, training and continuing learning.

The layout for the ILP/PDP should allow identification of specific development areas. For example, don't just write, 'Attended Multidisciplinary Team' as an entry in the ILP, as at this level of practice, more is expected, and a greater depth of discussion and analysis is required. Box 13.1 provides an example of what to explore and capture from attending an MDT.

Breaking down the learning experience allows for a greater depth of understanding, to identify development more easily as seen in Box 13.1.

PIT STOP!

Review and reflect upon a piece of evidence submitted as part of your postregistration portfolio. Does this capture the analysis and self-reflection to support your development?

The template for the ILP should allow for identification of learning opportunities, development, impact and outcome. All practitioners working at this level of practice will be expected to show the impact of the role, to justify its need and how it improves service delivery and, ultimately, patient care. This is important to embed into the development and training from the outset. Box 13.2 is an example of an ILP.

BOX 13.1 ■ Example of How to Gain Depth to Evidence

What do you want to gain from the MDT?

To

- Understand the roles of the individuals attending the MDT.
- Understand the scope of the roles represented and what they bring to the decision-making process.
- Experience how to debate opinion in a professional setting.
- Expand knowledge of disease within scope of practice.
- Develop anatomy and physiology skills in diagnostics.
- Understand why different diagnostics are requested.
- Experience how the patient is involved in the decision-making process.

BOX 13.2 ■ Example of an Individual Learning Plan

ADVANCED CLINICAL PRACTITIONER INDIVIDUAL LEARNING PLAN

Name _____ Job Title_____

Mentor _____ Job Title _____ Additional Mentor _____

Timeline _____

Document meeting with clinical oncologist and service manager to identify how your role fits with the MDT and draft ideas for your ILP

Training objectives (agreed with mentor, line manager and head of service)

Activity	Dates/ venue/ online etc	Main learning outcomes	Priority High/ med/long term	Completed/ signed off (date)	Evaluation/contribution to role

How to Develop Critical Thinking and Reflection Within the Portfolio

Developing critical thinking and reflection includes assessing the evidence base within the roles defined by your individual scope of practice. It is important that you define your scope of practice, and its relation to your local job description. This supports you in working within your scope and safeguards in relation to clinical governance. The evidence should show the advanced practitioner's development, competency and capability at master's level. Often, practitioners fall into the trap of being very descriptive of the situation. To develop your critical thinking, see Box 13.3. It is the quality of the evidence, not the quantity, that is important. Those who may review the portfolio do not wish to see a list of certificates; what assessors want to see is the development of the advanced practitioner, critical application of knowledge to practice and evidence of work within the defined scope of practice at this level (Eddy et al., 2015).

BOX 13.3 ■ Critical Thinking Example

Documenting a patient's history, examination findings and differentials in a portfolio could be viewed as descriptive; furthermore, it is important that you can demonstrate that this was your work as opposed to someone else's.

In relation to the example of documenting a patient consultation, questions can be asked to help develop criticality to what has been presented. For example:

- How did you make the clinical decision?
- What information from the history and/or examinations supported the diagnostic thinking?
- What information did you require?
- Why did you obtain this information?
- How did this help with the diagnostic process?
- If information is missing, how do you gain it (referral for additional diagnostics)?
- Knowing the boundary of their scope of practice (when to refer on).

What Types of Evidence Might Be Collected?

There is a move away from learning and development being assessed entirely by academic assessment to the inclusion of assessments within the workplace to assess competency and professionalism with the presence of the patient and the true clinical environment (Wallis et al., 2022). Overall assessment of practice should be inclusive of the constructively aligned tent of competency assessment as seen in Fig. 13.1. This image (Fig. 13.1) includes Miller's prism of clinical competence, Biggs' constructive alignment and Dreyfus and Dreyfus' development of expertise model (Dalia et al., 2020).

> **PIT STOP!**
>
> Consider what evidence you collate, and how you have collated this evidence, through assessment to support your learning and ongoing development, according to the tent of competence earlier.

As well as the traditional critical reflections, there are other ways to collate evidence to demonstrate capability in practice. These can be dependent on frameworks and speciality requirements (FICM, 2023; RCEM, 2022). Please note that in some frameworks, there are a set number of different types of evidence required, so always refer to the specificity training framework (RCEM, 2022).

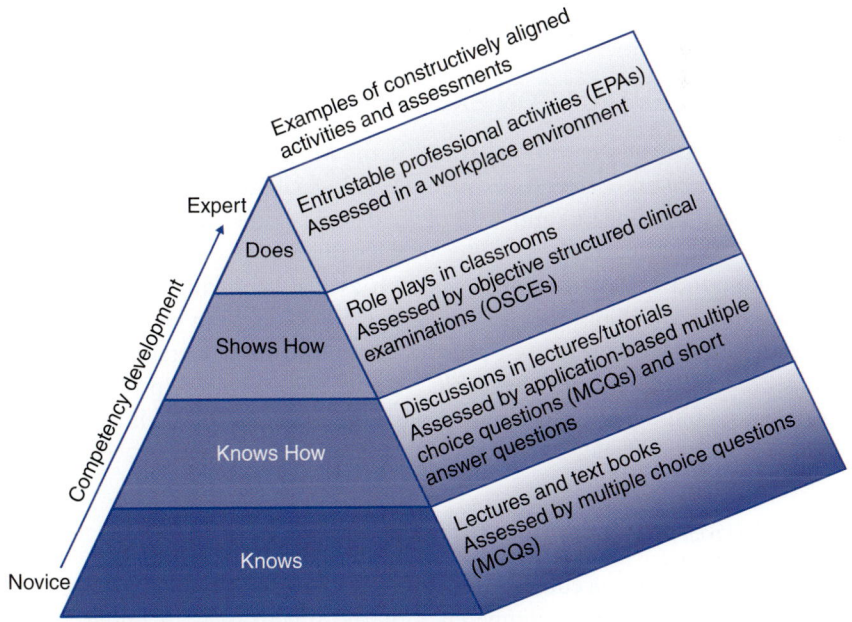

Fig. 13.1 Tent of competency assessment. *(From Dalia, B., Chaar, B., & Moles, R. (2020). Rethinking competence: A nexus of educational models in the context of lifelong learning. Pharmacy 8(2), 81. https://doi. org/10.3390/pharmacy8020081)*

It is expected that all assessors will be competent to assess the area of practice being evidenced and able to provide constructive feedback. The assessors should understand the training regime of the practitioner and the role of assessment in the individual's development. Please consider your own professional body requirements for supervision. For example, the NMC (2023) has specific standards for student supervision and assessment (SSSAs). Please do review the PSRB requirements and wider literature for further information.

Workplace-Based Assessments

Workplace-based assessments (WPBAs) can be aligned or integrated into the advanced practitioner's academic training programme or their clinical training. This assessment is seen as an evaluation of day-to-day practice within the individual's scope of practice. Reflection and feedback are an important component to enhance and drive learning (Eddy et al., 2015). The use of WPBA should not be seen as a tick box exercise or something that needs to be passed. It should be seen as a learning opportunity to work closely with the associated supervisor to identify strengths and any areas for further development (Liu, 2012). It is important that the assessment activities are mutually agreed upon in advance, and it is often the responsibility of the trainee advanced practitioner to arrange this. As with all assessments, the WPBA should be spread appropriately throughout the practitioner's training and ongoing development to show progression. A variety of assessment types should be demonstrated throughout the portfolio. It should also be noted that these assessments should form part of CPD and learning once training has been completed, examples of which can be found in the next sections.

MINI CLINICAL EVALUATION EXERCISE

As stated by Grime and Thomson (2013 p13), the Mini-Clinical Evaluation eXercise (Mini-CEX) is a Work-Based Assessment (WBA) facilitating supervision and feedback on essential components and skills of good clinical care. The use of a mini-CEX allows evaluation of a clinical encounter with a patient to assess clinical competency in providing good clinical care in areas such as history taking, examination and clinical reasoning (Wilkinson et al., 2008). The mini-CEX can be used at any time and in any setting when there is a practitioner and patient interaction, and an associate workplace supervisor is available. To encourage ownership of training, the practitioner should agree on the timing with the assessor, although assessors may also conduct unscheduled assessments.

DIRECT OBSERVATION OF PRACTICE

Direct observation of procedural skills (DOPS) is an assessment tool intended to assess the performance and competency of the practitioner in undertaking an element of practice against a structured checklist (Wilkinson et al., 2008). Unlike the mini-CEX, the DOPS assesses the whole procedure and not just a 'snapshot' of a clinical experience (Loerwald et al., 2018). The required DOPS will depend on the individual's scope of practice. The practitioner then receives immediate feedback to feed forwards in their development.

CONSULTATION OBSERVATION TOOL

A consultation observation tool (COT) is a recorded holistic observational assessment used to provide feedback and assessment on the consultation process (consent must be sought). It can be:

1. *In person (live)*
2. *In person (recorded)*
3. *Virtual consultation (live)*
4. *Virtual consultation (recorded)*

(Royal College of General Practitioners (RCGP), 2024)

The consultation should be no longer than 15 minutes in duration, as one of the assessment areas is the efficient and effective use of time (Skills for Health, 2023). Evidence suggests a COT is better linked to a formative assessment process; however, triangulation of assessment and feedback with a DOPS should be encouraged (Gillam et al., 2009).

CLINICAL EXAMINATION PROCEDURES

When completing clinical examinations, you may complete a clinical examination procedure (CEP) to allow for wider learning. The CEP is part of the COT or the multisource feedback (MSF) and is related to the appropriateness of choice of examination (HEE, 2020a). This may not only be the physical procedure but also the wider consideration of concepts such as consent, the use of a chaperone and individual requirement for the examination as examples. This WPBA was included as part of the COT and MSF in 2015, to increase good clinical practice by the appropriate interpretation of clinical signs (RCGP, 2024).

CASE-BASED DISCUSSION

Case based discussions (CBD) offer a method of exploring critical thinking and clinical reasoning and capability. It is a structured way to assess professional judgement based on real patient cases that you will deal with, within your scope of practice (HEE, NHSE and Skills for Health 2020). The assessment should indicate the level of competency within areas inclusive of clinical reasoning, decision-making and application of medical knowledge in relation to patient care. The discussion will also include assessment of a written record, such as written case notes, outpatient letters or discharge summaries. The full discussion should be documented, and the feedback should include feed-forward principles to allow the individual to develop (Skills for Health, 2023). CbDs are often a favoured assessment method, due to the ease of assessment and the validity of the process (Johnson et al., 2011)

ACUTE CARE ASSESSMENT TOOL

The Acute Care Assessment Tool (ACAT) is intended to provide feedback to practitioners on supervised aspects of delivering acute care. This should be over a period of time and not specific to an individual patient, for example, assessment immediately post ward round. The assessor will provide feedback on clinical assessment and management, decision-making, teamworking, time management, record keeping and handover, which may cover multiple patients (Johnson et al., 2011). In a review of WPBA by Johnson et al. (2011), ACATs were favoured by both the practitioner and the assessor, with the opportunity for assessment and teaching, although there are some weaknesses considered with the assessment of leadership.

SIGNIFICANT EVENT ANALYSIS (SEA)

This tool provides the opportunity to critically reflect on a learning situation that can further enhance and support development in practice. This does not need to be a negative event; it could be a positive one where you have been involved, which was significant to you, as it made you think and reflect about your practice. Using a reflective model, an in-depth review of the event should indicate learning on the mitigation and management of risk and learning from the event (NES, 2022).

MULTIPLE TRAINER REPORT

The multiple trainer report (MTR) captures the feedback of the supervisor and other senior staff who have been involved in the development of the practitioner's clinical skills. The feedback should be from those who have worked directly with the practitioner in the previous 12 months. The MTR provides a more structured opportunity of feedback from the consultancy team and other leaders (Royal College of Anaesthetists, 2021). A summary sheet is developed to highlight areas of excellence and where further support is required. It would be appropriate to complete this evidence at the end of a training period.

MULTISOURCE FEEDBACK (MSF)/360-DEGREE FEEDBACK

This tool is a method of assessing 'soft' skills such as communication, leadership, teamworking and reliability, across the four pillars of practice. The aim is to gain objective feedback from several colleagues who will 'rate' the practitioner's performance. The colleague group should be inclusive of medical consultants, specialist registrars, qualified advanced practitioners, administration staff and other nursing and allied healthcare professionals and total a minimum of 12 individual views (Wilkinson et al., 2008). Within Wilkinson et al.,'s (2008) study, they also recommend consideration of the balance of gender and roles in the selection of the 'raters' identified by the supervisor, at the start of the training year. The practitioner will not see individual responses, only the collated feedback. The practitioner will then act upon this feedback within their ILP to further aid their development.

Patient feedback should also be sought and included within a portfolio as a source of feedback to support self-reflection and development. This rich feedback can aid and support the development of communication skills which are essential to the consultation (see Chapter 4).

Evidence Against the Remaining Pillars of Professional Practice

To evidence against the four pillars of practice, other more appropriate tools can be used to collate evidence against the education, leadership and research pillar. Please note that Multi-Source Feedback (MSF)/360-degree feedback can also be used as evidence against these pillars of practice.

QUALITY IMPROVEMENT PROJECT AND AUDIT ASSESSMENT TOOL

A quality improvement project and audit assessment tool (QIPAT) is designed to assess a practitioner's capability in completing an audit or quality improvement (QI) project. It can be used in the programme of study, or in ongoing development to aid the development in this area, but the final evidence will be collated at the end of the training period on completion of the project. The assessment should be inclusive of verbal feedback and discussion to ensure an action plan for development is completed.

TEACHING OBSERVATION

The teaching observation (TO) form is designed to provide structured, formative feedback to practitioners about their competence at teaching. This should be a practitioner-led activity where the assessor is present throughout to provide feedback. This could include a wide variety of teaching activities inclusive of formal educational delivery such as seminars, tutorials, one-on-one training, micro-teaching sessions and patient teaching sessions. The TO has no scale of assessment, and therefore, care should be given to bias in feedback. Inclusion of criteria would help the validity of this tool; however, study results by Wilkinson et al. (2008) show positive support of the use of the TO.

LEARNING LOG (LL)

This should include critical reflection and identify further learning, linking to capabilities and progression. The log can form part of the personal development review (PDR) and is inclusive of:

- *Critical thinking and analysis*
- *Self-awareness*

- *Evidence of learning*
- *Links to specific curriculum*
- *Professionalism and appropriate behaviours*

(HEE, 2020b)

SUPERVISOR'S ANNUAL REVIEW AND REPORT (AR)

This is a formal annual report from the supervisor/assessor/mentor who will collate all the information from the practitioner's training that year to compile a report. This should be completed on an annual basis with a review of the previous year to demonstrate progress.

Other Essential Evidence

With your portfolio, you should also include:
- Current job plan, scope of practice and job description
- Up-to-date curriculum vitae (CV)
- Current training records for clinical competency and up-to-date mandatory training
- Statement of completion of successful modules, programmes and CPD completed to complement training
- Anonymous compliments or complaints

PIT STOP!

With all these examples of evidence, review your current portfolio and identify how you could capture some of these examples. The RCGP provides some excellent examples of these data collection tools.

https://www.rcgp.org.uk/mrcgp-exams/wpba/assessments

Applying Evidence to Each of the Four Pillars

Within the next section, we will discuss how to collect evidence for each of the pillars of AP. MSc AP programmes might require the collection of evidence during training; however, this might vary depending on the university/programme you are attending. As highlighted within this chapter and throughout other chapters of this book, once qualified, the need to maintain and further develop a professional portfolio linking to the pillars of AP is ongoing, in relation to revalidation e.g., NMC, (2021), but also as best practice.

HOW TO COLLECT EVIDENCE FOR THE CLINICAL PILLAR

For some advanced practitioners, the collection of evidence for the clinical pillar might be the most favourable of all pillars to collect and develop. Many opportunities will present themselves without much provocation and will often be opportunistic.

Choosing the ideal form to present this evidence is key to showcasing knowledge, skills and behaviours.

The recommended choice of forms could include a COT, and as outlined earlier, this tool allows the supervisor to rate, assess and provide feedback on individual performance when observing a consultation. Box 13.4 provides an example of performance feedback.

BOX 13.4 ■ Example of Performance Feedback

Assessment of Performance

Based on this observation, please rate the overall competence the Practitioner has shown*:

○ Significantly below the level expected for the completion of training

○ Below the level expected for the completion of training

○ At the level expected for the completion of training

○ Above the level expected for the completion of training

○ Significantly above the level expected for the completion of training

○ Not observed

Observation and feedback on performance*: ❶

Agreed actions for further development*:

An example of a COT could be that you visited an elderly lady with advanced dementia following a fall who has been discharged from the emergency department with no management plans in place. You had a discussion with the family and agreed that further surgical intervention would not be in the patient's best interest. You discussed palliative care options and supported the family and carers to understand what to expect and how to manage the individual and prevent further hospital admissions. You would recognise the level of complexity and highlight which clinical experience group this covered, for example, older people including frailty and/or people at the end of life. Your trainer will then rate you and provide feedback on your performance.

Alternatively, mini-CEX is often utilised for a similar purpose and the topic is jointly chosen by the trainee advanced practitioner and the educational/clinical supervisor or mentor. From this, there will be a period of observation of the consultation and then feedback and suggestion of recommendations for further learning.

These opportunities will be readily available when you are working with your supervisor/assessor/mentor, and it is ideal to record these events as soon as possible.

Using an e-portfolio can assist you to complete these in a timely manner and enable convenient access for your supervisor.

As reflective practitioners developing critical thinking and clinical reasoning skills, this is an ideal way to evidence those elements of the clinical pillar which are not simply just 'demonstrating a skill'. Reflection is not just describing the situation; it is a systematic process that allows the context to be explored and analysed. This allows you to learn and consider new knowledge and how you will improve or change your practice in the future. Writing reflective accounts will provide rich evidence clearly presenting evidence of your expertise within the clinical pillar (HEIW, 2023b).

Recording of DOPS enables you to evidence competence of performing a practical procedure, which can include all manner of skills ranging from taking a blood pressure to performing fundoscopy, mini-mental test, radiotherapy planning or an abdominal examination. Again, the focus is on receiving feedback and you as the practitioner's personal reflection as highlighted in Box 13.5.

Finally, a CbD is an ideal tool for evidencing your clinical knowledge, skills and behaviours. The professional discussion takes place after the event. It is a structured conversation discussing a case that has been agreed upon by the student and supervisor to address a range of topics to reflect the learning needs. Having regular

---

BOX 13.5 ■ Example of Feedback for a DOPS

Feedback based on the behaviours observed*: ❶

Agreed action*:

Practitioner's Reflection: ❶

Trainer's Position*:

○ GP

○ Consultant

○ ST3 or above/SPR

○ ACP

○ Pharmacist

○ Other

meetings with the supervisor will allow for time to have such discussions away from the immediate situation.

In addition to consultation skills and the obvious clinical skills, it is worth noting that there is overlap with the other pillars. For example, an audit of antibiotic pre-scribing in children with symptoms of a urinary tract infection would evaluate the data against best practice and then disseminate findings to colleagues. This would be evidencing not only the research pillar but the clinical and educational pillars too, and it may lead onto a service improvement project (for an in-depth discussion, Chapter 6 explores research within the AP pillar).

HOW TO COLLECT EVIDENCE FOR THE LEADERSHIP PILLAR

There are many opportunities to capture the leadership skills identified within this pillar; often, they might go unrecognised. Contributing to team meetings and service delivery is a good way of recognising that you are working collaboratively and utilising your leadership skills. Using compassionate/shared leadership (Bailey & West, 2022) can be an enabler for achieving goals and implementing new practice. Writing about an experience such as this as a reflection and/or pub-lishing the work is an excellent source of evidence and should be included in the portfolio.

In England, the NHS Leadership Academy produced an evidence-based model in 2013 which allows for self-assessment and identification of areas for develop-ment (NHS Leadership Academy, 2013). Participating in such an activity would be a suitable method to demonstrate commitment to developing your leadership skills. The other four nations of the UK also have valuable resources for developing lead-ership skills (see Chapter 5).

An example, within Wales, the focus is on fostering compassionate and collective leadership practices which is based on the overarching vision outlined in the Social Care Wales (2020) 'A Healthier Wales' Strategy for Health and Care. The strategy articulates that by 2030, leaders within the health and social care domain will dem-onstrate a collective and compassionate leadership ethos. HEIW has since devel-oped the NHS Wales Leadership portal, named Gwella (HEIW, n.d.), which offers inclusive free access to a range of evidenced-based leadership resources, providing a range of articles, toolkits and webinars which can be used when developing your leadership pillar.

Critically reflecting on your experiences as a leader allows for further self-awareness and exploration into the varying methodologies that allow for growth and develop-ment. Such evidence should be visible in your portfolio.

Clinical leaders often find themselves in a position of managing staff which normally would include rota planning, attendance management, appraisals, pastoral and clinical support. Advanced practitioners need to have the skills to deliver this and evidence such as case studies, courses, and multisource (MSF)/360 feedback can all demonstrate a student's commitment to supportive leadership or compas-sionate leadership (Box 13.6).

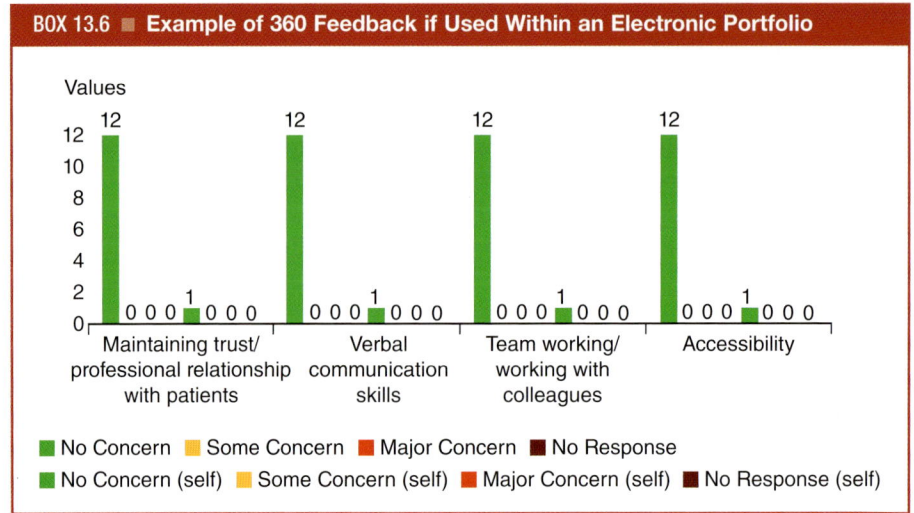

BOX 13.6 ■ Example of 360 Feedback if Used Within an Electronic Portfolio

HOW TO COLLECT EVIDENCE FOR THE RESEARCH PILLAR

Research is part of every NHS organisation; it provides assurance of continued advancing/improving clinical practice. Research led by AP helps to drive change and influences and shapes healthcare professions, informing and underpinning policy and professional decision-making (NHS England, 2021).

The advanced practitioner's role requires the application of relevant research to provide efficient, optimal, evidence-based practice (NHSE, 2025). However, a recent review undertaken by Stewart-Lord et al., (2020) around AP research concluded that research is often a neglected pillar, with advanced practitioners only spending an average of 8% of their role on research, which resulted in only 22% of the advanced practitioners questioned feeling confident in this pillar.

Collecting evidence for the research pillar might appear challenging at first for those who might feel less confident with research; however, this does not need to be an onerous task. This pillar is often steeped in confusion to what evidence is required and what defines research, often with the misunderstanding that this is solely related to undertaking a research project. It is about challenging professional boundaries and pioneering innovations, evaluating what is going well and what needs to change, ensuring that practice is based on the best available evidence. For an in-depth discussion, Chapter 6 explores research within the AP pillar.

PIT STOP!

Think about what research or QI projects you have been involved in.

Here are some examples of how you can evidence this pillar in your portfolio:

Academic Modules

Reviewing the evidence base when completing academic assignments. This is a good way of recognising that in critically reviewing the current literature and evidence surrounding a topic/protocol/clinical tool, you have developed and maintained research and QI skills.

Within academic modules, trainee advanced practitioners are supported to examine the evidence base critically before making well-reasoned decisions and recommendations. This type of activity can take place in classroom settings and within the assessment process. Furthermore, trainee advanced practitioners are encouraged to have critical and evidence-based conversations with clinical supervisors which can be recorded within the portfolio. This method encourages the synthesis of different data to answer challenging questions which are important to practise.

Journal Reviews

Reading a journal and then reflecting upon how this has added to your understanding and created new knowledge and understanding. Develop a journal club within your organisation to share ideas and resources. Journal clubs have been found to enhance the implementation of evidence-based practice (Kopf et al., 2018).

Audit and Service Improvement Projects

Most of you will have been involved in service evaluation and audit. To meet the research pillar requirements, what you need to think about is the extent to which you were involved and what this means. The completion of a strengths, weaknesses, opportunities and threats (SWOT) analysis is useful to help inform your decision-making when you need to decide between implementing and testing a new solution or improvement project to help change the way you are currently working. If you have a range of different options to choose from, a SWOT analysis can help to choose the right one to test or implement. It is a useful and structured way of assessing and evaluating an improvement solution, project or initiative. It can be carried out in a range of different environments and helps to identify a preferred or better solution where different options are available (Benzaghta et al., 2021). The tool focuses on understanding the following (Benzaghta et al., 2021):

- **Strengths:** What are the elements of your solution, project or initiative that give it an advantage over others?
- **Weaknesses:** What elements give your solution, project or initiative a disadvantage relative to others?
- **Opportunities:** When considering your solution, project or initiative in the context of your environment, what opportunities might present themselves?
- **Threats:** When considering your solution, project or initiative in the context of your environment, what could cause problems and threaten the success of what you are trying to achieve?

PIT STOP!

Complete a SWOT analysis.

Clinical audits are ways in which you can seek to improve the quality of patient care by examining your own practice against a predetermined standard, for example, National Institute for Health and Clinical Excellent (NICE) guidelines. It can aid your questions around current practice and evaluate the effectiveness and cost (Foy et al., 2020). Box 13.7 highlights an example of an advanced practitioner and their application of research to an identified problem.

BOX 13.7 ■ Example of Research in Practice

In general practice for many years, it has been accepted practice that patients, if they think they have a urine infection (or in some cases patients just wanted it checked!), will collect a specimen of urine and leave it with the receptionist for testing. There was an expectation that the patient would then receive a prescription for antibiotics depending on the urinalysis results.

The impact of this practice included extra workload for the receptionist, multiple samples for a healthcare assistant to test with no facts behind why the sample required testing and then the 'positive' samples would be referred to the on-call clinician. This practice was lending itself to many misdiagnoses and inappropriate antibiotic prescribing.

The practice decided that this required a change in policy and would involve educating all practice staff and patients as to why this was no longer safe and appropriate practice.

The new policy was very clear: no urine samples to be left at reception unless a clinician had requested this and provided appropriate labels. Any patient who believed they had symptoms of a urinary tract infection would need at minimum a telephone call to assess the symptoms.

Implementing this took time as it required engagement from all staff and patients, but the outcome did result in fewer urine samples being left and patients receiving appropriate treatments.

Development and Review of Policies/Protocols and Guidelines

In developing and reviewing policies, protocols and/or guidelines, it demonstrates your ability to implement research findings into practice. These policies, protocols and guidelines can be local, national and international.

It is vital that as an advanced practitioner, you keep abreast with the developing and constantly expanding evidence base to your practice. To do this, you will use critical appraisal skills to understand different strengths and weaknesses of methodologies, results and findings, evaluate the quality and identify bias, to truly assess its value to clinical practice and the generalisability or transferability of the results. As an advanced practitioner, you are well placed to synthesise the results/findings of research evidence and look at a problem from different paradigm perspectives (Fielding et al., 2022).

HOW TO COLLECT EVIDENCE FOR THE EDUCATION PILLAR

The formats identified earlier in this chapter provide a comprehensive review of forms of evidence that can be included in the education as well as the clinical pillar.

Throughout the training period, and once you are qualified, you will be exposed to various learning, teaching and assessment pedagogies, from formal face-to-face teaching to asynchronous and synchronous distance learning. Simulation and technology enhanced learning (TEL) are also a commonplace in developing practitioners not only in the training phase, but also within lifelong learning which should be embedded into professional practice. Together with formal training, independent self-directed learning plays an important role in expanding knowledge; throughout learning and future development, you should engage with independent study to ensure currency of practice.

All staff, including students working in the NHS and being educated by partner institutions such as universities, are identified as having a responsibility for ensuring continual improvement in the quality of care delivered to patients. The education pillar enables you as an advanced practitioner to evidence your master's level education and CPD, in improving the quality of care (NHSE, 2025; HEIW, 2023a).

Practitioners are often concerned about developing and capturing evidence within the education pillar. However, there are a wide variety of ways to highlight your knowledge and skills within the education and learning pillar. Each devolved nation (DHNI, 2019; NHSE, 2025; HEIW, 2023b; NES, 2018) provides guidance on the requirements of each pillar. You will therefore need to cross-reference and check the requirements of your nation.

It is important that you can highlight an ability to self-assess and recognise learning opportunities and knowledge deficits related to your role. Self-assessment can be captured using a self needs analysis form and the use of critical reflection. Self needs analysis templates may either be provided by your university or can easily be found on the internet. One example is the Development Needs Analysis Tool (DNAT) developed by NES (2018). The template is designed to help practitioners reflect on their current job role and to identify areas where they may benefit from further training, education and development to enhance or develop the role.

To support your portfolio development in relation to education, see Chapter 12 for further guidance and reading. Throughout the development of the portfolio, it is essential that the evidence you provide highlights that practice development is evidence-based and implemented in a patient-focussed and caring manner.

Post-AP Training

It is expected within advanced clinical practice that the clinical pillar will be the most significant in each individual practitioner. The other pillars will be evidenced at a threshold level, but some practitioners will find that some pillars are stronger than others. Therefore, even on completion of training, further development is required to keep up-to-date with the ever-changing practice and develop to further roles and opportunities.

It is expected after qualification that once you are qualified as advanced practitioners, you will then become the assessors of the trainees. It is important that the standard of this assessment is maintained to provide mitigation and management of risk to the patient, practitioner and service. Assessor training should be sought to ensure that as a practitioner, you have developed an understanding of what the assessment process is aiming to achieve, the appropriate assessment at each level, how to identify excellence in practice and how to provide constructive feedback for development. Strategic development should also be considered for those wishing to progress to consultant level practice.

Conclusion

This chapter has provided a broad overview of portfolios, and their importance in your development as an advanced practitioner. The codependencies on the other pillars should be clearly defined and apparent within your portfolio, which should be maintained from trainee through your entire career as an advanced practitioner. A portfolio is not a collection of certificates but should be a narration through a critical evaluation of your professional development. The evidence submitted needs to reflect professional development and have meaning; it is no good just submitting a patient history clerking sheet or a PowerPoint of a teaching session that has been delivered, since this does not capture the professional learning and development from these activities. Cross-referencing to other chapters within the book should support your understanding and ability to demonstrate your learning and continuing development.

References

Bailey, S., & West, S. (2022). *What is compassionate leadership?* The King's Fund. https://www.kingsfund.org.uk/insight-and-analysis/long-reads/what-is-compassionate-leadership (Accessed April 27, 2024)

Benzaghta, M. A., Elwalda, A., Mousa, M., Erkan, I., & Rahman, M. (2021). *SWOT analysis applications: An integrative literature review.* ANAHEI Publishing, LLC.

Bridge, P., & Eddy, D. (2006). The virtual portfolio: From conception to reality. *Journal of Radiotherapy in Practice, 5*(1), 1–7. https://doi.org/10.1017/S146039690600001X

Dalia, B. Chaar, B., & Moles, R. (2020). Rethinking competence: A nexus of educational models in the context of lifelong learning. *Pharmacy, 8*(2), 81. https://doi.org/10.3390/pharmacy8020081

Department of Health and Social Care (DHSC). (2021). *Regulating healthcare professionals, protecting the public.* service.gov.uk (Accessed April 22, 2024)

Department of Health Northern Ireland (DHNI). (2019). *Advanced practice AHP framework.* https://www.health-ni.gov.uk/sites/default/files/publications/health/AHP-Framework.pdf (Accessed March 18, 2024)

Eddy, A. Eddy, D., & Doughty, J. (2015). Evidencing continual professional development: Maximising impact and informing career planning. *Journal of Medical Imaging and Radiation Sciences, 46*(4). https://doi.org/10.1016/j.jmir.2015.07.006

Faculty of Intensive Care Medicine (FICM). (2023). *ACCP curriculum: Training for advanced critical care practitioners.* https://www.ficm.ac.uk/careersworkforceaccps/accp-curriculum (Accessed March 18, 2024)

Fielding, A., Moad, D., & Tapley, A. (2022). *Prevalence and associations of rural practice location in early-career general practitioners in Australia: A cross-sectional analysis.* BMJ Open, 12, e058892. doi:10.1136/bmjopen-2021-058892

Forte, M., de Souza, W. L., da Silva, R. F., do Prado, A. F., & Rodrigues, J. F. (2013). A ubiquitous reflective E-portfolio architecture. *International Journal of Medical Informatics, 82*(11), 1111–1122. doi:10.1016/j.ijmedinf.2013.06.005

Foy, R., Skrypak, M., Alderson, S., Ivers, N. M., McInerney, B., Stoddart, J., et al. (2020). Revitalising audit and feedback to improve patient care. *BMJ (Online), 368*, m213. doi:10.1136/bmj.m213

Gillam, S. Hays, R. Lyons, N., & Sackin, P. (2009). Round up. *Education for Primary Care*, *20*(3), 190–194. do i:10.1080/14739879.2009.11493791

Grime, C., & Thomson, A. (2013) Getting the best out of Mini-Clinical Evaluation eXercise (Mini-CEX) – tips for trainers and trainees. *Paediatrics and Child Health*, *23*(2), 85–89

Hamilton, A., Downer, T., Flanagan, B., & Chilman, L. (2023). The use of ePortfolio in health profession education to demonstrate competency and enhance employability: A scoping review. *Journal of Teaching and Learning for Graduate Employability*, *14*(1), 154–166.

Health Education and Improvement Wales (HEIW). (n.d.). *Compassionate leadership hub*. https://nhswales-leadershipportal.heiw.wales/compassionate-leadership-hub# (Accessed April 27, 2024)

Health Education and Improvement Wales (HEIW). (2023a). *Professional framework for enhanced, advanced and consultant clinical practice in Wales*. https://heiw.nhs.wales/files/enhanced-advanced-and-consultant-framework/ (Accessed March 18, 2024)

Health Education and Improvement Wales (HEIW). (2023b). *Portfolio guidance for enhanced, advanced, and consultant clinical practice in Wales*. https://heiw.nhs.wales/files/portfolio-guidance/ (Accessed March 18, 2024)

Health Education England. (2020a). *Core capabilities framework for advanced clinical practice (nurses) working in general practice/primary care in England*. (hee.nhs.uk) (Accessed April 26, 2024)

Health Education England. (2020b). *A guide to completing the e-Portfolio Learning Log*. https://kss.hee.nhs.uk/wp-content/uploads/sites/15/2020/06/A-Guide-to-Completing-the-E-Portfolio-Learning-Log.pdf (Accessed April 21, 2024)

Health Education England, National Health Service England and Skills for Health. (2020). *Core Capabilities Framework for Advanced Clinical Practice (Nurses) Working in General Practice/Primary Care in England*. https://www.hee.nhs.uk/sites/default/files/documents/ACP%20Primary%20Care%20Nurse%20Fwk%202020.pdf

Johnson, G., Booth, J., Crossley, J., & Wade, W. (2011). Assessing trainees in the workplace: Results of a pilot study. *Clinical Medicine (London, England)*, *11*(1), 48–53. doi:10.7861/clinmedicine.11-1-48.

Kennedy, C., Brooks Young, P., Nicol, J., Campbell, K., & Gray Brunton, C. (2015). Fluid role boundaries: Exploring the contribution of the advanced nurse practitioner to multi-professional palliative care. *Journal of Clinical Nursing*, *24*, 21–22. https://doi.org/10.1111/jocn.12950

Kopf, R. S., Watts, P. I., Meyer, E. S., & Moss, J. A. (2018). A Competency-based curriculum for critical care nurse practitioners' transition to practice. *American Journal of Critical Care*, *27*(5), 398–406.

Langridge, N., Welch, H., Jones, D., Small, C., Lynch, G., & Ganatra, B. (2023). Portfolios in practice: Developing advancing practice within a musculoskeletal competency-based model. *Musculoskeletal Science and Practice*, *63*. https://doi.org/10.1016/j.msksp.2022.102689

Loerwald, A. C., Lahner, F. M., Nouns, Z. M., Berendonk, C., Norcini, J., Greif, R., & Huwendiek, S. (2018). The educational impact of Mini-Clinical Evaluation Exercise (Mini-CEX) and Direct Observation of Procedural Skills (DOPS) and its association with implementation: A systematic review and meta-analysis. *PloS One*, *13*(6), e0198009. https://doi.org/10.1371/journal.pone.0198009

Janssens, O., Haerens, L., Valcke, M., Beeckman, D., Pype, P., & Embo, M. (2022). The role of ePortfolios in supporting learning in eight healthcare disciplines: A scoping review. *Nurse Education in Practice*, *63*. https://doi.org/10.1016/j.nepr.2022.103418

Murray, C., Pellow, A., Hennessy, S., Currant, N., & Higgison, C. (2006). User perspectives on the pedagogical differences between electronic and paper portfolios. Paper presented at the Networked Learning Conference. https://www.lancaster.ac.uk/fss/organisations/netlc/past/nlc2006/abstracts/pdfs/02Murray.pdf (Accessed April 22, 2024)

NHS Education Scotland (NES). (2018). *Advanced practice toolkit*. https://learn.nes.nhs.scot/63343 (Accessed March 18, 2024)

NHS Education Scotland (NES). (2022). *Scottish Medical Appraisal Toolkit*. https://www.appraisal.nes.scot.nhs.uk/resources/toolkits/scottish-medical-appraisal-toolkit/domain-2/significant-event-analysis/#:~:text=Significant%20Events%20Analysis%20(SEA)%20is,inform%20and%20develop%20future%20practice (Accessed April 21, 2024)

NHS England. (2021). *Making research matter. Chief Nursing Officer for England's strategic plan for research*. https://www.england.nhs.uk/wp-content/uploads/2021/11/B0880-cno-for-englands-strategic-plan-fo-research.pdf (Accessed March 18, 2024)

NHS England. (2022). *Clinical Academic Support Panel* (CASP). https://advanced-practice.hee.nhs.uk/wp-content/uploads/sites/28/2021/11/Clinical-Academic-Support-Panel-V1.0-1.pdf (Accessed April 27, 2024)

NHS England. (2025). Multi-professional framework for advanced Practice in England. Birmingham: Centre for Advancing Practice.

NHS Leadership Academy. (2013). *The Healthcare Leadership Model*. Version 1.0, Leeds: NHS Leadership Academy. Available at: https://www.leadershipacademy.nhs.uk/wp-content/uploads/2014/10/NHSLeadership-LeadershipModel-colour.pdf (Accessed March 22, 2024)

Nursing and Midwifery Council. (2021). *Revalidation*. https://www.nmc.org.uk/revalidation/overview/what-is-revalidation/ (Accessed April 7, 2024)

Nursing and Midwifery Council. (2023). *Standards for student supervision and assessment*. https://www.nmc.org.uk/standards-for-education-and-training/standards-for-student-supervision-and-assessment/ (Accessed April 7, 2024)

Orland-Barak, L. (2005). Portfolios as evidence of reflective practice: What remains 'untold'. *Educational Research, 47*(1), 25–44. doi:10.1080/0013188042000337541

Royal College of Anaesthetists. (2021). *Acute Care Common Stem curriculum*. https://www.accs.ac.uk/2021-curriculum/curriculum-overview (Accessed April 21, 2024)

Royal College of Emergency Medicine. (2022). *Advanced Clinical Practitioner curriculum*. https://rcem.ac.uk/acp-curriculum/ (Accessed March 18, 2024)

Royal College of General Practitioners. (2024). *Work based assessment*. https://www.rcgp.org.uk/mrcgp-exams/wpba/assessments

Royal College of Paediatrics and Child Health (RCPCH). (2023). *Advanced practitioner (AP) paediatric curricular framework*. https://www.rcpch.ac.uk/education-careers/supporting-training/AP-curriculum (Accessed March 18, 2024)

Skills for Health. (2023). *Portfolio and assessment materials: Core Capabilities Framework for ACP (Nurses) Working in General Practice/Primary Care*. https://www.skillsforhealth.org.uk/info-hub/core-capabilities-framework-for-advanced-clinical-practice-nurses-working-in-general-practice-primary-care/ (Accessed March 18, 2024)

Social Care Wales. (2020). *10 year workforce strategy for health and social care*. https://heiw.nhs.wales/workforce/10-year-workforce-strategy-for-health-and-social-care/ (Accessed April 23, 2024)

Stewart-Lord, A., Beanlands, C., Khine, R., Shamah, S., Sinclair, S., Woods, S., et al. (2020). The role and development of advanced clinical practice within allied health professions: A mixed method study. *Journal of Multidisciplinary Healthcare, 13*, 1705–1715. https://doi.org/10.2147/jmdh.s267083

The Scottish Government. (2017). *Transforming nursing, midwifery and health professions roles: advanced nursing practice*. Chief Nursing Officer Directorate. http://www.gov.scot/Publications/2017/12/3061/1 (Accessed March 18, 2024)

Wallis, L., Locke, R., Sutherland, C., & Harden, B. (2022). Assessment of advanced clinical practitioners. *Journal of Interprofessional Care, 36*(6), 946–950. https://doi.org/10.1080/13561820.2021.1997950 (Accessed April 27, 2024)

Wilkinson, J. R., Crossley, J. G. M., Wragg, A., Mills, P., Cowan, G., & Wade, W. (2008). Implementing workplace-based assessment across the medical specialties in the United Kingdom. *Medical Education, 42*, 364–373. https://doi.org/10.1111/j.1365-2923.2008.03010.x

CHAPTER 14

Emotional and Spiritual Well-Being and Resilience for Advanced Practitioners

Elisabeth Gulliksen ■ Melanie Rogers ■ Angela Windle

CHAPTER OUTLINE

This chapter presents and discusses some of the current stressors that advanced practitioners may face along their professional journey. It also discusses recent work around spirituality and emotional and physical well-being to provide suggestions on how advanced practitioners can overcome these challenges and build resilience in their professional careers.

Introduction

Most of you will have worked in healthcare and are aware of the long hours, chronic staff shortages and stressful working environments. To add to this, over the last few years, the 'perfect storm' of a global pandemic, union strikes, lack of financial investment and Brexit has led to unrivalled clinical challenges for all healthcare professionals and strained the funds that are available to the National Health Service (NHS, 2017; Department of Health, 2022). Now, more than ever before, those in our care and the public are also aware of the demands on the NHS, the need for structural change and the support that healthcare staff require. If we delve a little deeper into these issues, we can see that not only are advanced practitioners affected by the aforementioned problems, but that they also form part of the solution (Mann et al., 2023).

> **PIT STOP!**
> Before reading about the stressors that advanced practitioners face, consider what stressors you have faced in your work or are aware of in your area of practice.

Stressors Facing Advanced Practitioners in Healthcare

STAFFING

The NHS spends the largest proportion of its budget on staff, describing them as 'its most valuable asset' (NHS & Public Health England, 2017). Yet, despite reports of increased staff numbers across many professions, it recognises that at times it 'doesn't feel like it' (NHS & Public Health England, 2017). The United Kingdom (UK) has just 2.9 doctors and 7.78 nurses per thousand of the population, which is significantly lower than many European Union countries (NHS England (NHSE), 2023c). The NHS employs more than 1.5 million staff; however, in 2022, there were over 130,000 empty healthcare posts in secondary care (Nuffield Trust, 2021, 2023) and the same picture is reflected across the UK (Royal College of Nursing Wales, 2023). Without urgent changes, this is expected to develop into a workforce gap of over 260,000 staff by 2036 (NHSE, 2023c). Chronic understaffing is compounded by staff continuing to leave their roles, and a worrying number of healthcare professionals consider doing so in the near future (Nuffield Trust, 2023). With an increasing and aging population, the demand on the NHS is only expected to continue (NHSE, 2023c; Welsh Government, 2023). In an attempt to combat this problem, alternative approaches to developing the health and social care workforce have been sought (NHSE, 2020b).

The national workforce strategy (Scottish Government (SG), 2022) and NHS Long Term Workforce Plan (NHSE, 2023c) stated key priorities as to how the NHS must evolve, which included retaining existing staff, increasing education to support new healthcare roles and increasing productivity. The new roles (including advanced practitioners) aim to develop a rich skill mix within clinical teams by training-up existing multidisciplinary staff to provide advanced or extended practice (NHSE, 2023c; SG, 2022). By providing apprenticeship-based education (see Chapter 1) and new career pathways for health professionals, it supports the existing workforce to reach its full potential and it is hoped that this will therefore improve staff retention (NHSE, 2020b, 2023c). Advanced practitioners also bring a consistent and skilled workforce to the healthcare system, improving the morale for the whole team and therefore exponentially improving staff retention and well-being on a wider level (Evans et al., 2020). Consequently, several of the UK's health service plans aim to increase advanced practitioner training to harness the strengths they bring to the workforce (NHSE, 2023c; SG, 2021a).

The relatively new role of advanced practitioners has been warmly embraced and accepted by many (Evans et al., 2020; Fothergill et al., 2022). The clinical experience and practical 'know-how' of experienced multidisciplinary professionals gives advanced practitioners a strong foundation for assessing and communicating with patients, whilst working across traditional organisational boundaries (National Health Service England (NHSE) 2025). Working in both physical and mental health specialities as part of multiprofessional teams means that advanced practitioners are at the forefront of workforce development plans to embrace a new model of working (NHS Employers, 2020; NHSE, 2020b; SG, 2021a, 2021b). Yet, there is still much confusion as to the level of practice to which they operate at, and the seniority to which they may attain (Fothergill et al., 2022; Murphy & Mortimore, 2020). This is likely to be partially due to a lack of an advanced practice (AP) regulatory body and also that many AP standards and resources are still being developed

(Campbell, 2020; HEE, 2023). There is also the concern that advanced practitioners may be used to fill a rota gap that should have been covered by junior doctors, rather than resolving the wider issues of medical training and staffing (NHS, 2017). Consequently, on qualifying as an advanced practitioner, you may be left feeling potentially misunderstood or undervalued.

STAFF WELL-BEING

People leaving the healthcare profession due to a poor work–life balance and personal health issues has significantly increased in the last decade (NHSE, 2023b; Nuffield Trust, 2023). Between 2011 and 2018, over 56,000 NHS staff left due to an unbalanced work–life ratio (NHSE, 2020b). Forty-four percent of NHS staff report suffering from work-related stress, with mental health conditions being the biggest reason for sickness (NHSE, 2022; NHS Wales, 2022). These worrying statistics have prompted a transition from trying to limit staff sickness to promoting a more sustainable well-being culture for healthcare professionals. There is now a keen focus on supporting emotional, mental and physical well-being in healthcare professionals (NHSE, 2022; SG, 2021a). This starts with ensuring that the basic physical needs of staff are met, for example, regular breaks, adequate rest periods and safe work environments. However, it goes further to advocate that staff must be supported to reach their full potential to be satisfied with their work (Maslow, 1943; NHS Employers, 2022b). This can be achieved through regular staff well-being checks (NHS Employers, 2022a) and ensuring that a sense of value and belonging is being embedded into the workplace ethos (NHSE, 2020b, 2023b; SG, 2024).

Protection for health professionals from violence and abuse is well stated and implemented (NHSE, 2020a), yet there is a recognition that there is a need not only for physical safety but also for a compassionate work environment (McSherry & Pearce, 2018; NHSE, 2020b). Policies are beginning to reflect a culture shift in improving working environments for NHS employees. These include developing a 'just culture' which advocates a fair and constructive approach to staff when they are involved with serious incidents, rather than a blame culture (NHSE, 2023a). Another example includes compassionate and inclusive leadership training for senior leaders in healthcare to foster increased compassion throughout healthcare services and towards healthcare professionals themselves (NHSE, 2023b; Sinclair et al., 2016; Welsh Government, 2023).

Despite these policies, the lived experience of many employees, including advanced practitioners, may not always be positive. There is increasing recognition of the impact of moral distress, and the potential for moral injury. Moral distress is a psychological experience that occurs in response to an event where a person is prevented from doing what they felt was right based on their personal values (Jameton, 1993). In a clinical setting, this occurs as a violation of professional, rather than personal, values, such as not being able to care for patients to the expected standards, witnessing poor care, the lack of resources, chronic understaffing, clinical complexity and lack of recognition (Riedel et al., 2022). The resulting challenge to one's personal values and the resulting unease about the quality of care that is either being delivered (or witnessed) is moral distress (BMA, 2021). If episodes of moral distress accumulate and are left unresolved, moral injury may occur. Moral injury can result in psychological harm, including loss of self-trust, self-depreciation and social withdrawal. Ultimately, this can lead to problems with a clinical relevance, including depression, anxiety and substance abuse (Riedel et al., 2022).

Burnout is a similar condition that results from prolonged exposure to occupational stress and is particularly common in healthcare professionals (Conversano et al., 2020), with up to one-third of UK healthcare practitioners experiencing high levels of burnout (De Hert, 2020; Hall et al., 2019; Hunter et al., 2019; NHSE, 2023b). It results in exhaustion, increased cynicism and poor work efficiency (World Health Organization, 2019). The underlying cause of burnout is the chronic excessive workload resulting from staff shortages (Health and Social Care Parliamentary Committee, 2021), and the prevalence of burnout is such that the Nursing and Midwifery Council (2021) states that it has been exacerbated by the pandemic to now reaching an emergency level. The impact of burnout is multifaceted. You may feel a reduced job satisfaction and experience negative consequences in your personal life, including anxiety and depression. This results in increased staff turnover and poorer quality of care for patients, as well impacting the organisation's performance (De Hert, 2020).

Consequently, actively encouraging staff well-being, encouraging leaders to model healthy work patterns and the early recognition of burnout are key priorities (NHSE, 2020b). When burnout does occur, its management is two-fold. It requires organisational level changes to support a more manageable working environment, as well as supporting the individual to develop healthy coping strategies to readjust their work–life balance (De Hert, 2020).

WORK PATTERNS

Workload within healthcare has also significantly shifted from the vast majority of the work being carried out during week-day hours to a comprehensive out-of-hours service (NHS, 2017). There has also been a transition to most NHS care being provided by primary care: with an increasing public expectation that this should be convenient and personalised to their needs (NHS, 2017). NHS and Public Health England (2017) acknowledged that over 50% of NHS staff work unpaid overtime every week. In 2021 the NHS Staff survey found 21% of respondents stated that every hour they worked felt tiring (NHS Employers, 2023). Consequently, a focus on meeting basic well-being needs (including regular hydration and sleep) is highlighted as a priority, as well as looking at how to support staff to reach their full potential in their chosen careers (NHS Employers, 2022b). There is also increasing awareness that many healthcare professionals are being forced to choose between working as a professional or fulfilling personal commitments (Welsh Government, 2023). To overcome this problem, and to improve staff retention, the NHS is trialling opportunities for variable working patterns and the use of e-rosters. The aim is to provide a more flexible work–life balance and to support people to work when, and how, they prefer (NHSE, 2023c).

TECHNOLOGY

Before the COVID-19 pandemic, the use of technology to access healthcare was increasing (NHS, 2017); however, the pandemic triggered an accelerated digital transformation across the health service. This has resulted in shifting workloads to a technology-reliant pattern including telephone appointments, remote consultations, virtual wards and remote clinics (NHSE, 2021). Within the first 8 weeks of the pandemic lockdown, the average number of weekly remote consultations rose from approximately 13,000 to over 90,000 (NHSE, 2020b). Whilst being an essential measure to protect the public and health service during the pandemic, it also supports the NHS long-term plans to increase capacity within healthcare more generally (NHS & Public Health England, 2017). The use of artificial intelligence is also being explored to further improve efficiency (NHSE, 2023c). Remote working and consultations using the improved technology have been welcomed by some patients and staff (Welsh Government, 2023). For some patients, it improves accessibility to healthcare services, and for staff, it can help their work–life balance (NHSE, 2020b). However, the potential negative impact on clinicians must also be considered. This includes the stress felt by practitioners making potentially life-changing decisions remotely, without the assurance (or benefits) of a face-to-face assessment. Training and support must be provided to help practitioners cope with this new style of consultation and reduce the burden they experience (Bakhai & Atherton, 2020; van Galen et al., 2019).

IMPOSTER SYNDROME

Imposter syndrome is the inability to internalise success and therefore causes a feeling of obtaining a role (in this case a health professional role) fraudulently. This leads to ongoing self-doubt and a feeling of being unworthy of the associated responsibility (Bravata et al., 2020). Imposter syndrome is recognised throughout all healthcare specialities, and advanced practitioners are no exception. Chapter 11 explored students' perspective of undertaking AP education and training, recognising imposter syndrome as a common feature of this journey. Trainee advanced practitioners may have entered training programmes from relatively senior positions in their prior disciplines, but on commencing AP training, they often become novices again and face a steep learning curve of new skills and knowledge. This can potentially result in reduced self-confidence and imposter syndrome (Benner, 1984; Murphy & Mortimore, 2020).

JOB SATISFACTION

Little has been studied about advanced practitioners' job satisfaction apart from studies mainly with nurse practitioners (NPs). However, we know that job satisfaction is also key to well-being. Most studies have been conducted in the United States (Athey et al., 2015; Bae, 2016; Bumbach & Weber, 2014; Bush & Lowery, 2016; De Milt et al., 2011; Faris et al., 2010; Goolsby, 2011; Judge et al., 2016; Shea, 2015) and suggest that NPs become dissatisfied with their work when they are unable to offer the holistic care that is foundational to their clinical practice. If care compromises patient safety, then NPs become dissatisfied with their work and role. Additionally, NPs who are unable to practice at their full level of autonomy also become dissatisfied with their roles.

An international study by Steinke et al. (2017) mirrored some of the US findings. A total of 1680 NPs from 19 countries responded and participated in the study. New findings suggested that where NP roles were new and where NPs were not valued, job satisfaction decreased. Additionally, those who had been in the role longer were more likely to be less satisfied with their work than newly qualified NPs (Steinke et al., 2017). NPs who felt respected, supported and able to work to a full scope of practice have more job satisfaction. Therefore, for you to thrive as an advanced practitioner, you need workplaces that value your role, that facilitate you working to the full scope of practice and which provide you with adequate support.

> **PIT STOP!**
>
> Can you relate to the stressors mentioned earlier? Reflect on which of these stressors have impacted you most. How did you deal with these or what help would you have wanted at that time?

What Can Help?

Unpacking the difficulties that face advanced practitioners can make the future seem a little bleak. Yet, advanced practitioners are in a unique position to help support changes in the healthcare system; but to do so, they too must be protected, valued and supported. Whilst organisational level improvements are welcomed, you must also be equipped and empowered to protect your own health and well-being.

Recent studies during the COVID-19 pandemic explored emotional and spiritual well-being and resilience of advanced practitioners, NPs and advanced practice nurses (Rogers et al., 2022a, 2022b). The UK study (Rogers et al., 2022a) identified that advanced practitioners working during the pandemic had lower levels of spiritual and emotional well-being. Their resilience had been greatly impacted. Support is needed from colleagues, employers and government level to support well-being and resilience. Interestingly, in the global study, Rogers et al. (2022b) found that UK advanced practitioners had the lowest well-being and resilience scores compared to other countries. Only speculative reasons can be attributed to this, but considering the state of the NHS, reduced workforce and unmanageable demands may be some of the causes.

A factor that seems to support well-being and resilience is spirituality. Advanced practitioners who report higher levels of spirituality also report greater resilience in their work. Consequently, increased resilience leads to increases in well-being.

PIT STOP!

What does spirituality mean to you? Is it an area you have considered in your personal and professional life?

So, knowing this, how can advanced practitioners support and increase their well-being and resilience in a demanding role and culture? Spiritual well-being, self-compassion and resilience are several factors that can help.

SPIRITUAL WELL-BEING

Spirituality is simply what gives each person hope, meaning and purpose; it is inherently human (Rogers, 2016). Pink (2009) talks about three aspects that drive us as people: autonomy, mastery and purpose. Throughout this book, the authors have discussed autonomy as an advanced practitioner, which is vital at advanced levels of practice. When considering mastery, it is clinical practice which most advanced practitioners will want to develop mastery in (a caveat being that we will never become a master, or know it all, as our roles necessitate continual learning, reflection and development!). However, it could be argued that finding one's purpose as an advanced practitioner is an aspect of spirituality which leads to complete AP embodiment.

Many healthcare practitioners conflate spirituality and religion, despite each being a differing concept. However, for some people, their faith is what gives them purpose and symbolises their spirituality. Nevertheless, many people's spirituality comes from their work, their family, their pets and nature, for example (Rogers, 2021). Wattis et al., (2017) identify spirituality as the way we live, the way we relate and how we perceive the world around us. Being aware of our own spirituality, nurturing our spiritual well-being and integrating spirituality into our practice can have significant positive impacts. Rogers' (2021) book has examples of how advanced practitioners across the world integrate spiritualty into holistic care.

Working as advanced practitioners consistently necessitates the development of relationships with those we work with, those we care for, families, carers and the wider organisation and communities. Showell Nicholas (2021) suggests that advanced practitioners can develop their spirituality by integrating the skills of empathy, congruence and unconditional positive regard. Using these skills will help us integrate spirituality into our practice. She goes on to say in addition to honing these skills, advanced practitioners' own spiritual well-being is paramount; if this reduces, advanced practitioners will become prone to burnout and compassion fatigue. We commend you for being honest about your well-being. If you are struggling, ask for help; if something is worrying you, talk to a colleague or supervisor; if you don't know something, don't pretend you do, ask for a colleague's opinion/ help. It is a brave advanced practitioner who holds their hand up and says I am struggling; it is highly likely that if you do this, then you will be more resilient, have higher levels of spiritual well-being and flourish in your work.

So how do advanced practitioners (including trainees) support and develop their spiritual well-being? We suggest a number of simple practices:

Firstly, take time now to consider what gives your life meaning and purpose. This may be your work as an advanced practitioner, seeing the difference the care you give has for your patients and being part of a team/organisation. It may have little to do with work; it could be your partner, your friends or the community you live in. Or it may be faith, nature, your pets or hobbies, for example. There are no right answers here. Each of us is a unique individual; we are human. However, we hope that you will view AP as a vocation and not just a job. Many of us go into healthcare because we want to make a difference. We want to care for patients and see the positive impact we can have with every patient whether it is treating a chest infection, supporting someone through depression or supporting an end-of-life patient to die with dignity.

Secondly, reflect upon the aspects that give you meaning and purpose. Is the way you are working/living congruent with this? If not, it is likely your spiritual well-being will reduce. Take time to rebalance and reconnect, and sometimes take time off work to address some of the issues that may be impacting your well-being. This may involve seeing a professional for support.

Thirdly, in your work, look for cues from patients about what gives them meaning and how their illness is impacting them. Give your patients time to explore this and let them know this is important. Remember to be fully present with your patients, listening to them and showing that you do care. This will help you to be more holistic and more person-centred. Integrating spirituality into practice leads to greater well-being and resilience for clinicians as well as for patients.

Finally, consider exploring and using the Advanced Practice Framework of Spiritualty, as highlighted in Table 14.1 (Rogers, 2021). The framework was developed by Melanie Rogers after 7 years of doctoral study looking at advanced NP perceptions of spirituality, as well as many years studying spirituality and integrating spirituality into practice.

The premise of the framework is for advanced practitioners to integrate working in a way which is both available and vulnerable, within the boundaries of healthcare. It is integrated with all advanced practitioners' skills and competencies to provide truly holistic care and is a way of ensuring spirituality is embedded in practice. In-depth understanding of this framework can be read about in Rogers' (2021) book and understood through case studies presented there.

Availability starts with being available to yourself first as an advanced practitioner. It requires reflection on your own spirituality and your own practice. It includes being self-aware and recognising what gives you meaning and purpose. Secondly, it is being available to those in our care, not just being physically available. Emotional availability with our patients is a choice. It means welcoming patients into your care, offering them time, presence, acceptance and understanding as they open up to you as an advanced practitioner and trust you to help them. It is about making space for patients to voice their concerns in a safe place. Finally, availability also involves

TABLE 14.1 ■ Rogers' Availability and Vulnerability Framework for Operationalising Spirituality

Availability	
Availability to self	Self-reflection and self-awareness; this will help you to embrace spirituality by understanding your own meaning, purpose and direction in life.
Availability to others	Welcome people into your care, be hospitable by offering your time, acceptance and understanding. This involves being truly 'present' and listening attentively. It necessitates providing care and demonstrating concern through active participation in therapeutic relationships with patients.
Availability to community	Develop your practice in response to the needs of the community and those in your care. The community may be your colleagues, organisation or the community as a whole.
Vulnerability	
Vulnerability to self	Embrace the vulnerability of your role and the reality that you can never 'know it all'.
Vulnerability to others	Embrace accountability, engage in supervision and reflection, and accept constructive criticism. Allow yourself to be vulnerable in your approach to practice, acknowledging your mistakes and limitations. Be willing to share your uncertainty with patients to reveal your openness, honesty and transparency.
Vulnerability to the community	Advocate for those in your care; question authority where necessary, keeping the interests of your patients at the centre of care.

From Rogers, M. (Ed.) (2021). Spiritual dimensions of advanced practice nursing – Stories of hope. Springer.

being willing to develop yourself as an advanced practitioner in response to the needs of those you care for. This includes being willing to keep learning, to recognise your limitations and to ask for help when need.

Vulnerability is often viewed in a negative way. However, in this setting, it is a positive intentional attribute. It involves us as advanced practitioners recognising that we will never 'know it all'. If you think you do know it all, you need to stop practicing! It involves advanced practitioners continually seeking supervision throughout their work life, reflecting on practice and admitting when things go wrong. It is a healthy practitioner who can hold their hand up and say they have made a mistake. Additionally, when patients tell us something that has upset or hurt them, or when they are complaining, do not become defensive. Say that you are sorry about their experience; this approach often diffuses difficult situations and develops trust with your patients.

As an advanced practitioner, you will frequently have consultations where you may be uncertain about a diagnosis or management, share your uncertainty with your patients and ask for help from colleagues/supervisors. Patients often feel more comfortable with a practitioner who is willing to be honest. It also takes the pressure off you from thinking you have to know and do it all!

Finally, be willing to be vulnerable in the way you work and authentic in your approach to patients. It is a sign of true humility and great leadership (Brown, 2018) and she suggests that a true leader is one who has the courage to be vulnerable, to turn up, be willing to develop and learn. She quotes Theodore Roosevelt by saying:

> 'It is not the critic who counts; not the man who points out how the strong man stumbles, or where the doer of deeds could have done them better. The credit belongs to the man who is actually in the arena, whose face is marred by dust and sweat and blood; who strives valiantly; who errs, who comes short again and again...who at the best knows in the end the triumph of high achievement, and who at the worst, if he fails, at least fails while daring greatly.'

PIT STOP!

Do you think the framework in Table 14.1 could be integrated into your practice?

SELF-COMPASSION

Compassion is the engagement with another's suffering (Oxford English Dictionary, 2022), but at its very core, an element of action, separating it from empathy (Goetz et al., 2010). Perez-Bret et al. (2016, p. 605) define compassion as:

> 'the sensitivity shown to understand another person's suffering, combined with a willingness to help and promote well-being of that person, to find a solution to their problem.'

Healthcare delivered with a compassionate approach benefits both the patient (as it alleviates their distress) (Malenfant et al., 2022) and the practitioners themselves (Sinclair et al., 2017). It is also known that the organisational structure of institutions goes a long way to developing a compassionate culture towards both staff and patients (Braithwaite et al., 2017). Consequently, the emphasis of compassion as a core component of the NHS ethos is evident in many of its latest policies and standards (NHSE, 2020b, 2023b; SG, 2017).

Healthcare professionals are often (quite rightly) very focused on delivering compassionate care to patients, but rarely stop to reflect on the care they offer to themselves (NHSE, 2020b), or are perhaps are more generous with the failings and suffering of others than their own (Neff, 2003). If advanced practitioners are encouraged and taught how to provide compassionate care to themselves, it can protect and promote their well-being and health. This type of compassion is termed 'self-compassion', and Neff (2003 p. 224) defines it as:

> 'being open to and moved by one's own suffering, experiencing feelings of caring and kindness to oneself, taking an understanding, non-judgemental attitude toward one's inadequacies and failures, and recognising that one's own experience is part of the common human experience.'

Or simply, it is compassion that is offered inwards to the self (Germer & Neff, 2013). Self-compassion is not to be confused with self-pity because that causes immersion in our own woes. Rather, when we offer self-kindness and self-compassion to ourselves, we are gentle and encouraging to ourselves, acknowledging that we suffer, just as others do (Germer & Neff, 2013). It utilises negative emotions to allow the development of positive emotions (Germer & Neff, 2013). Consequently, self-compassion increases, psychological well-being and emotional resilience improve (Gilbert & Procter, 2006) and the fear of failure is reduced (Neff et al., 2005), allowing the practitioner to keep delivering compassionate care to patients in a sustainable manner (Conversano et al., 2020).

PIT STOP!

How self-compassionate do you think you are? Consider taking the self-compassion assessment:

https://self-compassion.org/self-compassion-test/

RESILIENCE

Resilience refers to the ability to adapt and recover when faced with challenges, Wiig et al., (2020, p. 1) define resilience in healthcare as:

> *'...the capacity to adapt to challenges and changes at different system levels, to maintain high quality care.'*

Healthcare professionals working in AP roles encounter demanding and emotionally charged situations. They are often pivotal in managing these interactions by making critical decisions in high-pressure environments. Promoting resilience for an advanced practitioner is therefore a key strategy to enhance personal well-being and the ability to continue providing quality patient care.

To become a resilient practitioner involves the ability to recognise, understand and manage your own emotions, as well as managing the emotions of others to cope with adversity and the ability to bounce back from failures (Pahwa & Khan, 2022). Therefore, the attributes of self-compassion, acceptance of vulnerability and the implementation of a support structure (from the workplace or home life) are necessary tools. These tools can enable you to deal with the day-to-day challenges of clinical practice as well as the complex ethical challenges that frequently occur, especially those recently seen during the COVID-19 pandemic. Stress management and well-being considerations are key practices to support a higher degree of emotional intelligence as a mechanism to support the building of a resilient practitioner. Apart from the peer support and mentorship of colleagues within the workplace, the use of reflective practice and clinical supervision are widely practiced in psychotherapeutic settings. These methods may also be applied to AP clinical supervision, either through group or 1:1 supervision (Yegdich, 1998). Finding the method that works well for you or your organisation can be complex especially within healthcare environments. This is due to conflicting priorities of managers and supervisees, or tensions between healthcare workers, which can influence the success of a supervision relationship (Milne & Reiser, 2023).

Healthcare organisations need to invest in clinical supervision models and reflective practice initiatives that specifically address the emotional well-being of staff alongside the flexible workplace arrangements. The modelling of good practice in leadership, peer support programmes and rewarding staff will all foster a positive workplace culture. Supportive and collaborative workplace environments should work towards reducing workplace adversity both as individual practitioners in healthcare and collectively as organisations to build the emotional intelligence of the staff (Tabakakis et al., 2022). In the context of AP within England, the clinical supervision model is guided by the HEE (2021) framework, which outlines the principles, standards and outcomes for effective supervision. It is, however, just one example of a clinical supervision framework and different countries will have different frameworks and models. The HEE framework aims to promote a culture of continuous improvement, reflection and feedback, as well as to ensure consistency and quality across different settings and professions.

The main components of this clinical supervision relationship are:

- Contracting: establishing the purpose, goals, expectations, roles and responsibilities of the supervision relationship. It is vital to clarify who forms this relationship in terms of the supervisor and supervisee.
- Reflection: exploring the supervisee's experiences, thoughts, feelings, actions and outcomes in relation to their practice.
- Analysis: identifying the strengths, weaknesses, opportunities and challenges of the supervisee's practice, as well as the learning needs and objectives.
- Action planning: developing and implementing strategies to address the learning needs and objectives, as well as to improve the quality and safety of care.
- Evaluation: assessing the effectiveness and impact of the supervision process and the action plan on the supervisee's practice and outcomes (HEE, 2021).

Effective clinical supervision is a valuable tool for enhancing your professional development and contributing to a culture of patient safety through the development of a resilient, emotionally intelligent practitioner. As a concept, emotional intelligence was first described in the 1990s (Salovey & Mayer, 1990). An emotionally intelligent practitioner is someone who can understand and navigate their own emotions (Nightingale et al., 2018). Emotional intelligence is the ability to identify and express your emotions, so that you can manage these emotions to motivate oneself despite challenges during daily life (Herland, 2022). The successful employment of emotional intelligence for healthcare workers involves utilising the skills of personal competence by being self-aware, motivated and self-regulating, along with social competence, which includes using social skills and empathy (Goleman, 2006). The promotion of integrating an understanding of becoming an emotionally intelligent practitioner and exploring this concept as a component of resilience may empower building an understanding of one's own, and others', emotions (Herland, 2022).

This focus should contribute to building positive workplace relationships and surviving increasingly demanding healthcare environments.

Conclusion

Providing healthcare has become increasingly complex, particularly following the global COVID-19 pandemic. The delivery of challenging, complex care has had a negative impact on the well-being and resilience of healthcare staff, including advanced practitioners. To improve the lived experiences of advanced practitioners, the focus must be on building resilient teams that work collaboratively and improving our work–life balance and self-care. Sharing experiences and role modelling good practice through clinical supervision have the potential to improve the job satisfaction of advanced practitioners, but other initiatives are also necessary. Flexible rostering and the use of technology have the potential to improve job satisfaction, which may go some way to reduce the feelings of burnout that have been reported recently.

Overall, it is now much more recognised that we must care for the workforce, in order for them to provide compassionate care for the population. There is an increased urgency to reduce burnout and improve the retention and recruitment of healthcare staff. Advanced practitioners are both the leaders of this compassionate approach to the workforce, as well as needing to be the recipients of support to develop their personal well-being and resilience in challenging clinical environments.

References

Athey, E., Leslie, M., Briggs, L., Park, J., Falk, N., Pericak, A., El-Banna, M., & Green J. (2015). How important are autonomy and work setting to nurse practitioners' job satisfaction? *Journal of the American Association of Nurse Practitioners, 28*(6), 320–3266. https://doi.org/10.1002/2327-6924.12292

Bae, S. H. (2016). Nurse practitioners' job satisfaction in rural versus nonrural areas. *Journal of the American Association of Nurse Practitioners, 28*(9), 471. https://doi.org/10.1002/2327-6924.12362

Bakhai, M., & Atherton, H. (2020). *Using online consultations in primary care.* National Health Service England. https://www.england.nhs.uk/wp-content/uploads/2020/01/online-consultations-implementation-toolkit-v1.1-updated.pdf (Accessed April 1, 2023)

Benner, P. (1984). *From novice to expert: Excellence and power in clinical nursing practice.* Menlo Park, CA: Addison-Wesley.

Braithwaite, J., Herkes, J., Ludlow, K., Testa, L., & Lamprell, G. (2017). Association between organisational and workplace cultures, and patient outcomes: Systematic review. *British Medical Journal Open, 7*, e017708. doi:10.1136/bmjopen-2017-017708

Bravata, D. M., Watts, S. A., Keefer, A. L., Madhusudhan, D. K., Taylor, K. T., Clark, D. M., Nelson, R. S., Cokley, K. O., & Hagg, H. K. (2020). Prevalence, predictors, and treatment of impostor syndrome: A systematic review. *Journal of General Internal Medicine, 35*(4), 1252–1275. doi:10.1007/s11606-019-05364-1

British Medical Association. (2021). *Moral distress and moral injury.* https://www.bma.org.uk/media/4209/bma-moral-distress-injury-survey-report-june-2021.pdf (Accessed April 3, 2023)

Brown, B. (2018). *Daring to lead.* Vermillion.

Bumbach, M., & Weber, B. (2014). *Nurse practitioner job satisfaction: A systematic review.* Proceedings at the 11th Annual Research and Scholarship Day & Malasanos Lectureship, Gainesville, FL, 2014. https://www.researchgate.net/publication/261562212_Nurse_Practitioner_job_satisfaction_A_systematic_review

Bush, C. T., & Lowery, B. (2016). Original research: postgraduate nurse practitioner education: Impact on job satisfaction. *The Journal for Nurse Practitioners, 12*(4), 226–234. https://doi.org/10.1016/j.nurpra.2015.11.018

Campbell, J. (2020). Regulation of advanced critical care practitioners: Past, present and future. *Journal of the Intensive Care Society*, 21(1), 7–11. doi:10.1177/1751143718809682

Conversano, C., Ciacchini, R., Graziella, O., Mariagrazia, D. G., Gemignani, A., & Poli, A. (2020). Mindfulness, compassion and self-compassion among health care professionals: What's new? A systematic review. *Frontiers in Psychology*, 11, 1683. https://doi.org/10.3389/fpsyg.2020.01683

De Hert, S. (2020). Burnout in healthcare workers: Prevalence, impact and preventative strategies. *Local and Regional Anesthesia*, 13, 171–183. doi:10.2147/LRA.S240564

De Milt, D., Fitzpatrick, J., & McNulty, S. (2011). Nurse practitioners' job satisfaction and intent to leave current positions, the nursing profession, and the nurse practitioner role as a direct care provider. *Journal of the American Academy of Nurse Practitioners*, 23, 42–50. https://doi.org/10.1111/j.1745-7599.2010.00570.x

Department of Health. (2022). *Health and social care workforce strategy 2026 – Delivering for Our People. Second Action Plan* (2022–23 to 2024–25). https://www.health-ni.gov.uk/publications/health-and-social-care-workforce-strategy-2026 (Accessed April 11, 2024)

Evans, C., Pearce, R., Greaves, S., & Blake, H. (2020). Advanced clinical practitioners in primary care in the UK: A qualitative study of workforce transformation. *International Journal of Environmental Research and Public Health*, 17(2), 4500. doi:10.3390/ijerph17124500

Faris, J., Douglas, M., Maples, D., Berg, L., & Thrailkill, A. (2010). Job satisfaction of advanced practice nurses in the Veterans' Health Administration. *Journal of the American Academy of Nurse Practitioners*, 22, 35–44. https://doi.org/10.1111/j.1745-7599.2009.00468.x.

Fothergill, L. J., Al-Oraibi, A., Houdmont, J., Conway, J., Evans, C., Timmons, S., Pearce, R., & Blake, H. (2022). Nationwide evaluation of the advanced clinical practitioner role in England: a cross-sectional survey. *British Medical Journal Open*, 12, e055475. doi:10.1136/bmjopen-2021-055475

Germer, C. K., & Neff, K. D. (2013). Self-compassion in clinical practice. *Journal of Clinical Psychology*, 69(8), 856–867. https://doi.org/10.1002/jclp.22021

Gilbert, P., & Procter, S. (2006). Compassionate mind training for people with high shame and self-criticism: Overview and pilot study of a group therapy approach. *Clinical Psychology & Psychotherapy*, 13(6), 353–379. https://doi.org/10.1002/cpp.507

Goetz, J. L., Keltner, D., & Simon-Thomas, E. (2010). Compassion: An evolutionary analysis and empirical review. *Psychological Bulletin*, 136(3), 351–374. doi:10.1037/a0018807

Goleman, D. (2006). *Working with emotional intelligence*. Bloomsbury.

Goolsby, M. (2011). 2009–2010 AANP national nurse practitioner sample survey: An overview. *Journal of the American Academy of Nurse Practitioners*, 23(5), 266–268. https://doi.org/10.1111/j.1745-7599.2011.00611.x

Hall, L., Johnson, J., Watt, I., & O'Conner, D. (2019). Association of GP wellbeing and burnout with patient safety in UK primary care, a cross sectional study. *British Journal of General Practice*, 69(684), 507–514.

Health and Social Care Parliamentary Committee. (2021). *Workforce burnout and resilience in the NHS and social care*. United Kingdom Parliament.

Health Education England. (2021). *Workforce supervision for advanced clinical practice*. https://advanced-practice.hee.nhs.uk/workplace-supervision-for-advanced-clinical-practice-2/

Health Education England. (2023). *Advanced practice – About us*. https://advanced-practice.hee.nhs.uk/about-us/ (Accessed April 8, 2023)

Herland, M. D. (2022). Emotional intelligence as a part of critical reflection in social work practice and research. *Qualitative Social Work*, 21(4), 662–678. https://doi.org/10.1177/14733250211024734 (Accessed April 1, 2023)

HS England (2025) *Multi-professional framework for advanced Practice in England*. Birmingham: Centre for Advancing Practice.

Hunter, B., Fenwick, J, Sidebotham, M., & Henley, J. (2019). Midwives in the United Kingdom: Levels of burnout, depression, anxiety and stress and associated predictors. *Midwifery*, 79, 102526.

Jameton, A. (1993). Dilemmas of moral distress: Moral responsibility and nursing practice. *AWHONN's Clinical Issues in Perinatal and Women's Health Nursing*, 4(4), 542–551.

Judge, S., Boursaw, B., & Cohen, S. (2016). Trends in the supply and practice environment of nurse practitioners in New Mexico. *Nursing Economics*, 34(1), 35–43.

Malenfant, S., Jaggi, P., Hayden, K., & Sinclair, S. (2022). Compassion in healthcare: An updated scoping review of the literature. *BMC Palliative Care*, 21, 80. https://doi.org/10.1186/s12904-022-00942-3

Mann, C., Timmons, S., Evans, C., Pearce, R., Overton, C., Hinsliff-Smith, K., & Conway, J. (2023). Exploring the role of advanced clinical practitioners and their contribution to health services in England: A qualitative exploratory study. *Nurse Education in Practice, 67,* 103546. https://doi.org/10.1016/j.nepr.2023.103546

Maslow, A. H. (1943). A theory of human motivation. *Psychological Review, 50(4),* 370–396. https://doi.org/10.1037/h0054346

McSherry, R., & Pearce, P. (2018). Measuring health care workers' perceptions of what constitutes a compassionate organisation culture and working environment: Findings from a quantitative feasibility survey. *Journal of Nursing Management,* 26(2), 127–139. https://doi-org.libaccess.hud.ac.uk/10.1111/jonm.12517

Milne, D. L., & Reiser, R. P. (2023). *Resolving critical issues in clinical supervision: A practical, evidence-based approach.* John Wiley & Sons.

Murphy, K., & Mortimore, G. (2020). Overcoming the challenges of role transition for trainee advanced clinical practitioners. *Gastrointestinal Nursing,* 18(5), 35–41. https://doi.org/10.12968/gasn.2020.18.5.35

National Health Service. (2017). *Next steps on the NHS five year forward view.* National Health Service.

National Health Service Employers. (2022a). *NHS staff wellbeing needs poster.* https://www.nhsemployers.org/system/files/2022-04/Basic_NHS_staff_needs_poster.pdf (Accessed April 1, 2023)

National Health Service Employers. (2022b). *Supporting the wellbeing needs of NHS staff.* National Health Service. https://www.nhsemployers.org/articles/supporting-wellbeing-needs-nhs-staff (Accessed April 1, 2023)

National Health Service Employers. (2023). *NHS Staff Survey 2021: Health and wellbeing.* National Health Service. https://www.nhsemployers.org/articles/nhs-staff-survey-2021-health-and-wellbeing (Accessed April 1, 2023)

National Health Service England. (2020a). *Violence prevention and reduction standard.* National Health Service.

National Health Service England. (2020b). *We are the NHS: People plan for 2020/21.* National Health Service England.

National Health Service England. (2021). *Digital and technology.* https://www.england.nhs.uk/mat-transformation/matrons-handbook/digital-and-technology/ (Accessed April 1, 2023)

National Health Service England. (2022). *NHS health and wellbeing framework.* National Health Service England.

National Health Service England. (2023a). *A just culture guide.* https://www.england.nhs.uk/patient-safety/a-just-culture-guide/ (Accessed April 1, 2023)

National Health Service England. (2023b). *Compassionate and inclusive leadership.* https://www.england.nhs.uk/culture/what-does-compassionate-and-inclusive-leadership-mean-to-us/ (Accessed April 1, 2023)

National Health Service England. (2023c). *NHS long term workforce plan.* https://www.england.nhs.uk/publication/nhs-long-term-workforce-plan/. (Accessed September 30, 2023)

National Health Service and Public Health England. (2017). *Facing the facts, shaping the future. A draft health and care workforce strategy for England to 2027.* Public Health England.

National Health Service Wales. (2022). *NHS Wales workforce trends* (as at 31st March 2022). https://heiw.nhs.wales/files/nhs-wales-workforce-trends-as-at-31-march-2022/ (Accessed April 11, 2024)

Neff, K. D. (2003). Development and validation of a scale to measure self-compassion. *Self and Identity,* 2(3), 223–250. https://doi.org/10.1080/15298860309027

Neff, K. D., Hsieh, Y. P. & Dejitterat, K. (2005). Self-compassion, achievement goals, and coping with academic failure. *Self and Identity,* 4(3), 263–287. https://doi.org/10.1080/13576500444000317.

Nightingale, S., Spiby, H., Sheen, K., & Slade, P. (2018). The impact of emotional intelligence in health care professionals on caring behaviour towards patients in clinical and long-term care settings: Findings from an integrative review. *International Journal of Nursing Studies,* 80, 106–117. https://doi.org/10.1016/j.ijnurstu.2018.01.006

Nuffield Trust. (2021). *The NHS workforce in numbers.* https://www.nuffieldtrust.org.uk/resource/the-nhs-workforce-in-numbers (Accessed April 1, 2023)

Nuffield Trust. (2023). *The long goodbye? Exploring rates of staff leaving the NHS and social care.* Nuffield Trust. https://www.nuffieldtrust.org.uk/resource/the-long-goodbye-exploring-rates-of-staff-leaving-the-nhs-and-social-care (Accessed April 1, 2023)

Nursing and Midwifery Council. (2021). *NMC comments on the "Workforce burnout and resilience in the NHS and social care" report.* https://www.nmc.org.uk/news/news-and-updates/health-social-care-burnout-comment/ (Accessed April 1, 2023).

Oxford English Dictionary. (2022). *Compassion*. Oxford University Press. https://www.oed.com/viewdiction-aryentry/Entry/37475 (Accessed April 1, 2023)

Pahwa, S., & Khan, N. (2022). Factors affecting emotional resilience in adults. *Management and Labour Studies*, *47*(2), 216–232.

Perez-Bret, E., Altisent, R., & Rocafort, J. (2016). Definition of compassion in healthcare: A systematic literature review. *International Journal of Palliative Nursing*, 22(12), 599–606. doi:10.12968/ijpn.2016.22.12.599.

Pink, D. (2009). *Drive: The surprising truth about what motivates us*. Riverhead Books.

Riedel, P. L., Kreh, A., Kulcar, V., Lieber, A., & Juen, B. (2022). A scoping review of moral stressors, moral distress and moral injury in healthcare workers during COVID-19. *International Journal of Environmental Research and Public Health*, 19(3), 16. doi: 10.3390/ijerph19031666. PMID: 35162689; PMCID: PMC8835282.

Rogers, M. (2016). *Spiritual dimensions of advanced nurse practitioner consultations in primary care through the lens of availability and vulnerability. A hermeneutic enquiry*. Doctoral thesis, University of Huddersfield.

Rogers, M. (Ed.). (2021). *Spiritual dimensions of advanced practice nursing – Stories of hope*. Springer.

Rogers, M., Windle, A., Wu, L., Taylor, V., & Bale, C. (2022a). Emotional well-being, spiritual well-being and resilience of advanced clinical practitioners in the United Kingdom during COVID-19: An exploratory mixed method study. *Journal of Nursing Management*, *30*(4), 883–891. https://doi.org/10.1111/jonm.13577

Rogers, M., Lamarche, K., Miller, M., Moore, K., Spies, L., Taylor, J., & Staempfli, S. (2022b). Global emotional and spiritual well-being and resilience of advanced practice nurses during the COVID-19 pandemic: A cross-sectional study. *Journal of Advanced Nursing*, *78*(5), 1483–1492.

Royal College of Nursing Wales. (2023). *RCN nursing in numbers 2023*. https://www.rcn.org.uk/news-and-events/Press-Releases/rcn-wales-publishes-nursing-in-numbers-2023-report-260923 (Accessed April 11, 2024)

Salovey, P., & Mayer, J. D. (1990). *Emotional intelligence. Imagination, cognition and personality*, *9*(3), 185–211. https://doi.org/10.2190/DUGG-P24E-52WK-6CDG (Accessed November 1, 2023)

Scottish Government. (2017). *Nursing 2030 vision*. https://www.gov.scot/publications/nursing-2030-vision-9781788511001/pages/6/ (Accessed April 17, 2024)

Scottish Government. (2021a). *NHS recovery plan 2021–2026*. https://www.gov.scot/binaries/content/documents/govscot/publications/strategy-plan/2021/08/nhs-recovery-plan/documents/nhs-recovery-plan-2021-2026/nhs-recovery-plan-2021-2026/govscot%3Adocument/nhs-recovery-plan-2021-2026.pdf (Accessed April 11, 2024)

Scottish Government. (2021b). *Advanced nursing practice – Transforming nursing roles: Phase two*. https://www.gov.scot/publications/transforming-nursing-roles-advanced-nursing-practice-phase-ii/ (Accessed April 17, 2024)

Scottish Government. (2022). *Health and social care: National workforce strategy* https://www.gov.scot/publications/national-workforce-strategy-health-social-care/pages/1/ (Accessed April 17, 2024)

Scottish Government. (2024). *Staff governance*. https://www.staffgovernance.scot.nhs.uk/improving-employee-experience/working-well/ (Accessed April 11, 2024)

Shea, M. (2015). Determined persistence: Achieving and sustaining job satisfaction among nurse practitioners. *Journal of the American Association of Nurse Practitioners*, *27*(1), 31–38. https://doi.org/10.1002/2327-6924.12119

Showell Nicholas, W. (2021). Personal spirituality and self-compassion in advanced practice nursing. In Rogers, M. (Ed.), *Spiritual dimensions of advanced practice nursing- stories of hope* (pp. 61–79). Springer.

Sinclair, S., Norris, J. M., McConnell, S. J., Chochinov, H. M., Hack, T. F., Hagen, N. A., McClement, S., & Bouchal, S. R. (2016). Compassion: A scoping review of the healthcare literature. *BMC Palliative Care*, 15, 6. https://doi.org/10.1186/s12904-016-0080-0

Sinclair, S., Russell, L. B., Hack, T. F., Kondejewski, J., & Sawatzky, R. (2017). Measuring compassion in healthcare: A comprehensive and critical review. *The Patient*, 10(4), 389–405. https://doi.org/10.1007/s40271-016-0209-5

Steinke, M., LaMarche, K., Lehwaldt, D., & Rogers, M. (2017). An examination of nurse practitioners/advanced practice nurses' job satisfaction internationally. *International Nursing Review* 65(2), 162–172 https://doi:10.1111/inr.12389

Tabakakis, C., McAllister, M., & Bradshaw, J. (2022). Exploring resilience and workplace adversity in registered nurses: A qualitative analysis. *Nursing & Health Sciences*, *24*(1), 174–182.

van Galen, L. S., Wang, C. J., Nanayakkara, P. W. B., Paranjape, K., Kramer, M. H. H., Car, J. (2019). Telehealth requires expansion of physicians' communication competencies training. *Medical Teacher,* 41(6), 714–715. https://doi.org/10.1080/0142159X.2018.1481284

Wattis, J., Curran, S., & Rogers, M. (2017). Spirituality competent practice in health care. CRC.

Welsh Government. (2023). *National Workforce Implementation Plan: Addressing NHS Wales workforce challenges.* https://www.gov.wales/sites/default/files/publications/2023-01/national-workforce-implementation-plan.pdf (Accessed April 11, 2024)

Wiig, S., Aase, K., Billett, S., Canfield, C., Roise, O., Nja, O., et al. (2020). Defining the boundaries and operational concepts of resilience in the resilience in healthcare research program. *BMC Health Serv Res, 20,* 330. https://doi.org/10.1186/s12913-020-05224-3

World Health Organization. (2019). *Burn-out an "occupational phenomenon": International Classification of Diseases.* https://www.who.int/news/item/28-05-2019-burn-out-an-occupational-phenomenon-international-classification-of-diseases (Accessed April 1, 2023)

Yegdich, T. (1998). How not to do clinical supervision in nursing. *Journal of Advanced Nursing, 28*(1), 193–202. https://doi.org/10.1046/j.1365-2648.1998.00706.x

CHAPTER 15

Advanced Practice Beyond the UK: An International Context

Melanie Rogers ▪ Colette Henderson ▪ Jonathan Thomas

CHAPTER OUTLINE

This chapter brings together some of the international perspectives related to advanced practice. As the United Kingdom (UK) is the only country to have integrated multiprofessional advanced practice, the focus internationally will be on how nursing has developed advanced practice roles. It is hoped that as the UK approach continues to demonstrate impact on patient care, service delivery and workforce, that will allow other countries to consider how they develop their healthcare practitioners. The chapter begins with an overview of advanced practice nursing, followed by a discussion about advanced practitioners being ideally placed to impact universal health coverage and Sustainable Development Goals. This chapter will end with examples of advanced practice nursing in each of the World Health Organization regions of the world.

Introduction

This chapter brings together some of the international perspectives related to advanced practice (AP). As the United Kingdom (UK) is the only country to have integrated multiprofessional AP, the focus internationally will be on how nursing has developed advanced practitioner roles; both Chapters 1 and 2 cover the history of AP from an international perspective. It is hoped that as the UK approach continues to demonstrate impact on patient care, service delivery and workforce, that will allow other countries to consider how they develop their healthcare practitioners. The chapter begins with an overview of AP nursing, followed by a discussion about advanced practitioners being ideally placed to impact universal health coverage (UHC) and Sustainable Development Goals (SDG) (World Health Organization (WHO), 2024). This chapter will end with examples of AP nursing in each of the WHO regions of the world.

In the UK, England, Scotland, Northern Ireland and Wales have moved towards a multiprofessional approach for the integration of AP into the health and social care sectors. To date, there is little international development akin to the UK; therefore, a focus on the main AP role of the advanced practice nurse (APN) provides exemplars of how AP has changed healthcare. APN numbers have increased exponentially across the globe in recent years. Pulcini et al., (2010) stated that in 2008,

24 countries had formal educational programmes for APNs. Maier et al., (2017) conducted an analysis of APN roles in 37 countries and identified that many countries have worked hard to develop these roles. More recently, Miller et al., (2024) identify the presence of APN in over 80 countries.

Poghosyan and Maier (2022) recognise that APN evolution has mainly occurred in response to increased patient need and the complexity of that need, inequitable access to services as well as the shortages within the medical workforce. APNs have consistently been shown to be key to meeting the healthcare needs of diverse populations and healthcare systems (Rogers et al., 2024; Thomas & Rowles, 2023). Ongoing shortages of clinicians, the global challenges related to ageing populations and noncommunicable and communicable diseases will continue to force countries to look at diversifying their healthcare workforce (Heale & Rieck Buckley, 2015, Laurant et al., 2018; Maier et al., 2017). There has been significant research comparing APNs with medical staff and it has been acknowledged that equivalent care is provided by APNs; it has even, at times, been seen as superior. Additionally, patients are satisfied with the APN role and improved healthcare it supports (Laurant et al., 2018; Martin-Misener et al., 2015; Poghosyan et al., 2017; Poghosyan & Maier, 2022). Poghosyan and Maier (2022) recognise APNs' continual commitment to addressing healthcare inequalities and ensuring that care is person-centred and holistic. Internationally, however, there is marked variation in regulation, title protection, education and scope of practice (Rogers et al., 2024).

To address global variation, the International Council of Nurses (ICN) published its revised guidelines for APNs (ICN, 2020). APNs are defined as:

> 'a generalist or specialised nurse who has acquired, through additional graduate education (minimum of a master's degree), the expert knowledge base, complex decision-making skills and clinical competencies for Advanced Nursing Practice, the characteristics of which are shaped by the context in which they are credentialed to practice.'
>
> (ICN, 2020, p. 6)

The two most common AP roles globally are that of the nurse practitioner (NP) and the clinical nurse specialist (CNS) (ICN, 2020). NPs are:

> 'educated to diagnose and treat conditions based on evidence-informed guidelines that include nursing principles' with a focus on holistic care.
>
> (ICN, 2020, p. 18)

They have the advanced clinical skills needed to care autonomously for patients and have been educated to master's level, as a minimum (ICN, 2020; Ljungbeck et al., 2021). Key to APN roles globally is that the role and scope of practice are shaped by the context and/or country in which they are credentialed to practice (ICN, 2020). The NP role globally correlates closely with the role of the advanced practitioner seen across the four UK nations of England, Scotland, Wales and Northern Ireland.

Advanced Practice Across the Globe

Across the world, AP has developed and integrated into the clinical environment to various degrees, but as highlighted, this is mainly confined to nursing practice. To capture AP globally, the WHO member states are grouped into six regions. The narrative in the next sections will provide exemplars of APN role development in each of the regions. These are exemplars only and each region has significant APN developments in many countries.

REGION OF THE AMERICAS (AMR)

United States

The origin of advanced nursing practice dates back to 1960s in the United States, where a shortage of medical staff, evolving healthcare needs and economic challenges inspired the development of this expanded nurse role (Silver et al., 1968). The role was seen to combine characteristics of nursing and medicine, holistic assessment with clinical examination and decision-making skills (Silver et al., 1968).

The American Association of Nurse Practitioners (AANP) (2022) report identified that there are currently 385,000 licensed NPs in the United States. Currently, the route of entry to AP nursing is a master's degree that encompasses modules that include pathophysiology, pharmacology, physical assessment, leadership, quality improvement and health technologies (Moore et al., 2024). Individual states regulate full, reduced or restricted authority APN practice. Reduced and restricted authority practice controls the amount of physician oversight of APN practice ultimately confining NP practice (Mackavey et al., 2024).

Of note, the American Association of Colleges of Nursing (AACN) and The National Organization of Nurse Practitioner Faculties (NONPF) have endorsed the doctor of nursing practice (DNP) as an entry level to AP in the United States by 2025. This requirement for doctoral education as a route of entry to APN roles continues to provoke an ongoing debate (Moore et al., 2024).

Chile

In Latin American countries, Chile is one of the countries that have been actively developing AP nursing roles. There has been MSc nurse education since 2011; initially for the CNS, this has now been expanded to include NP education. Jaman-Mewes et al., (2021) identified specific challenges to role development, including issues with the scope of practice and regulation being unstandardised. There is a significant amount of collaborative work ongoing between the countries in Latin America which recognises the role of APNs, and how they can contribute to meeting UHC (Cassiani et al., 2018; Zug et al., 2016). The Pan American Health Organization (PAHO, 2015) has worked hard to support the development of AP nursing in Latin American countries, developing many networks supporting this. Currently, APN roles are being developed in Chile, Mexico, Columbia and Brazil (Cassiani et al., 2018). Aguirre-Boza et al., (2019) and Espinoza et al., (2021) have identified specific aspects of CNS roles in Chile and discuss in depth the development of networks which support the effective implementation of APN roles.

AFRICA (AFR)

The Anglophone Africa Advanced Practice Nurse Coalition (AAAPNC) was established in 2018 with the goal of developing a global strategy to enable the integration of APNs into the healthcare workforce in Africa. This coalition serves to provide educational leadership and create the network and collaboration required to develop a regional Family Nurse Practitioner Curriculum Framework in Africa (Gray et al., 2023a). Subsequently, this coalition work has culminated in the development of a proposal to the WHO (Africa) to ensure that the development of the APN role in Africa was a policy priority (Gray et al., 2023a; Moosa, 2021; Sibanda & Stender, 2018).

Across Africa, many nurses work in APN roles despite these often not being recognised (Christmals, 2021). Countries that have progressed well with APN developments include Botswana, Ghana, Eswatini, South Africa and Kenya. These countries have specific APN roles, for example, CNS/NP, and are licensed to practice (Christmals & Armstrong, 2019; Dlamini et al., 2020; Geyer & Christmals, 2020). Additionally, some African countries like Sierra Leone, Namibia and the Seychelles have APNs practicing; however, these APNs have to train in other countries as there are no educational programmes available for nurses in their own countries.

Botswana

Family nurse practitioners (FNPs) are a key priority in terms of workforce development as they are considered vital to support African primary healthcare (PHC) and the progression to achieve the United Nations' (UN's) SDGs of UHC in Africa.

In their 2023 publication, Gray et al., (2023a) detail the progress made within Africa in their achievement towards UHC. AP nursing has existed in Botswana since the 1980s, and consequently, Botswana functions as a role model for the APN role development in Africa. Botswana currently has the highest number of NPs in Africa and offers a diploma and master's degree (Gray et al., 2023b). Most AP work is in outpatients and inpatients, with the majority of NPs working in primary care, including remote and rural settings, health posts, roadside mobile clinics, schools as well as urban health centres (Gray et al., 2023b).

EUROPEAN REGION (EUR)

The APN role was first established in the Netherlands in 1998. Legal frameworks have existed since 2008, stipulating that unsupervised and autonomous NPs in the Netherlands can assess, diagnose and manage presenting complaints including prescribing medications within their scope of practice (Mackavey et al., 2024). APNs must be registered nurses who have completed a 2-year master of advanced nursing practice (MANP) degree programme and registered with the Dutch registry as a certified nurse specialist (V&VN, 2023). Several European countries such as Switzerland and Norway have a reciprocal agreement with the Netherlands for transferrable qualifications. However, if nurses undertake AP education outside these countries and wish to work in the Netherlands, they will need to undertake the MANP degree. Rotterdam University of Applied Sciences requires APN students to gain an understanding of AP internationally. To achieve this, Rotterdam University has collaborated with Swansea University (Wales), University of Texas (United States), Texas Women's University (United States), University of Minnesota (United States) and University of Dundee (Scotland) to develop international student placements. The main aim of this collaboration is to support development of critical thinking, cultural competence and understandings of global healthcare systems and has been welcomed by students and faculty (Mackavey et al., 2024).

Finland

Suutarla et al., (2023) advise that registered nurses are typically very autonomous in Finland. The authors indicate that there is variation between employing organisations, but as an example, in primary care settings, the registered nurse may be the only point of contact for patients. Finland is fortunate to have the highest proportion of registered nurses per head of population (Suutarla et al., 2023), indicating the reliance on appropriately qualified nurses to support the country's healthcare requirements.

AP roles began to emerge in 2000, with programmes materialising in 2006. Suutarla et al., (2023) indicate that although the role has been considered, the approach to AP has not been fully realised. Similar to the UK, prescribing regulations exist having come into force in 2010, but as yet, AP nursing is not regulated. Suutarla et al., (2023) advise that an APN expert group was organised and assembled in 2021 to elucidate the APN role and support this role development, and this work continues to be enacted.

EASTERN MEDITERRANEAN REGION (EMR)

Across the Eastern Mediterranean Region, the role of the APN remains in its infancy but is evolving (Al-Maaitah et al., 2020; Nahari et al., 2023). The definition of the role, scope of practice and title protection remain ambiguous and unclear, challenging role progression (Al-Maaitah et al., 2020; Nahari et al., 2023).

Israel

Although still in its infancy, Israel has made good progress with APN role development. In 2013, Israel approved and enacted the Advanced Practice Nursing Degree Regulations, which provided speciality definitions, prerequisites and licensing rules and requirements (Fighel & Hefetz, 2023). Areas identified as priority for role development were within care of the elderly, surgery and neonatology. Originally, there were 6 specialities, and now there are 11 nursing specialties, with another speciality being planned for development. Interestingly, 10 of these specialties are clinically focused roles, with the 11th speciality being a managerial/administrative role. APN speciality programmes are master's or postmaster's level and require 700 to 1240 hours of study with 4 to 700 hours of supervision from a specialist physician and, for registration, a written and oral licensing examination (Fighel & Hefetz, 2023). Fighel and Hefetz (2023) report that the impact of the APN role on availability, continuity and quality of care is already being detected.

Pakistan

In Pakistan, nursing is often viewed as a subservient profession, which has repercussions on the desirability of joining the profession. As such, AP nursing has struggled to develop despite desperate healthcare needs due to poverty, overpopulation and a high number of vulnerable people (Jan et al., 2023). Lalani and Ali (2021) reported that emerging APN roles include CNS roles in most specialities. These nurses have master's level education to prepare them for the roles and are usually employed at large hospitals in urban regions (Lalani & Ali, 2021), not in rural areas, where there is a desperate need for UHC. In 2022, the first MSc APN programme began at Aka Khan University (Aga Khan, 2022).

SOUTHEAST ASIAN REGION (SEAR)

Sri Lanka

Maithreepala and Konara Mudiyanselage (2023) advise that Sri Lanka is considered to be a low–middle-income country and the state provides free public healthcare services for the population. Nurse education has been influenced by the British model, and currently, five universities offer a BSc nursing programme (Maithreepala & Konara Mudiyanselage, 2023).

Maithreepala and Konara Mudiyanselage (2023, p. 283) describe nurses as the 'backbone' of the Sri Lankan healthcare system; however, as yet the role of the APN is yet to evolve. Changing healthcare needs have provided an opportunity to provide additional and specialised nursing education such as surgical care and neonatal care which is restricted to nurses who have at least 5 years postqualification experience (Maithreepala & Konara Mudiyanselage, 2023). A pilot project was operationalised in 2017 which observed 100 registered nurses enrol in additional education programmes. These nurses consequently received authorisation to prescribe pain relief and provide care for wounds, ostomies and noncommunicable diseases. It is anticipated that these nurses will, in the future, become NPs (Maithreepala & Konara Mudiyanselage, 2023).

WESTERN PACIFIC REGION (WPR)

Australia

In Australia, AP nursing has been well established since 2000. The only regulated APN role in Australia is the NP (Chief Nursing and Midwifery Officers Australia, n.d.), whose registration is endorsed by the Nursing and Midwifery Board of Australia to enable practice within their scope using the legally protected title of NP.

There are over 2500 NPs in Australia (Australian College of Nurse Practitioners, 2023). NPs have an expanded scope of practice that includes autonomous decision-making, advanced clinical skills and the ability to diagnose, treat and prescribe medications within their scope of practice and area of expertise.

Singapore

The APN role first developed in Singapore in 2003, and in 2006 the APN register was established (Tracy & Tan, 2014). An APN in Singapore is seen as a hybrid combination of both the NP and CNS roles. The title and role are regulated by the Singapore Nursing Board (SNB), and there are specific regulatory requirements. An APN is a registered nurse who must have completed a specific accredited master of nursing (MN) programme. Nurses applying for the MN programme must have 3 years postregistration experience in their speciality area (Moore et al., 2024). The MN programme is fully funded by the Singapore Ministry of Health and takes 18 months to complete, with a minimum 2500 hours. The core programme includes modules in pathophysiology, clinical assessment, pharmacology and prescribing. Once graduated from an accredited programme, 1 year supervised clinical practice encompassing a minimum of 1280 hours of direct patient care precedes formal assessment by the SNB. To maintain AP certification, there is an annual review of practice and continuous professional development. The APN role also has opportunities for doctoral level programmes which emerged in 2014 (Tracy & Tan, 2014).

Global Impact of Advanced Nursing Practice: Policy to Practice

In 2015, all UN member states agreed to the adoption of the 17 SDGs to ensure growth of people and the planet by 2030 (Fig. 15.1).

Although the third SDG focuses upon health and well-being, all the SDGs are dependent upon each other; for example, SDG1 focuses on the elimination of poverty, and this has been closely linked to improved health outcomes (WHO, 2024). In relation to the third SDG, there are 13 specific targets, with target 3.8 focussing on the achievement of UHC. Specifically, target 3.8 advises we need to:

'Achieve universal health coverage, including financial risk protection, access to quality essential health-care services and access to safe, effective, quality and affordable essential medicines and vaccines for all'.

(WHO, 2024)

Target 3.8 sets the ambition to provide all states with access to quality healthcare including essential medicines and vaccines with no financial hardship. Whilst healthcare is free at the point of delivery in the UK, the UK government has committed to building global partnerships to support developing countries' work to achieve UHC, including supporting a reform to the international financial system (Foreign, Commonwealth and Development Office, 2023).

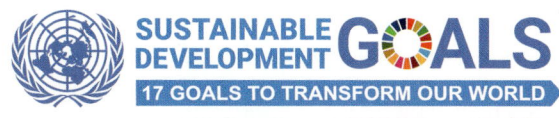

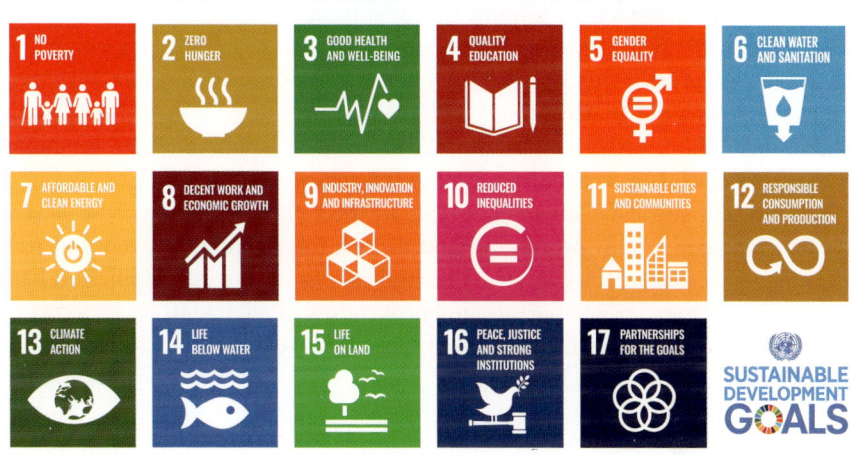

Fig. 15.1 Sustainable Development Goals. *(UN Department of Economic and Social Affairs. THE 17 GOALS. https://www.un.org/sustainabledevelopment/.* (The content of this publication has not been approved by the United Nations and does not reflect the views of the United Nations or its officials or Member States.)

Despite these targets, the UN's annual report (United Nations, n.d.) highlighted that progress to achievement has been slow. This was particularly noted within areas of disease preventable vaccinations and financial spending on healthcare. There were some reports of achievement particularly around HIV treatment, but overall, the third SDG is not on track to be achieved by 2030. The global pandemic of COVID-19 has been cited as one potential instigator for the reduction in available financial resources and spending, thus impacting on achievement of UHC. However, the UN report (United Nations, n.d.) also notes that there will be a global shortage of healthcare workers by 2030. Madigan et al., (2024) identify many areas in which advanced practitioners can impact and influence SDG achievement, including providing access to the most vulnerable, challenging inequalities, tackling antibiotic resistance and advocating for climate change for example. They also identify how you as an advanced practitioner (or trainee) can become more involved globally, for example, with the UN, WHO or the World Bank.

Within the 2019 World Bank Group report, there is a recognition that significant investment is needed by all UN countries to achieve the UHC target (World Bank, 2019). This investment needs to be both financial and workforce related. The ICN recognises that nurses have a central role to play with the achievement of the SDGs through various interventions (ICN, 2017). This can range from health promotion intervention, through to improved patient access to healthcare, to pandemic management (Aiken et al., 2021; Morley et al., 2022; Ziegler et al., 2023).

Rosa et al., (2020) argue that NPs have been underutilised in the achievement of SDGs, especially within the lower economic countries, and this could be reflective of AP role recognition, development and implementation, which has been highlighted earlier. With comparison between the UK's NHS and the healthcare systems in lower-income countries, Friebel et al., (2018) recognise that there are significant staffing challenges around labour shortages, retention and recruitment. However, strategic plans have been developed amongst many lower-income countries to try and address this workforce challenge (Republic of Zambia Ministry of Health, 2022) in a bid to achieving UHC.

The World Bank (2021) report on education and labour markets for nursing recognised that PHC services are central to the achievement of UHC, with nursing at advanced and specialist roles being able to meet these demands. Key activities identified included health promotion and disease management/prevention. Acorn (2023) recognises that NPs can play a central role in improving population health outcomes but argues for greater investment in terms of education.

Table 15.1 provides some examples of how APNs can help achieve the SDGs, including UHC within a PHC setting.

PIT STOP!

Review the UN's SDG website and review how you and the country you practice in are working to achieve these goals for 2030.
https://unstats.un.org/sdgs/

TABLE 15.1 ■ **Examples of APNs' Work on Achieving SDGs and UHC Goal**

Target	APN Examples
3.1 Reducing maternal mortality	Ensuring adequate education for those caring for pregnant women, including the recognition of complications in pregnancy. APNs offer contraception services and preconception counselling and specialist referral especially for high-risk births such as those patients with comorbidities such as diabetes mellitus or epilepsy. The APN working within the primary care setting may be ideally placed for recognising early complications of pregnancy, for example, gestational diabetes or preeclampsia.
3.2 End preventable deaths of newborns and those under 5 years of age	APNs are well placed to provide health promotion advice to parents. They can act as first point of contact for assessment and management of common childhood illnesses, especially within the primary and community healthcare settings. APNs undertake newborn health checks to screen for potential pathologies.
3.3 End epidemics of AIDS, tuberculosis, malaria and neglected tropical diseases, combat water-borne disease, hepatitis and other communicable diseases	APNs undertake specialist roles within the care and management of patients with HIV and TB. This includes patient education, disease monitoring and recognition of potential complications, as well as the therapeutic management of the disease (prescribing and monitoring medications).
3.4 Reduced one-third premature mortality and promote mental health and well-being	APNs screen for physical and psychological health issues. This aids early diagnosis and intervention in which the APNs could manage from assessment through to diagnosis and management. APNs may recognise the signs of deteriorating mental health within a patient but may need to escalate and refer on to more specialist services.

TABLE 15.1 ■ Examples of APNs' Work on Achieving SDGs and UHC Goal—cont'd

3.5 Prevention and treatment of substance abuse	APNs undertake substance misuse roles within their scope of practice. This includes assessment, diagnosis, prescribing and long-term monitoring of clients with addiction issues.
3.6 Halve number of deaths and injuries from road traffic accidents	This can be achieved through health promotion and those APNs working in prehospital care settings such as primary care.
3.7 Universal access to sexual and reproductive healthcare	APNs working within sexual health services can assess, diagnose and manage family planning intervention; this includes sexual health screening and management. Within the UK, this represents a common practice area for APNs.
3.8 Achieve UHC	This can be achieved with APNs being ideally placed within primary care settings. The key being around access to healthcare, with APNs providing a valuable resource and being well placed to support patient access which includes assessment, diagnosis, and management of episodes of patient care.
3.9 Reduce number of deaths and illnesses from hazardous chemicals and air, water and soil pollution	APNs offer health promotion and screening for potential hazards. For example, APNs may be employed within industry within an occupational health role.
3.a Strengthen and implement WHO framework on tobacco control	Achieved through health promotion and making every APN patient encounter an opportunity to provide health promotion intervention. The APN can also influence and be involved with policy development, which can contribute to the achievement of this target.
3.b Support research and development of vaccines	APNs must integrate the research pillar into their practice; this may include supporting research into the development of vaccines.
3.c Increase health financing and the development, training and retention of health workforce in developing countries	Many APNs are integral to the workforce and can ensure data are collected which recognise the impact of their roles. This can be translated to policy and support AP workforce development. Organisations like the ICN Nurse Practitioners/Advanced Practice Nurse Network use these data and their expertise to support the development of AP in developing countries.
3.d Strengthen capacity to early warning, risk reduction and management of national and global health risks.	APNs during the pandemic worked to their full scope of practice in many settings. They are now being utilised to support the development of systems that strengthen risk reduction for future health risks.

AP, Advanced practice; *APN,* advanced practice nurse; *HIV,* human immunodeficiency virus; *SDGs,* Sustainable Development Goals; *TB,* tuberculosis; *UHC,* universal health coverage; *WHO,* World Health Organisation.

The International Council of Nurses (ICN)

The ICN represents nurses across the globe. The aim of the ICN is to advance the profession of nursing whilst supporting the well-being of nurses and being influential in the development of health, social, educational and economic policies (ICN, 2023). The ICN is a federation of members from most of the world's national nursing associations (N = 130), representing more than 28 million nurses globally. The ICN has published key documents related to AP, prescribing and nurse anaesthetists (ICN, 2023). In addition to this, the ICN works with many key organisations such as WHO and the UN and provides consultants who can contribute to policy making (ICN, 2023). The ICN supports the ongoing work to address the SDGs. The ICN also provides development and leadership opportunities for nurses. One such leadership opportunity is the ICN NP/APN Network, discussed in the next section.

The ICN Nurse Practitioner/Advanced Practice Nurse Network

The ICN NP/APN Network was launched at the 8th International Conference of NPs in San Diego in 2000. The title was used to encompass the wide diversity of AP nursing roles globally. The network has grown to almost 4000 members from 141 countries reflecting the interest in AP (Miller et al., 2024). The ICN NP/APN Network was established to be an international resource for APNs and those with an interest in AP whether working in policy, education or research. Although the network recognises that regulation and titles of advanced roles vary across the globe, these roles all have largely consistent education and training requirements (ICN NP/APN Network, 2023).

The ICN NP/APN Network (2023, p. 1) identifies the following key goals:
'Making relevant and timely information about practice, education, role development, research, policy and regulatory developments, and appropriate events widely available.

Providing a forum for sharing and exchange of knowledge, expertise and experience.

Supporting nurses and countries who are in the process of introducing or developing NP or ANP roles and practice.

Accessing international resources that are pertinent to this field.'

The network contributes to all areas of AP nursing, including policy, clinical practice, education, research and education. It is led by the chair and deputy chair, who work with a Core Steering Group (CSG) composed of 12 members from across the globe.

The ICN NP/APN Network comprises of the CSG, five subgroups, the ICN NP/APN Network Academy of Global Research and Enterprise and the Alumni. Each of these groups develops a 4-year strategic plan to enhance and develop APNs in their specific areas of expertise.

PIT STOP!

Membership is free to all interested in AP. You can join the Network via: https://icnnpapnnetwork.wildapricot.org/page-1075400

International Academy for Global Research and Enterprise

Within the structure of the ICN NP/APN Network is the Academy for Global Research and Enterprise. The Academy oversees and supports a number of large and collaborative AP projects. It provides a strategic direction for research projects under the auspices of the ICN NP/APN Network. The research priorities focus on informing and facilitating the ongoing development of APNs globally. Key to this is research that enhances role clarity, service provision and workforce planning.

The Academy priorities are:

'Priority 1: To grow and develop Network members to contribute to Academy activities, projects and research.

Priority 2: To develop research, projects and initiatives that assist the Network to advocate for the APN role, and to support ICN NP/APN Network goals and missions.

Priority 3: To acknowledge outstanding, long-lasting contributions of Network members to APN global developments, implementation, and evaluation through the development of a Fellowship of the ICN NP/APN Network Academy' (Rogers et al., 2024).

Over the past 4 years, the Academy has been working on four global projects:

- It has been supporting the development of APNs in Africa (Gray et al., 2023a).
- It has researched Emotional and Spiritual Wellbeing and Resilience of APNs globally through the COVID-19 pandemic, providing data from over 1400 APNs (Rogers et al., 2022). This project is now in the implementation phase offering resilience-based clinical supervision to network members with the aim of offering this to 400 network members over the upcoming years.
- It is finishing a project researching APN Perceptions of Spirituality Globally with the aim of supporting holistic, person-centred care.
- It has recently completed the largest and first Review of Systemic Reviews of APNs looking at APN research globally over the past 2 years. The Review of Systematic Reviews led by Dr Kelley Kilpatrick from McGill has been a seminal piece of work to determine the APN research gaps globally.

These projects have included broad participation of ICN NP/APN Network members. Over 2000 APN participants have been reached globally from 53 countries. Each of these projects has included researchers in all stages of their careers, APNs, educators, policy makers and interested parties. Many of these projects have led to further projects which early career researchers are leading.

In 2021 the network commenced a systematic review of reviews. This is the biggest piece of work the network has undertaken but it was considered necessary to identify the current gaps in AP nursing research globally. The aim of the systematic review of systematic reviews, which may also be referred to as an umbrella review, is to provide a description of the current state of research, including gaps, on AP nursing globally. This umbrella review will be published in 2024 and will support AP researchers to identify and fill research gaps. The protocol has been published and is available (Kilpatrick et al., 2023).

Conclusion

Internationally, AP nursing continues to develop to meet the healthcare needs of populations. Research evidence supports the impact of the APN.

The ICN NP/APN network, developed to support the growth and sustainability of AP nursing, offers membership to individuals and nursing organisations (including other allied health professionals). Membership in this network provides opportunities for individual and country-wide exchanges and collaboration to enhance practice and achieve UHC and the SDGs. Opportunities to collaborate together as a community of practitioners are welcomed and should be seized.

Do consider how you can connect globally with other advanced practitioners. Being aware of global concerns and AP developments will help you be more outward facing professionally. It will also bring lots of opportunities to become more involved in driving policy which impacts our patients.

References

Acorn, M. (2023). Commentary: Investing in advance practice nurses is a global health system solution. *International Nursing Review, 70*, 97–99. doi.org/10.1111/inr.12804

Aga Khan University. (2022). *AKU to launch first advanced practice nursing training in Pakistan.* https://www. aku.edu/news/Pages/News_Details.aspx?nid=NEWS-002769

Aguirre-Boza, F., Cerón, M., Pulcini, J., & Bryant-Lukosius, D. (2019). Implementation strategy for advanced practice nursing in primary health care in Chile. Acta Paul Enferm *32*(2), 120–128.

Aiken, L., Sloane, D., Brom, H., Todd, B., Barnes, H., Cimiotti, J., et al. (2021). Value of nurse practitioner inpatient hospital staffing. *Medical Care, 59*(10), 857–863. doi:10.1097/MLR.0000000000001628

Al-Maaitah, R., AbuAlRub, R., & Honig, J. (2020). Exploration of advanced practice nurses' competencies necessary for achievement of universal health coverage in Jordan. *Nursing Forum, 55*(4), 711–722. doi: 10.1111/nuf.12488

American Association of Nurse Practitioners (AANP). (2022). *NP fact sheet.* https://tinyurl.com/yk7ppufb (Accessed November 26, 2023)

Australian College of Nurse Practitioners. (2023). *Nurse practitioners and advanced practice nurses.* https:// www.acnp.org.au/home (Accessed November 26, 2023)

Cassiani, S. H., de B., Aguirre-Boza, F., Hoyos, M. C., Barreto, M. F. C., Peña, L. M., Mackay, M. C. C., et al. (2018). Competências para a formação do enfermeiro de prática avançada para a atenção básica de saúde. *Acta Paulista de Enfermagem, 31*(6), 572–584. https://doi.org/10.1590/1982-0194201800080

Chief Nursing and Midwifery Officers Australia. (n.d.). *Advanced nursing practice guidelines for the Australian context.* https://www.health.gov.au/sites/default/files/documents/2020/10/advanced-nursing-practice-guidelines-for-the-australian-context.pdf (Accessed November 26, 2023)

Christmals, C. (2021). Global advanced practice nurse case study in spirituality. Stories of hope from Africa. In M. Rogers (Ed.), *Spiritual dimensions of advanced practice nursing – Stories of Hope* (pp. 99–112). Springer.

Christmals, C. D., & Armstrong, S. J. (2019). The essence, opportunities and threats to advanced practice nursing in Sub-Saharan Africa: A scoping review. *Heliyon, 5*(10). https://doi.org/10.1016/j.heliyon.2019. e02531

Dlamini, C. P., Khumalo, T., Nkwanyana, N., Mathunjwa-Dlamini, T. R., Macera, L., Nsibandze, B., et al. (2020). Developing and implementing the family nurse practitioner role in Eswatini: Implications for education, practice, and policy. *Annals of Global Health, 86*(1), 50. doi:10.5334/aogh.2813

Espinoza, P., Troncoso, B., Jacobson, L., & Schober, M. (2021). Advanced practice nursing in Chile and the role of the registered nurse: Integrating 2 realities through continuous education. *Clinical Nurse Specialist, 35*(5), 264–270. doi:10.1097/NUR.0000000000000622

Fighel, H., & Hefetz, T. (2023). From dream to reality: Nurse practitioners in Israel. *Nurse Leader, 21*(1), 113–117.

Foreign, Commonwealth and Development Office. (2023). *UK statement at the UN Universal Health Coverage High-level Meeting, 21 September 2023.* https://www.gov.uk/government/speeches/the-uk-calls-for-international-financial-system-reform-to-make-universal-health-coverage-a-reality-uk-statement-for-the-un-universal-health-coverage (Accessed January 3, 2024)

Friebel, R., Molloy, A., Leatherman, S., Dixon, J., Bauhoff, S., & Chalkidou, K. (2018). Achieving high-quality universal health coverage: A perspective from the National Health Service in England. *BMJ Global Health, 3.* doi:10.1136/bmjgh-2018-000944

Geyer, N., & Christmals, C. D. (2020). Advanced practice nursing in Africa. In S. B. Hassmiller & J. Pulcini (Eds.), *Advanced practice nursing leadership: A global perspective,* 63–76. Springer. https://link.springer.com/chapter/10.1007/978-3-030-20550-8_6

Gray, D., Rogers, M., & Miller, M. (2023a). Advanced practice nursing initiatives in Africa, moving towards the nurse practitioner role: Experiences from the field. International Nursing Review. E-Pub. doi:10.1111/inr.12835

Gray, D., Kgositau, M., & Lubina-Sinombe, G. (2023b). The nurse practitioner role and practice in Botswana. In S. Thomas & J. Rowles (Eds.), *Nurse practitioners and nurse anesthetists: The evolution of the global roles* (pp. 225–234). Springer.

Heale, R., & Rieck Buckley, C. (2015). An international perspective of advanced practice nursing regulation. *International Nursing Review, 62*(3), 421–429. doi:10.1111/inr.12193

International Council of Nurses. (2017). Nurses: A voice to lead. Achieving the SDG's. https://www.icnvoicetolead.com/wp-content/uploads/2017/04/ICN_AVoiceToLead_guidancePack-9.pdf

International Council of Nurses. (2020). Guidelines on advanced practice nursing. https://www.icn.ch/system/files/documents/2020-04/ICN_APN%20Report_EN_WEB.pdf (Accessed March 6, 2024)

International Council of Nurses. (2023). *The global voice of nursing.* https://www.icn.ch/ (Accessed November 1, 2023).

International Council of Nurses Nurse Practitioner/Advanced Practice Nurse Network. (2023). The International Council of Nurses Nurse Practitioner/Advanced Practice Nurse Network. https://icnnpapnnetwork.wildapricot.org (Accessed November 1, 2023)

Jaman-Mewes, P., Troncoso Valenzuela, B., & Cerón Mackay, M. (2021). Global case studies in spirituality – Stories of hope from Chile. In M. Rogers (Ed.), *Spiritual dimensions of advanced practice nursing – Stories of hope* (pp. 223–236). Springer.

Jan, R., Lakhani, A., Musaddique, A., & Nadeem Parpio, Y. (2023). Why Pakistan needs advanced nurse and advanced midwife practitioners. In S. Thomas & J Rowles (Eds.), *Nurse practitioners and nurse anesthetists: The evolution of the global roles* (pp. 293–302). Springer.

Kilpatrick, K., Savard, I., Audet, L. A., Kra Friedman, A., Atallah, R., Jabbour, M., et al. (2023). A global perspective of advanced practice nursing research: A review of systematic reviews protocol. PLOS ONE, 18(1). https://journals.plos.org/plosone/article?id=10.1371/journal.pone.0280726

Lalani, N., & Ali, G. (2021). Global advanced practice nurse case study in spirituality – Stories of hope from Pakistan. In M. Rogers (Ed.), *Spiritual dimensions of advanced practice nursing – Stories of Hope* (pp. 181–194). Springer.

Laurant, M., van der Biezen, M., Wijers, N., Watananirun, K., Kontopantelis, E., & van Vught, A. (2018). Nurses as substitutes for doctors in primary care. *Cochrane Database of Systematic Reviews, 7*(7). doi:10.1002/14651858.CD001271

Ljungbeck, B., Sjögren Forss, K., Finnbogadóttir, H., & Carlson, E. (2021). Content in nurse practitioner education – A scoping review. *Nurse Education Today, 98,* 104650. doi:10.1016/j.nedt.2020.104650

Mackavey, C., Henderson, C., de Zwart van Leeuwen, E., & Maas, L. (2024). The APN role development: A struggle for identity. *International Journal for Advancing Practice, 2,* 1.

Madigan, E., Shaw, H., Chui, P., & Anders, L. (2024). WHO, UN, WB strategic plan and national declinations. In M. Rogers, D. Lehwaldt, J. Roussel, & M. Acorn (Eds.), *Influencing and shaping Policy Agendas: Advanced Practice Nurses Engagement with Global Organisations* (pp. 191–214). Springer.

Maier, C., Aiken, L., & Busse, R. (2017). Nurses in advanced roles in primary care: Policy levers for implementation. *OECD Health Working Papers,* No. 98, OECD Publishing. https://doi.org/10.1787/a8756593-en

Maithreepala, S. D., & Konara Mudiyanselage, S. P. (2023). The nurse practitioner (NP) role in Sri Lanka. In S. Thomas & J. Rowles (Eds.), *Nurse practitioners and nurse anesthetists: The evolution of the global roles* (pp. 279–286). Springer.

Martin-Misener, R., Harbman, P., Donald, F., Reid, K., Kilpatrick, K., Carter, N., et al. (2015). Cost-effectiveness of nurse practitioners in primary and specialised ambulatory care: Systematic review. *BMJ Open*, *5*(6), e007167. doi:10.1136/bmjopen-2014-007167

Miller, M., Roussel, J., Rogers. M., & Lehwaldt, D. (2024). The global phenomenon of advanced practice nurses. In M. Rogers, D. Lehwaldt, J. Roussel, & M, Acorn (Eds.), *Advanced practice nurse networking to enhance global health* (pp. 19–42). Springer.

Moore, K., Lockwood, E., Henderson, C, & Li, M. (2024). Advanced practice nurses. A global overview of education. In M. Rogers, D. Lehwaldt, J. Roussel, & M. Acorn (Eds.), *Advanced practice nurse networking to enhance global health* (pp. 105–132). Springer.

Moosa, S. (2021). Development of African forum for primary health care. *African Journal of Primary Health Care & Family Medicine*, *13*(1), e1-e2. https://doi.org/10.4102/phcfm.v13i1.2973

Morley, D., Kilgoreb, C., Edwards, M., Collins, P., Scammella, J., Fletcherz, K., et al. (2022). The changing role of advanced clinical practitioners working with older people during the COVID-19 pandemic: A qualitative research study. *International Journal of Nursing Studies*, *130*. doi:10.1016/j.ijnurstu.2022.104235

Nahari, A., Alhamed, A., Moafa, H., Aboshaiqah, A., & Almotairy, M. (2024). Role delineation of advanced practice nursing: A cross-sectional study. *Journal of Advanced Nursing*, *80*, 366–376. https://doi.org/10.1111/jan.15797

Pan American Health Organization (PAHO). (2015). *Report on universal access to health and universal health coverage: Advanced Practice Nursing Summit. Hamilton-CA April 15-17*, https://www.observatoriorh.org/es/report-universal-access-health-and-universal-health-coverage-advanced-practice-nursing-summit (Accessed December 17, 2024)

Poghosyan, L., Liu, J., Shang, J., & D'Aunno, T. (2017). Practice environments and job satisfaction and turnover intentions of nurse practitioners: Implications for primary care workforce capacity. *Health Care Management Review*, *42*(2), 162–171. doi:10.1097/HMR.0000000000000094

Poghosyan, L., & Maier, C. (2022). Advanced practice nurses globally: Responding to health challenges, improving outcomes. *International Journal of Nursing Studies*, *132*, 104262. doi:10.1016/j.ijnurstu.2022.104262

Pulcini, J., Jelic, M., Gul, R., & Loke, A. (2010). An international survey on advanced practice nursing education, practice, and regulation. *Journal of Nursing Scholarship*, *42*(1), 31–39. doi:10.1111/j.1547-5069.2009.01322.x

Republic of Zambia Ministry of Health. (2022). *2022–2026 National health strategic plan: "Towards attainment of quality universal health coverage through decentralisation"*. https://www.moh.gov.zm/wp-content/uploads/2023/02/National-Health-Stratergic-Plan-for-Zambia-2022-to-2026-revised-February-2023-lower-resolution.pdf (Accessed January 10, 2024)

Rogers, M., Lamarche, K., Miller, M., Moore, K., Spies, L., Taylor, J., et al. (2022). Global emotional and spiritual well-being and resilience of advanced practice nurses during the COVID-19 pandemic: A cross-sectional study. *Journal of Advanced Nursing*, *78*(5), 1483–1492.

Rogers, M., Lehwaldt, D., Roussel, J., & Acorn, M. (2024). *Advanced practice nurse networking to enhance global health*. Springer.

Rosa, W., Fitzgerald, M., Davis, S., Farley, J., Khanyola, J., Kwong, J., et al. (2020). Leveraging nurse practitioner capacities to achieve global health for all: COVID-19 and beyond. *International Nursing Review*, *67*(4), 554–559.

Sibanda, B., & Stender, S. C. (2018). *Anglophone Africa Advanced Practice Nurse Coalition Project* (AAAPNC): A proposal to WHO (Africa) Health Systems Leadership Team. https://afrophc.org/wp-content/uploads/2020/11/africa-apn-coalition-project_final-draft.pdf

Silver, H. K., Ford, L. C., & Day, L. R. (1968). The Pediatric Nurse-Practitioner Program expanding the role of the nurse to provide increased health care for children. *JAMA*, *204*(4), 298–302.

Suutarla, A., Sulosaari, V., & Heikkilä, J. (2023). The NP role and practice in Finland. In S. Thomas & J. Rowles (Eds.), *Nurse practitioners and nurse anesthetists: The evolution of the global roles* (pp. 181–196). Springer.

Thomas, S., & Rowles, J. (2023). *Nurse practitioners and nurse anesthetists: The evolution of the global roles*. Springer.

Tracy, C., & Tan, S. (2014). Advanced practice nursing in Singapore. *Proceedings of Singapore Healthcare*, *23*, 269–270. https://www.researchgate.net/publication/285018729_Advanced_Practice_Nursing_in_Singapore (Accessed November 21, 2023)

V&VN. (2023). *The nurse practitioner in the Netherlands.* https://www-venvn-nl.translate.goog/registers/ver-pleegkundig-specialisten-register/registratie/buitenslands-gediplomeerden/?_x_tr_sl=auto&_x_tr_tl=en&_x_tr_hl=en&_x_tr_pto=wapp (Accessed November 26, 2023)

United Nations. (n.d.). *Sustainable Development Goals. Decade of Action.* https://www.un.org/sustainabledevel-opment/decade-of-action (Accessed March 5, 2024)

UN Department of Economic and Social Affairs. (n.d.). *The 17 goals.* THE 17 GOALS | Sustainable Development (https://sdgs.un.org/goals)

World Bank. (2019). *High-performance health financing for universal health coverage (Vol. 2): Driving sustain-able, inclusive growth in the 21st century (English).* Washington, DC: World Bank. http://documents.worldbank.org/curated/en/641451561043585615/Driving-Sustainable-Inclusive-Growth-in-the-21st-Century

World Bank. (2021). *A labor market assessment of nurses and physicians in Saudi Arabia projecting imbalances between need, supply, and demand.* Washington, DC: World Bank. World Bank Document https://docu-ments.worldbank.org/en/publication/documents-reports/documentdetail/830511632373746956/a-labor-market-assessment-of-nurses-and-physicians-in-saudi-arabia-addressing-future-imbalances-be-tween-need-supply-and-demand

World Health Organization. (2024). *Universal health coverage.* https://www.who.int/news-room/fact-sheets/detail/universal-health-coverage-(uhc)

Ziegler, E., Martin-Misener, R., Rietkoetter, S., Baumann, A., Bougeault, I., Kovacevic, N., et al. (2023). Response and innovations of advanced practice nurses during the COVID-19 pandemic: A scoping review. *International Nursing Review,* 1–26. https://doi.org/10.1111/inr.12884

Zug, K. E., Cassiani, S. H. D. B., Pulcini, J., Bassalobre Garcia, A., Aguirre-Boza, F., & Park, J. (2016). Enfermagem de prática avançada na América Latina e no Caribe: Regulação, educação e prática. *Revista Latino-Americana de Enfermagem, 24.* https://doi.org/10.1590/1518-8345.1615.2807

INDEX

Note: Page numbers followed by '*f*' indicate figures, '*t*' indicate tables, and '*b*' indicate boxes.